Feline Anesthesia and Pain Management

Feline Anesthesia and Pain Management

Edited by

Paulo Steagall
Université de Montréal, Saint-Hyacinthe, Canada

Sheilah Robertson
Lap of Love Veterinary Hospice, Lutz, FL, United States

Polly Taylor
Taylor Monroe, Little Downham, Ely, United Kingdom

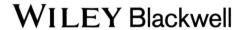

This edition first published 2018
© 2018 John Wiley & Sons, Inc.

The right of Paulo Steagall, Sheilah Robertson, and Polly M Taylor to be identified as the editors of the editorial material in this work has been asserted in accordance with law.

Registered Office
John Wiley & Sons, Inc., 111 River Street, Hoboken, NJ 07030, USA

Editorial Office
111 River Street, Hoboken, NJ 07030, USA

For details of our global editorial offices, customer services, and more information about Wiley products visit us at www.wiley.com.

Wiley also publishes its books in a variety of electronic formats and by print-on-demand. Some content that appears in standard print versions of this book may not be available in other formats.

Limit of Liability/Disclaimer of Warranty

Library of Congress Cataloging-in-Publication Data
Names: Steagall, Paulo V. M., author. | Robertson, Sheilah A., author. |
    Taylor, Polly M., author.
Title: Feline anesthesia and pain management / by Paulo V.M. Steagall,
    Sheilah A. Robertson, Polly Taylor.
Description: Hoboken, NJ : Wiley, 2018. | Includes bibliographical references
    and index. |
Identifiers: LCCN 2017026911 (print) | LCCN 2017027877 (ebook) | ISBN
    9781119167846 (pdf) | ISBN 9781119167877 (epub) | ISBN 9781119167808 (pbk.)
Subjects: | MESH: Cat Diseases–drug therapy | Pain Management–veterinary |
Anesthesia–veterinary
Classification: LCC SF985 (ebook) | LCC SF985 .S74 2018 (print) | NLM SF 985
    | DDC 636.8/089796–dc23
LC record available at https://lccn.loc.gov/2017026911

Cover images: Courtesy of the editors
Cover design by Wiley

Set in 10/12 pt WarnockPro-Regular by Thomson Digital, Noida, India

10 9 8 7 6 5 4 3 2 1

Dedication

Paulo Steagall
*To my mother Ilza who has always supported my
dreams. To my partner in crime Beatriz Monteiro
who accepted me to ride along in this journey. To
my father who taught me the love for cats. To Polly
Taylor and Sheilah Robertson for believing. This
book is for all cats and for people who dedicate
their lives to protect and help them. Cats gave me
a reason to become a veterinarian, and a job for
the rest of my life.*

Sheilah Robertson
*To my parents who always believed in education
and supporting my career choice. To Paulo Steagall
and Polly Taylor for their friendship, unwavering
patience, and dedication to detail during the
writing and editing process. To all the cats that
have owned me and all my feline patients, thank
you for everything you have taught me.*

Polly Taylor
*Thanks to Leslie Hall and Peter Lees who each in
their own way encouraged me in the pursuit of all
things feline – for cats in their own right, not as
"little dogs." To all cats, wonderful creatures,
especially those who have owned me over the
years, and particularly to Jasper, the current
incumbent, who typed enthusiastically, if
unhelpfully, some variations on the text herein.
And most of all to Paulo and Sheilah for making it
all happen, and to my family for their extreme
patience and well-timed glasses of wine.*

*We would like to thank all collaborators for
donating their time and expertise for this book.*

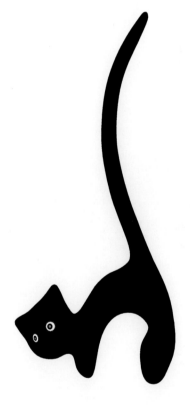

Contents

Foreword

It gives me enormous pleasure, and it is a great privilege, to be able to write a preface for the first edition of this new book, edited and coauthored by Drs. Paulo Steagall, Sheilah Robertson, and Polly Taylor. If you are reading this having just purchased the book, the first thing to say is congratulations! You have made a sound investment!

For many decades there has been a trend for growth in cat ownership, and in many countries throughout the world the pet cat population now exceeds that of dogs. Despite their rising popularity, cats are still often a "second class" veterinary patient. Cats are taken to the veterinarian less frequently than dogs, and, regrettably, veterinary publications on dogs still far outweigh those on cats. Things are changing though – many practitioners appreciate the real value in focusing on the differing (and sometimes unique) needs of cats, and there is a growing emphasis on a better understanding of cats as veterinary patients.

The welfare of patients under our care is, of course, the primary concern of every veterinarian. It is also true that, in terms of animal welfare, nothing is more important than pain relief, which is why I am so pleased to see the publication of this new book. It is nearly 25 years since the last veterinary book to focus on feline anesthesia was published (*Anaesthesia of the Cat*, edited by Hall and Taylor, published in 1994). As so much has changed in our knowledge in the past 25 years, this new publication is both timely and a very welcome addition to the literature.

This book takes a very practical approach to feline anesthesia and analgesia. It is designed to be a practical clinical tool, providing state-of-the-art information in accessible format enabling improved management of cats under our care. This book is equally relevant to veterinary practitioners, students, nurses and technicians, and with its emphasis on the management of both acute and chronic pain it will serve as an invaluable resource in any clinic.

The concise and clear layout of this book makes accessing information particularly easy for the busy practitioner. The text is concise, practical, relevant, and addresses exactly the sorts of questions and issues that occur in day-to-day veterinary practice. Chapters are well illustrated and authored by an outstanding collection of international experts in feline anesthesia and analgesia.

It is perhaps unusual to look at a book's table of contents and to look forward to reading every single chapter in the publication. I can honestly say that is the case with this book though. Much thought has gone into its structure, the subjects covered, and the way they are addressed. I hope and believe that this book will be very widely read and used. For anyone purchasing the book, it is destined to be something that is used on a daily basis in the clinic, and will not be a book that simply collects dust on the shelf!

On a personal note, I am passionate about feline welfare – I have also known Paulo, Sheilah, and Polly for a number of years and I know how passionate they are too about improving cat welfare through better clinical application of analgesia. With this book, any veterinarian or nurse/technician will find a wealth of practical information that will directly impact their everyday clinical work, and will improve the lives of the cats that are under their care. I can offer no higher recommendation – this book will improve your ability to care for your feline patients and improve their welfare, and as such it deserves to have a place in every small animal clinic.

Dr. Andy Sparkes BVetMed PhD DipECVIM MANZCVS MRCVS
Veterinary Director, International Cat Care and International Society of Feline Medicine
www.icatcare.org

Contributors

Graeme Doodnaught
Resident in Veterinary Anesthesia and
Analgesia
Department of Clinical Sciences
Faculty of Veterinary Medicine
Université de Montréal
3200 Rue Sicotte
Saint-Hyacinthe, QC J2S2M2
Canada

Craig B. Johnson
Professor of Veterinary Neurophysiology
Institute of Veterinary, Animal and
Biomedical Sciences
College of Sciences
Massey University Private Bag 11 222
Palmerston North
New Zealand

Duncan Lascelles
Professor of Small Animal Surgery and
Pain Management Comparative Pain
Research Laboratory
College of Veterinary Medicine
North Carolina State University
1060 William Moore Drive
Raleigh, NC 27607
United States

Beatriz Monteiro
PhD Candidate in Veterinary
Pharmacology
Vanier Scholar
Department of Biomedical Sciences
Faculty of Veterinary Medicine
Université de Montréal
3200 Rue Sicotte
Saint-Hyacinthe, QC J2S2M2
Canada

Daniel Pang
Associate Professor of Veterinary
Anesthesiology
Department of Clinical Sciences
Faculty of Veterinary Medicine
Université de Montréal
3200 Rue Sicotte
Saint-Hyacinthe, QC J2S2M2
Canada

Peter Pascoe
Professor of Anesthesia and Critical
Patient Care
Department of Surgical and Radiological
Sciences
School of Veterinary Medicine
1 Shields Ave
University of California
Davis, CA 95616
United States

Bruno Pypendop
Professor of Veterinary Anesthesiology
Department of Surgical and Radiological
Sciences
School of Veterinary Medicine
University of California
One Shields Avenue
Davis, CA 95616
United States

Sheilah Robertson
Senior Medical Director
Lap of Love Veterinary Hospice
17804 US-41, Lutz, FL 33549
United States

Bradley Simon
Assistant Professor of Veterinary
Anesthesiology
Department of Small Animal Clinical
Sciences
College of Veterinary Medicine and
Biomedical Sciences, Texas A&M
University
402 Raymond Stotzer Pkwy
College Station, TX 77843-4474
United States

Francesco Staffieri
Associate Professor of Veterinary
Anesthesiology
Department of Emergency and Organ
Transplantation, Section of Veterinary
Clinics and Animal Production
University of Bari
SP per Casamassima km 3, 70010
Valenzano
Bari
Italy

Paulo Steagall
Associate Professor of Veterinary
Anesthesiology
Department of Clinical Sciences
Faculty of Veterinary Medicine
Université de Montréal
3200 Rue Sicotte
Saint-Hyacinthe, QC J2S2M2
Canada

Polly Taylor
Independent Consultant in Veterinary
Anaesthesia
Taylor Monroe
Little Downham
Nr. Ely
Cambs CB6 2TY
United Kingdom

Eric Troncy
Professor of Veterinary Pharmacology
Department of Biomedical Sciences
Faculty of Veterinary Medicine
Université de Montréal
3200 Rue Sicotte
Saint-Hyacinthe, QC J2S2M2
Canada

1

Handling, Restraint, and Preanesthetic Assessment

Graeme Doodnaught and Paulo Steagall

Université de Montréal, Saint-Hyacinthe, Canada

Key Points

- Behavioral considerations
- Handling methods and physical restraint
- Routes of drug administration
- Airway management
- Preanesthetic evaluation
- Mortality and morbidity in feline anesthesia

Introduction

The pet cat population has grown over the last few decades, as has our understanding of disease prevention and treatment in this species. Despite population growth, fewer cats visit a veterinary clinic on a regular basis when compared with dogs. Cat owners often avoid veterinary visits as transportation of the cat to the clinic may be stressful. Handling, appropriate physical examination, knowledge of behavior, and preanesthetic assessment are essential components of feline anesthesia and analgesia.

Box 1.1: Cat-friendly techniques in clinical practice

Safe handling and cat-friendly practices minimize stress, fear, anxiety, and potential personnel injuries related to aggression. They are key components of veterinary care for the anesthetist and staff members.

A cat-friendly practice will provide an environment that reduces the stress of veterinary consultation and hospitalization. More information can be found at http://icatcare.org (June 24, 2017). These practices involve:

- A calm, safe, and quiet clinic with cat-designated areas or cat-only appointment times
- Gentle and efficient physical examination and treatment
- Client education on transporting the cat to and from the clinic
- Client communication about feline anesthesia and analgesia

Feline Anesthesia and Pain Management, First Edition. Edited by Paulo Steagall, Sheilah Robertson and Polly Taylor.

Handling and Restraint

Each cat is unique and can exhibit a wide range of behaviors. Experienced handlers will often adapt their approach and handling technique to suit each patient. While there is no substitute for "experience", some principles exist to aid in the restraint of *most* cats. The mantras "go slow to go fast" and "less is more" are commonplace. Good feline handling revolves around the premise of *de-escalation*, where the handler avoids potential actions that may elevate a patient's stress. *De-escalation* minimizes noxious visual, auditory, and olfactory stimuli that could lead to avoidance or aggressive behavior. It should be noted that the major cause of defensive or aggressive behavior is fear. Cats have limited appeasement behaviors, making it difficult to calm them once they are distressed. Thus, avoiding these behavioral triggers is critical to success.

To facilitate handling throughout life, kittens should be encouraged to interact with people, animals, and new environments between 2 and 7 weeks of age. With all ages of cats, positive reinforcement techniques (e.g. rewarding with food, play, brushing) along with behavioral therapy in difficult individuals, help to reduce the stress and anxiety associated with veterinary visits.

Most cats in a calm environment will readily explore their surroundings. Anxious or fearful individuals will tend to remain within their carriers. The cat should be handled with patience and a positive attitude throughout the physical examination. Minimal restraint is required to perform a full physical examination in most cats. Gentle touch and petting around the head and neck are generally well tolerated, and allow for minor manipulations without the need for physical restraint (*Figure* 1.1a, b, c). Timid or fearful individuals who choose to remain in the carrier should be allowed to do so. The top of a carrier may be removed and an examination can be performed with the cat still inside (*Box* 1.2).

Box 1.2: Safe handling in feline practice

Consider using top-opening carriers and baskets for transporting cats into the clinic. This allows for easy handling and provides a safe and secure environment.

It is understandable that most medical procedures in cats require some level of restraint. This makes treatments and procedures safer for both cat and handler. While immobilization is often required, the approach should still be gentle. *Figure* 1.2 shows common methods of control.

Scruffing

Scruffing is a controversial method of restraint. Many clinics have a "no-scruffing" policy. Scruffing should be regarded as a last resort for physical restraint to avoid injuries and accidents. For these exceptional cases, the cat is gently grasped by the skin over the dorsum of the neck and scapulae, and minimal (firm) pressure is maintained. The method should certainly not be used if there is already pain or discomfort present. It is important to highlight that scruffing may lead to fear-based aggression and further escalation of stress. The American Association of Feline

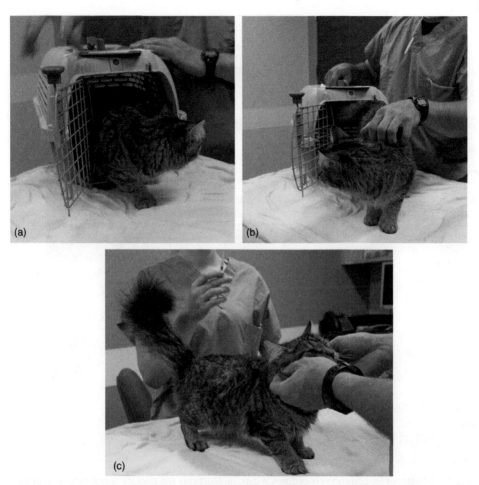

Figure 1.1 A cat-friendly approach in a hospital setting. (a) This cat explores the examination room and its surroundings. (b) The handler gently pets the cat to control its movement without using forcible restraint. (c) Placing the hands under the chin allows for better control of the head and neck.

Practitioners (AAFP) and the International Society of Feline Medicine (ISFM) state that the technique should be used sparingly. A cat should never have its full weight suspended from the scruff.

The Fearful Cat

Fear is the most common cause of aggression in hospitalized cats. De-escalation techniques do not always work in fearful individuals. These cats exhibit strong avoidance or aggressive behavior making handling difficult. In this situation, chemical restraint should be considered before any manipulation (Chapter 3). To assist in the physical restraint of these patients, use of appropriate handling equipment is recommended (description of techniques to follow). In these cases, the equipment for IV catheter placement, and for anesthetic induction, maintenance, and monitoring should be ready.

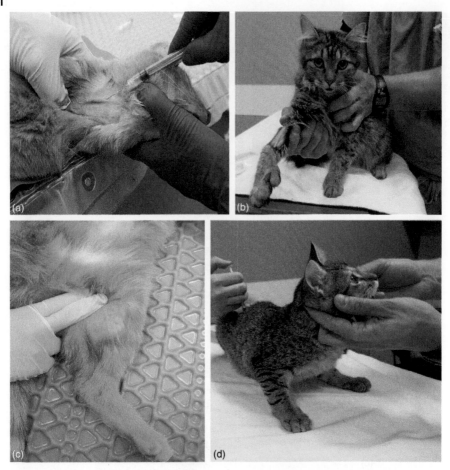

Figure 1.2 Restraint for common procedures in cats. (a) Most cats will tolerate gentle extension of the neck to expose the jugular veins for blood sampling. In this image the jugular vein is occluded with the cat in lateral recumbency. (b) Restraint of the forelimb for cephalic blood sampling or IV catheterization. The handler is preventing the cat from backward movement by applying gentle pressure over the cat's hind limbs. Using the same arm, the handler is extending the right limb forward with three fingers behind the elbow to prevent retraction of the limb, and rotating and raising the cephalic vein with their first and second digits. (c) Restraint of the hind limb for medial saphenous blood sampling or IV catheterization. The cat is restrained in lateral recumbency with the dependent limb intended for venous sampling. The handler uses one hand to restrain the contralateral (upper) hind limb and apply medio-lateral pressure over the vein proximal to the sampling site. Once the vessel is visualized, the clinician directs the needle in a distal to proximal direction while maintaining control of the lower limb with the opposite hand. (d) This cat is allowed to stand freely on the treatment table and is only restrained by gentle control of the head and neck. This allows free access to the epaxial muscles for intramuscular injection.

Box 1.3: The handling equipment

Handling equipment should be:

- Safe for the cat and handler
- In good working order with frequent "check ups"
- Easy to use and to clean
- Suitable for the intended task

Some techniques used for appropriate restraint of the fearful and/or aggressive cat are listed below:

- *Towels or blankets* are commonly used for restraining fearful cats. They are often successful in protecting the handler from injury. By covering the patient, they give the cat a place to hide, minimizing visual and auditory stimulation. The handler maintains good dexterity and can assist with the procedure
- *Synthetic feline facial pheromones* mimic natural pheromones that are secreted by cats via facial rubbing when they are comfortable and when they mark their territories. These products have been shown to decrease stress and facilitate handling of some cats
- *Masks* or *hoods* may assist with physical restraint of some cats by limiting visual stimulation. A well-fitted mask will also protect the handler from bites. They are variably tolerated and require judicious use
- *Bags* for restraint protect individuals from aggressive cats. Openings in these bags allow access to the limbs and head
- Feral cats may require the use of *squeeze cages, humane traps* or *nets* for drug administration. Their application is limited to capture and restraint of cats for injection. Nets are used in exceptional conditions such as when a cat escapes or where there are extremely limited facilities. Such equipment can easily cause trauma if not used properly
- *Anesthetic induction chambers* may be used to anesthetize cats. This requires minimal restraint but placing the cat inside the chamber can be a challenge. While the absence of restraint is arguably better for the cat, there is potential for environmental contamination and exposure of personnel with volatile anesthetics. A fearful cat can be briefly restrained using a towel or cat bag for mask induction using volatile anesthetic agents. Techniques for induction of general anesthesia are discussed in Chapters 4 and 6
- *Leather handling gauntlets* or *gloves* can protect the handler from an aggressive cat but they limit dexterity. They should be used only as a last resource for restraint. Leather is also difficult to clean and repeated disinfection is required

Blood Sampling

Restraint for blood sampling can be performed in many ways. The jugular vein is a common site as it is easily identified and allows rapid withdrawal of large volumes of blood compared with distal veins (*Figure* 1.2a). The handler extends the head and neck with the cat in a sternal or lateral position. The clinician approaches the vein with the needle directed either in a cranio-caudal (*Figure* 1.2a) or caudo-cranial direction. The use of a 23-G 1.6 cm (5/8th inch) needle and a small volume syringe (1–3 mL) is recommended.

Peripheral blood sampling, for example from the cephalic vein (*Figure* 1.2b), may be used for low-volume sample collection, or where jugular sampling is contraindicated (e.g. coagulopathies, increased intracranial or intraocular pressure). Another common site for sampling is the medial saphenous vein (*Figure* 1.2c). To limit repeated venipuncture, the blood that is collected in the hub of a catheter's stylet can be used for a basic blood panel during the preoperative period (*Table* 1.1).

Table 1.1   Values for basic blood panel in cats.

Hematocrit (packed cell volume)	30–50%
Total solids (total protein)	60–85 g/L
Blood urea nitrogen	170–320 g/L
Calcium	85–110 g/L
Potassium	3.7–5.4 mEq/L

Drug Administration

A number of routes of administration are available for drug delivery, and the choice will depend on both drug selection and intended purpose.

- *Intravenous (IV)* administration is the most efficacious and reliable method of drug delivery. It is commonly used for anesthetic induction, or for analgesic drugs when a catheter is in place
- The intramuscular (IM) route is commonly used for premedication. Any skeletal muscle may be used but large-bellied and superficial muscles are preferred. The epaxial and muscles of the cranial and caudal thigh are often chosen (*Figure* 1.2d); if using the hind limb, the cranial thigh is more reliable. When using the caudal thigh, it is easy to miss muscle tissue and inject into fascial planes. The location of major blood vessels and nerves is important when selecting an injection site. For example, the sciatic nerve runs beneath the *biceps femoris* in the caudo-lateral thigh, and may be inadvertently injured. Aspiration should precede injection to avoid unintended intravascular injection
- The *subcutaneous (SC)* route is used for perioperative administration of drugs such as nonsteroidal inflammatory drugs. This route can also accommodate large volumes of crystalloid fluids when intravenous fluid therapy is not possible. Most conscious cats will tolerate injection between the shoulder blades
- *Buccal or oral transmucosal* (OTM) administration is not commonly used in hospital settings, as other routes are usually an option. However, it can be used as a less invasive route of administration during long-term hospitalization or "home care." It is accomplished by inserting the syringe tip into the cat's mouth and gently squeezing the syringe contents into the cheek pouch; swallowing must be avoided to allow transmucosal absorption and prevent first-pass hepatic metabolism

IV Catheterization

A wide array of IV catheter types exists in veterinary practice. These are commonly inserted into the cephalic or medial saphenous veins. Catheterization of these vessels is often performed following premedication (Chapter 3). Intravenous catheterization allows easy drug titration during anesthetic induction, administration of fluids, emergency intervention, and minimizes the need for multiple SC or IM injections in the perioperative period. Use of topical local anesthetic creams can facilitate placement of catheters (*Box* 1.4). The ideal catheter material is inert, long-lasting, and atraumatic. Catheters should be placed using a sterile technique.

Silicone catheters are good choices for long-term cannulation. In cats requiring extended hospitalization, central venous catheters (18- or 21-G) are placed using the modified Seldinger method, peel-away introducers, or cut-down techniques. Aseptic technique is mandatory for the placement of long term catheters.

Box 1.4: Intravenous catheterization in clinical practice using local anesthetic creams

Smaller gauge ($\leq$ 22-G) catheters are commonly used for the cephalic and medial saphenous veins in cats. Application of topical anesthetics (e.g. EMLA; eutectic mixture of local anesthetics, a combination of lidocaine 2.5% and prilocaine 2.5%) at least 30 minutes before catheterization desensitizes the skin, thereby reducing the stress of the whole procedure. This technique can also be used for jugular venipuncture enabling minimal restraint. The cream is applied and covered with an impermeable and non-absorbent dressing. The use of gloves is recommended, as the cream will anesthetize human skin. IV catheters should be examined daily for signs of infection and skin irritation, and to confirm patency. Taping should not be overtight otherwise distal limb edema may occur.

Intubation and Airway Management

Induction of anesthesia is commonly followed by maintenance with a volatile anesthetic and oxygen. Endotracheal intubation protects the airway, minimizing the risk of aspiration if regurgitation occurs; it also enables delivery of oxygen and anesthetic, and facilitates ventilation. *Figure* 1.3 shows appropriate positioning for intubation in a cat.

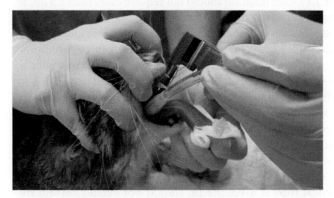

Figure 1.3 Restraint for intubation: with the cat in sternal recumbency, the handler gently extends the neck and head. Either the handler or the individual performing the intubation opens the mouth by exteriorizing the tongue. In this position the larynx is easily visualized with a laryngoscope enabling application of local anesthetic followed by intubation. The laryngoscope (or other instrument) should be used to exteriorize the tongue as intraoral manipulation of cats in a light plane of anesthesia may lead to a reflex bite.

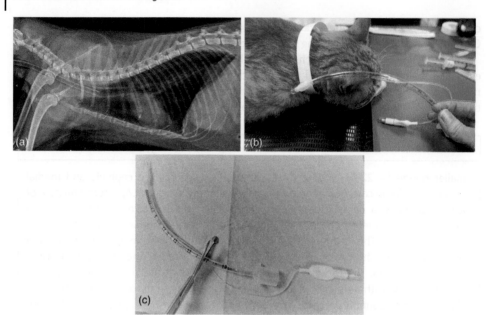

Figure 1.4 (a) The tip of the endotracheal tube should not reach further than the thoracic inlet. (b) Endotracheal tubes should be measured before use; they should reach from the tip of the shoulder (thoracic inlet) to the incisor teeth. (c) Endotracheal tubes should be cut to the correct length prior to use. Excess length adds dead space.

The challenges and complications (i.e. laryngospasm, laryngeal trauma, tracheal rupture or necrosis and airway obstruction) of intubation in cats (*Box* 1.5) are discussed in Chapters 2 and 10. Most adult cats can be intubated with a 3.5–5 mm internal diameter endotracheal tube (ETT). Cuff inflation should not require more than 1.5 mL of air using a small syringe. Small increments of air (0.5 mLs) should be injected at a time into the pilot balloon until a seal is achieved when the pressure in the breathing circuit is 16–18 cmH$_2$O. Pressure within the high-volume low-pressure cuff can be monitored using a special device (Posey Cufflator Endotracheal Tube Inflator and Manometer®). This will avoid high cuff pressures and the risk of airway trauma. Overlong ETT may cause a range of problems (Chapter 10) and should be cut to an appropriate length before insertion (*Box* 1.5; *Figure* 1.4a, b, c).

It is strongly recommended that the cat is disconnected from the breathing system when turning is required during anesthesia. This will prevent extubation and inadvertent trauma. All endotracheal tubes can damage the mucociliary apparatus, which moves particles in an orad direction, and can cause direct damage to the tracheal endothelium. If an endotracheal tube is used, the tip should not extend beyond the thoracic inlet (point of the shoulder); if a tracheal tear does occur, the prognosis is worse for an intrathoracic tear and it is more difficult to repair than an extrathoracic injury (Chapter 10).

Box 1.5: Endotracheal tubes

Cuffed tubes

- The inflatable cuff seals the airway but has the potential to cause damage
- The cuff and its pilot tube occupy a substantial proportion of the tube diameter, potentially reducing airway size. Modern tube construction minimizes this effect (e.g. soft silicone)
- Potential for damage caused by the cuff (Chapter 10)
- An inflated cuff may cause local pressure ischemia to the tracheal lining (Chapter 10)
- Lubricant gel on the cuff enhances the seal at a given pressure
- Cuffed tubes are required for IPPV (or a supraglottic airway device see below) and reduce the risks of fluid aspiration

Noncuffed tubes

- Used to be considered best for cats
- Avoid potential for cuff-induced tracheal damage but more difficult to seal the airway
- Require pharyngeal packing to prevent fluid entering the airway
- The Cole tube is cuffless; the seal is produced by advancing the shoulder until it impacts onto the larynx. These are difficult to place reliably without causing damage and are now rarely used

Supraglottic airway devices

- This device does not enter the trachea and ends above the larynx
- Distal elliptical component with an inflatable bladder on the dorsal aspect seals the airway
- The v-gel® developed for cats is easy to place
- Limited evidence so far suggests that the v-gel® is less likely to cause damage than standard ETT
- Suitable for IPPV

Endotracheal tube length

- Overlong tubes may cause excessive airway dead space, tracheal tears, and endobronchial intubation (Chapter 10)
- The length of the endotracheal tube should be measured in each cat before placement (*Figure* 1.4b) and cut as needed (*Figure* 1.4c)
- The endotracheal tube should reach from the incisor teeth to the point of the shoulder
- The tip should reach the mid to lower third of the trachea and not enter the thorax
- The connector end can be cut to shorten the tube

A stylet can be used cautiously to increase dexterity especially with silicone ETT. The tip of the stylet should never go through the distal part of the ETT.

Supraglottic airway devices (SGAD) (e.g. the v-gel®) are another option for airway management in cats. The device comprises a tube with a distal elliptical component that has an inflatable bladder on the dorsal aspect that is used when needed to create a better seal (*Figure* 1.5a). It is a practical alternative to endotracheal intubation in cats, leading to

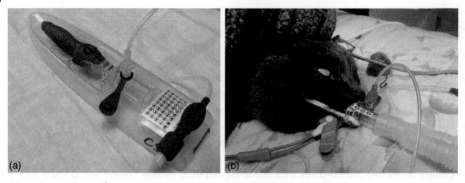

Figure 1.5 (a) A v-gel® has been selected, lubricated and is sitting in its cradle to avoid contamination; a side stream capnograph has been attached to confirm proper placement. (b) The v-gel® has been placed and secured in place.

a lower incidence of upper airway discomfort after extubation when compared with an endotracheal tube. The v-gel® can be inserted at a more superficial depth of anesthesia than an endotracheal tube. It can be used for mechanical ventilation and a variety of procedures. Placement is relatively easy and can be performed by inexperienced individuals. However, v-gels are much more expensive than endotracheal tubes.

Preanesthetic Assessment

The purpose of the preanesthetic examination is to assess the suitability of a patient for anesthesia, prevent complications, assess risks, and determine whether any special consideration, material, preparation or equipment is required. Planning is a key component to prevent anesthetic-induced complications such as hypothermia, hypoventilation, bradycardia, and hypotension.

A checklist for preanesthetic assessment is recommended. The Association of Veterinary Anaesthetists (AVA) have examples available for download at http://www.ava.eu.com/information/checklists/ (accessed June 24, 2017). The checklist should include:

- Patient identification, history, and signalment
  - A full history should be taken, with emphasis on previous anesthetic and surgical procedures, as well as current medication. Age is particularly important in identifying individuals at risk (pediatrics or geriatrics)
- Concomitant diseases/conditions
  - These have a potential impact on anesthesia and pain management. Particular considerations apply for managing anesthesia of neonatal, pediatric, and pregnant cats as well as for those with, for instance, diabetes, cardiomyopathy, and urinary tract obstruction (Chapter 9). Some cats may require stabilization before anesthesia
- Physical examination
  - Emphasis should be given to the cardiovascular, respiratory, hepatic, and renal systems as their roles in perfusion, oxygenation, and drug metabolism affect many aspects of anesthesia. Unfortunately, the hospital visit itself is stressful, generally elevating heart and respiratory rate, blood pressure, and body temperature (*Box* 1.6). Therefore, recognition of stress and anxiety is important in

clinical assessment of these values. Body condition scoring allows objective recognition of extremes in body weight, which may increase the patient's risk. An accurate weight should be obtained
- Risks associated with the surgical procedure
  - This includes planning for the potential of bleeding and perioperative pain, the effects of positioning, technique (e.g. laparoscopic procedures) and duration. Crossmatching and blood typing may be required for some cases and is discussed in Chapter 8. Certain surgical procedures require special equipment, materials or changes in the layout of the operating room. Team meetings prior to a nonroutine procedure prevent mistakes and misunderstandings, and save valuable time
- Fasting
  - Fasting has been recommended to allow time for gastric emptying, which should decrease the risk of vomiting, regurgitation, and aspiration. Withholding food for periods from 2 to 10 hours have been suggested; short fasting times are appropriate in some instances, for example pediatric patients and cats with diabetes mellitus. The anesthetist should never assume that fasting will result in an empty stomach and must be prepared to act if vomiting occurs in the perioperative period (Chapter 10)
- Risk assessment (ASA status)
  - Full discussion of all possible presenting conditions is beyond the scope of this chapter, but interpretation of clinical data should allow the patient's health status to be classified according to the American Society of Anesthesiologists (ASA). The five-point scale used in people is adapted in *Table* 1.2 for use in veterinary medicine. ASA status is correlated with risk of anesthetic death
- Set up
  - All materials and equipment should be tested and ready before general anesthesia is induced. Supplies include tape, catheters, eye lubricant, flush solution, airway devices, laryngoscope, stylet, anesthetic record, surgical preparation solutions, gauze and fluid bags. Monitors should be calibrated beforehand. Anesthetic machines and breathing systems must be in good working condition

---

Box 1.6: Normal physiological values in cats

- **Resting heart rate:** 120–200 beats per minute
- **Resting respiration rate:** 20–30 breaths per minute
- **Rectal Temperature:** 37.5–38.9 °C

Ancillary tests are recommended when abnormalities are identified from the history and physical examination. This may include a basic blood panel (*Table* 1.1). Low hematocrit may indicate anemia, limiting the patient's ability to carry oxygen. Decreases in total protein may increase the effect of highly protein bound drugs and may also require adjustment of the anesthetic dose and fluid therapy. Many clinicians extend their screening to include a complete blood count, biochemical panel, total thyroxin (T4), and a urinalysis in geriatric patients. The rationale behind geriatric screening is the detection of subclinical disease despite normal clinical findings. However, *it is important to highlight that blood collection may cause stress and results will not change the anesthetic plan in the majority of cases.*

Hypertrophic cardiomyopathy is often asymptomatic in cats and can be only diagnosed using echocardiography. A workup is recommended when murmurs are

Table 1.2 ASA physical status classification system.

ASA classification[a]	Definition
ASA I	A normal healthy patient
ASA II	A patient with mild systemic disease
ASA III	A patient with severe systemic disease
ASA IV	A patient with severe systemic disease that is a constant threat to life
ASA V	A moribund patient who is not expected to survive without the operation

Note:
a) Each classification is further subdivided with the inclusion of an "E" to represent an emergency surgery, where delay may affect outcome.
Source: ASA House of Delegates. (2014) ASA Physical Status Classification System, American Society of Anesthesiologists, www.asahq.org/resources/clinical-information/asa-physical-status-classification-system (accessed June 24, 2017).

auscultated and if cardiovascular disease is suspected as this could change the anesthetic protocol (Chapters 9 and 10).

Risk Factors, Morbidity, and Mortality

The risk of anesthetic-related death in cats varies between 0.1% and 0.3%. A study in the United Kingdom reported an overall mortality rate of 0.24% in cats, which was

Table 1.3 Timing, number, and percentage of anesthetic- and sedation-related deaths in dogs, cats, and rabbits.

Timing of death	Dogs (%)	Cats (%)	Rabbits (%)
After premedication	1 (1)	2 (1)	0
Induction of anesthesia	9 (6)	14 (8)	6 (6)
Maintenance of anesthesia	68 (46)	53 (30)	29 (30)
Postoperative death[a]	70 (47)	106 (61)	62 (64)
0–3 hours post-op	31	66	26
3–6 hours post-op	11	9	7
6–12 hours post-op	12	7	13
12–24 hours post-op	13	12	9
24–48 hours post-op	3	10	3
Unknown time	0	2	4
Total	148 (100)	175 (100)	97 (100)

Note:
a) Postoperative deaths were additionally categorized by time after anesthesia. The percentage values are given in parentheses.
Source: Brodbelt 2008. Reproduced with permission of John Wiley & Sons.

higher than the 0.17% reported in dogs. Healthy cats (ASA I to II) are >12 times more likely to survive anesthesia than those that are sick (ASA III to V). This demonstrates the importance of preanesthetic assessment and health-status classification. An ASA classification of ≥ 3 should not discourage clinicians from important procedural interventions, but the increased risk should be taken into account when the anesthetic protocol and monitoring are planned and should be discussed with the owner. Since disease increases the risk of anesthetic-related mortality, elective procedures should be delayed until the patient is stabilized and/or treated. Perioperative monitoring is crucial because it is associated with reduced anesthetic risk. *Almost two-thirds of all anesthetic-related deaths in cats occurred in the post-operative period, in particular during the first three hours after extubation (Table 1.3)* (Chapter 10).

Other risk factors associated with perioperative mortality in cats include:

- *Extremes of age*
  - Neonatal and geriatric cats are at higher risk of anesthetic-induced fatality (Chapter 9). However, healthy kittens over 1 kg tolerate general anesthesia remarkably well
- *Extremes of body weight*
  - Weight loss in cats may indicate underlying disease (e.g. hyperthyroidism, renal disease, lymphoma), which may affect drug metabolism, protein binding, and cardiovascular reserve. Small cats may be at a greater risk for becoming hypothermic. On the other hand, obesity may be associated with disease (e.g. cardiovascular disease, diabetes, lower urinary-tract disease). Obese cats (*Figure* 1.6) have increased intra-abdominal and thoracic fat, potentially limiting respiratory function when in dorsal recumbency and potentially putting them at higher risk of airway obstruction (Chapter 10). Obesity increases the volume of distribution for lipophilic drugs into tissues that do not actively participate in drug metabolism
- *Endotracheal intubation*
  - Endotracheal intubation protects the airway while providing means of oxygenation, ventilation, and administration of anesthetic gas mixtures. A study reported that 63% of cats that died after surgery were intubated compared to 48% of nonintubated cats. One of the most common causes of perioperative death in cats is airway obstruction, which may be a result of laryngeal trauma during intubation (Chapter 10)
- *Absence of, or excessive, fluid therapy*
  - The benefits and risks of fluid administration during anesthesia are discussed in Chapter 8. Cats are at higher risk of fluid overload when compared with dogs. Administration of fluids has been associated with increased anesthetic-induced fatality (Chapter 10)
- *Spay-neuter clinics*
  - A retrospective study from a large volume spay-neuter clinic reported the risk of mortality in cats as 0.05%, 5 times that of dogs in the same setting. The risk of mortality in females was twice that of males and most deaths occurred post-operatively. The lower mortality risk in these cats compared to the Confidential Enquiry into Perioperative Small Animal Fatality (CEPSAF) study is probably due to the young, healthy population and the skills of experienced veterinarians.

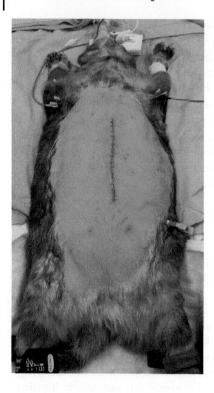

Figure 1.6 An obese cat (9.5 kg) immediately after the end of abdominal laparotomy for foreign body removal. Extremes of body weight are associated with increased risk of perioperative mortality in cats.

Further Reading

American Society of Anesthesiologists (2014) *ASA Physical Status Classification System,* www.asahq.org/resources/clinical-information/asa-physical-status-classification-system (accessed June 24, 2017).

Barletta, M., Kleine, S. A., and Quandt, J. E. (2015) Assessment of v-gel supraglottic airway device placement in cats performed by inexperienced veterinary students. *Veterinary Record* 177, 523.

Brodbelt, D. C., Blissitt, K. J., Hammond, R. A., *et al.* (2008) The risk of death: The Confidential Enquiry into Perioperative Small Animal Fatalities. *Veterinary Anaesthesia and Analgesia* 35, 365–373.

Brodbelt, D. C., Pfeiffer, D. U., Young, L. E., *et al.* (2007) Risk factors for anaesthetic-related death in cats: Results from the Confidential Enquiry into Perioperative Small Animal Fatalities (CEPSAF). *British Journal of Anaesthesia* 99, 617–623.

Carney, H. C., Little, S., Brownlee-Tomasso, D., *et al.* (2012) AAFP and ISFM feline-friendly nursing care guidelines. *Journal of Feline Medicine and Surgery* 14, 337–349.

Kronen, P. W., Ludders, J. W., Erb, H. N., *et al.* (2006) A synthetic fraction of feline facial pheromones calms but does not reduce struggling in cats before venous catheterization. *Veterinary Anaesthesia and Analgesia* 33, 258–265.

Levy, J. K., Bard, K. M., Tucker, S. J., *et al.* (2017) Perioperative mortality in cats and dogs undergoing spay or castration at a high-volume clinic. *Veterinary Journal* 224, 11–15.

Prasse, S. A., Schrack, J., Wenger, S., *et al*. Clinical evaluation of the v-gel supraglottic airway device in comparison with a classical laryngeal mask and endotracheal intubation in cats during spontaneous and controlled mechanical ventilation. *Veterinary Anaesthesia and Analgesia* **43**, 55–62.

Porters, N., de Rooster, H., Moons, C. P., *et al*. (2015) Prepubertal gonadectomy in cats: Different injectable anaesthetic combinations and comparison with gonadectomy at traditional age. *Journal of Feline Medicine and Surgery* **17**, 458–467.

Quimby, J. M., Smith, M. L., and Lunn, K. F. (2011) Evaluation of the effects of hospital visit stress on physiologic parameters in the cat. *Journal of Feline Medicine and Surgery* **13**, 733–737.

Rodan, I. (2010) Understanding feline behaviour and application for appropriate handling and management. *Topics in Companion Animal Medicine* **25**, 178–188.

Rodan, I., Sundahl, E., Carney, H., *et al*. (2011) AAFP and ISFM Feline-friendly handling guidelines. *Journal of Feline Medicine and Surgery* **13**, 364–375.

Thrall, M. A., Weiser, G., Allison, R. W., and Campbell, T. W. (2012) *Veterinary Hematology and Clinical Chemistry*, 2nd edn. Wiley-Blackwell, Ames, IA.

Turner, D. C., and Bateson, P. (2014) *The Domestic Cat: The Biology of its Behaviour*, 3rd edn. Cambridge University Press, New York, NY.

van Oostrom, H., Krauss, M. W., and Sap, R. (2013) A comparison between the v-gel supraglottic airway device and the cuffed endotracheal tube for airway management in spontaneously breathing cats during isoflurane anaesthesia. *Veterinary Anaesthesia and Analgesia* **40**, 265–271.

Wagner, K. A., Gibbon, K. J., Strom, T. L., *et al*. (2006) Adverse effects of EMLA (lidocaine/prilocaine) cream and efficacy for the placement of jugular catheters in hospitalized cats. *Journal of Feline Medicine and Surgery* **6**, 141–144.

Wallinder, E., Hibbert, A., Rudd, S., *et al*. (2012) Are hospitalised cats stressed by observing another cat undergoing routine clinical examination? *Journal of Feline Medicine and Surgery* **14**, 655.

2

Anatomy, Physiology, and Pharmacology

Bradley Simon[1] and Paulo Steagall[2]

[1]Texas A&M University, College Station, TX, United States
[2]Université de Montréal, Saint-Hyacinthe, Canada

Key Points

- Unique anatomical and physiological features of each organ system in the cat
- Overview of pharmacological effects of sedatives, analgesics, and anesthetics on each system
- Peculiarities of feline drug metabolism

Introduction

Assessment of physiological function can be difficult in cats due to their natural behavior, high sympathetic tone, disease, the effects of drugs, and lack of patient compliance in a hospital setting. This chapter describes specific features of normal feline physiology and anatomy, and includes a discussion of the effects of anesthetic and analgesic agents on body systems. Based on this information, the anesthetist may tailor an anesthetic protocol for the individual cat and prevent potential complications during anesthesia.

Cardiovascular System

Anatomy

The heart contains four chambers (right and left atria, right and left ventricle), and separates the arterial and venous systems. It is perfused by the right and left coronary arteries. The right ventricle pumps blood through the pulmonary valve into the pulmonary trunk and then into the pulmonary circulation where gas exchange takes place. The left ventricle pumps blood through the aortic valve into the aorta and out into the systemic circulation. Aortic blood enters arteries and then arterioles, which are heavily innervated and surrounded with smooth muscle to regulate tissue blood flow.

Feline Anesthesia and Pain Management, First Edition. Edited by Paulo Steagall, Sheilah Robertson and Polly Taylor.

The dorsal pedal artery is palpated on the dorsomedial aspect of the pelvic limb, distal to the tarsus, and the coccygeal artery on the ventral aspect of the tail. These arteries can be used for invasive blood pressure monitoring during anesthesia (Chapter 7). The radial artery is palpated on the palmar aspect of the forelimb, just distal to the carpal joint, and is often used for pulse detection and blood-pressure monitoring using Doppler ultrasound. Blood enters the capillaries where nutrient, waste, and fluid exchange occur. Arteriovenous (AV) anastomoses connect arterioles to venules and respond to α_1 and α_2 adrenergic stimulation. These AV anastomoses also play an intrinsic role in thermoregulation and are found in distal extremities and skin. Venules and veins transport blood from capillaries back to the heart and are a reservoir for 60–70% of the total blood volume during rest. They also possess α_1 and α_2 adrenergic receptors that alter vascular tone. The cephalic vein, medial saphenous, and the external jugular vein are used for venipuncture or intravenous catheter placement.

The chemoreceptors (pH, PCO_2, PO_2), baroreceptors (vascular and cardiac stretch receptors), local control mechanisms (PO_2, PCO_2, lactate, H^+), and the parasympathetic and sympathetic nervous systems play a fundamental role in acute blood pressure and heart-rate regulation.

Feline blood is unique when compared with other species, and this is further discussed in Chapter 8.

In cats, the heart sits in a more horizontal plane than in the dog, with greater sternal contact. Feline auscultation is best performed over the left and right parasternum, enabling the clinician to auscultate the following sounds (S):

- S1: "lub" is associated with closure of the tricuspid and mitral valves, and is best auscultated at the costochondral junction over the right apex of the heart at the fourth and fifth intercostal spaces (tricuspid) and over the left apex at the left fifth intercostal space (mitral)
- S2: "dub" is associated with closure of the pulmonary and aortic valves, and is loudest at the heart base, located medial to the triceps muscle on the left side at the third and fourth intercostal spaces
- S3 and S4 are considered abnormal in cats and constitute a "gallop rhythm". S3 may be associated with ventricular dilation or rapid ventricular filling during states of anemia, volume overload, dilated cardiomyopathy, and hypertrophic cardiomyopathy. S4 may be heard in patients with hypertrophic cardiomyopathy

The feline brain and retina receive the majority of their blood supply from the maxillary artery, which forms an arteriolar network known as the rete mirabile arteria maxillaris (*Figure 2.1*). *The prolonged use of a mouth gag or wide opening of the jaw may compress the maxillary artery via the angular process of the mandible, leading to blindness and neurological dysfunction* (Chapter 10). Opening the mouth narrows the distance between the medial aspect of the angular process of the mandible and the rostrolateral border of the tympanic bulla; the maxillary artery runs between these two osseous structures. In particular, spring-loaded mouth gags may reduce maxillary artery blood flow and compromise perfusion of the brain and retina. Mouth gags are no longer recommended in cats for dental procedures or endoscopy (*Figure 2.2*) (Chapter 10).

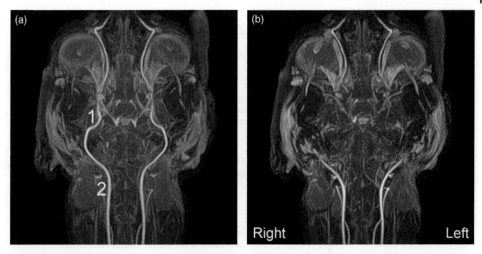

Figure 2.1 Magnetic resonance angiography of the head and neck of a cat. (1) maxillary artery; (2) external carotid artery. (a) normal blood flow with closed cat mouth; (b) severely decreased blood flow with open cat mouth.
Source: Barton-Lamb 2013. Reproduced with permission of Elsevier.

Cardiac Electrical Conductivity

The sinoatrial (SA) node contains specialized cardiac cells that allow spontaneous depolarization (automaticity) and is termed the "pacemaker". Automaticity depends on the slow influx of calcium and sodium into the cardiac myocyte, and is affected by temperature, pH, oxygen, carbon dioxide (CO_2), electrolytes, and hormones. Summation of the action potentials produced by all cardiac myocytes following SA node depolarization generates the electrocardiogram (ECG) (*Figure* 2.3a). The feline ECG (*Figure* 2.3b) can be difficult to interpret due to artifacts, rapid heart rate, and small

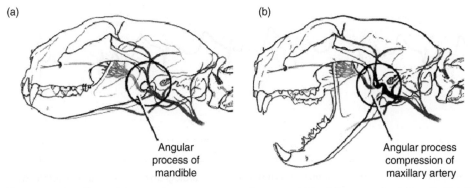

Figure 2.2 The effects of the angular process on maxillary arterial blood flow in cats with mouth closed (A) and mouth open (B).
Source: Barton-Lamb 2013. Reproduced with permission of Elsevier.

(a)

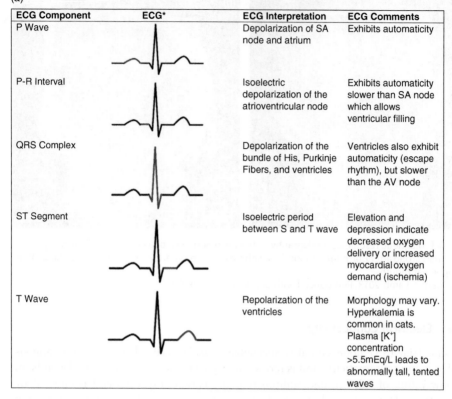

ECG Component	ECG*	ECG Interpretation	ECG Comments
P Wave		Depolarization of SA node and atrium	Exhibits automaticity
P-R Interval		Isoelectric depolarization of the atrioventricular node	Exhibits automaticity slower than SA node which allows ventricular filling
QRS Complex		Depolarization of the bundle of His, Purkinje Fibers, and ventricles	Ventricles also exhibit automaticity (escape rhythm), but slower than the AV node
ST Segment		Isoelectric period between S and T wave	Elevation and depression indicate decreased oxygen delivery or increased myocardial oxygen demand (ischemia)
T Wave		Repolarization of the ventricles	Morphology may vary. Hyperkalemia is common in cats. Plasma [K$^+$] concentration >5.5mEq/L leads to abnormally tall, tented waves

(b)

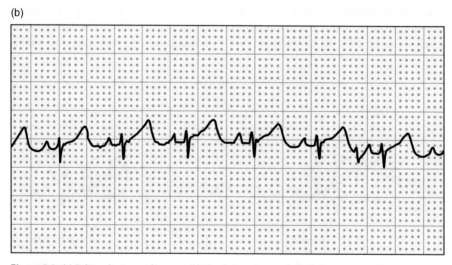

Figure 2.3 (a) Feline electrocardiogram. (b) The feline electrocardiogram can be difficult to interpret due to artifacts and electrical deflections.

electrical deflections. Electrolyte changes alter the ECG (for example in cats with hyperkalemia due to urinary tract obstruction) (Chapter 9).

Physiology

The volume of blood ejected from the left ventricle per contraction is termed the stroke volume (SV) and is affected by preload, afterload, and contractility. Stroke volume multiplied by the heart rate (HR) determines cardiac output (CO). This equation $(CO = SV \times HR)$ is of paramount importance in understanding and treating hypotension and hypertension in the clinical setting.

- The preload is the pressure of the blood creating stretch on the myocardium just before contraction. It is determined by the volume of blood returning from the systemic circulation (venous return)
- The afterload is the pressure in the wall of the left ventricle during ejection. It is directly related to the systemic vascular resistance (SVR). Increased systemic vascular resistance (i.e. after administration of agonists of α_2-adrenoreceptors) may decrease stroke volume
- Cardiac contractility depends on the availability of intracellular calcium. Sympathetic activation, afterload, circulating catecholamines, and heart rate affect ventricular contractility

Feline HR is affected by sympathetic and parasympathetic tone, mediated by norepinephrine and acetylcholine, respectively. Heart rates range from 140–200 beats per minute (bpm) in hospitalized cats while lower rates are reported in cats at home (120–140 bpm) (Chapter 1). Consensus statements of the American College of Veterinary Internal Medicine report that the mean (range) of systolic, mean, and diastolic arterial blood pressures (SAP, MAP, DAP) in conscious cats are 132 (115–162) mmHg, 102 (96–106) mmHg, and 83 (74–91) mmHg, respectively; these values may increase with age and are dependent on which device is used to measure blood pressure. Feline blood pressure may artificially increase when in hospital or stressed. This is termed "white-coat hypertension", and should be interpreted with caution. Values under anesthesia will be usually lower due to the depressant effects of general anesthetics.

Systemic hypertension is defined when SAP or MAP are persistently greater than 180 mmHg or 140 mmHg, respectively. Significant hypotension in cats occurs when SAP and MAP are below 80 mmHg and 60 mmHg, respectively. Blood pressure depends on CO and SVR (MAP = CO × SVR).

Under clinical conditions, hemodynamic changes during anesthesia are best evaluated as part of the whole picture. A combination of all variables such as HR, SAP, MAP, pulse pressure, oxygenation, and peripheral perfusion are integrated and considered before any therapeutic intervention is made. The ultimate goal is to deliver oxygen to the tissues.

Pharmacology

Table 2.1 summarizes the effects of sedatives and anesthetics on the cardiovascular system.

Respiratory System

Box 2.1 is a glossary of important terms relevant to anesthesia.

Box 2.1: Glossary of terms in anesthesia

- *Hypoxia* is the low oxygen tension *available to the tissues*. This includes hypoxic hypoxia (low arterial PO_2; pulmonary disease), anemic hypoxia (reduced oxygen carrying capacity in the blood; anemia or CO poisoning), circulatory hypoxia (decreased tissue blood flow; shock), and histotoxic hypoxia (poor ability for tissues to utilize oxygen; cyanide toxicity)
- *Hypoxemia* is the low oxygen tension *in the blood* ($PaO_2 < 60$ mmHg; normal $PaO_2 \geq$ 100 mmHg). Causes include low fractional inspired oxygen concentration, hypoventilation (when breathing room air), ventilation/perfusion mismatch (atelectasis, asthma, decreased pulmonary perfusion), anatomical shunting, and diffusion impairment
- Blood oxygenation may be measured as tension (pressure), hemoglobin saturation, and content. Most oxygen is carried by hemoglobin and very little is dissolved in plasma. Hemoglobin is 100% saturated above a PaO_2 of 150 mmHg (20 kPa). Any increase in PaO_2 above this adds very little to the total oxygen content. Higher tensions increase total content of oxygen in blood by increasing dissolved oxygen
- The volume of each normal breath (i.e. *tidal volume*) is approximately 8–9 mL/kg in cats. Normal *respiratory rate* varies from 20 to 30 breaths per minute in the adult; these values are lower during sedation and general anesthesia
- *Hyperventilation* leading to hypocapnia ($PaCO_2 < 30$ mmHg in cats) and *hypoventilation* leading to hypercapnia ($PaCO_2 > 50$ mmHg) are consequences of a change in minute volume (MV = tidal volume × RR). As CO_2 tension affects blood pH, hypercapnia causes respiratory acidosis (pH < 7.35), pulmonary vasoconstriction/hypertension, cerebral vasodilation, and increased sympathetic tone. Hypocapnia leads to respiratory alkalosis (pH > 7.45) and cerebral vasoconstriction
- *Cyanosis* is associated with extreme desaturation that renders a blue color to hemoglobin (Hb) (not detectable if Hb < 5 g/L). Indirectly, this is caused by low PaO_2 from sluggish peripheral circulation or admixture of venous blood, disruption of pulmonary ventilation or inadequate oxygen supply
- *Anatomical dead space* is contained in the conducting airways from the nares to the bronchi in which there can be no gas exchange. *Alveolar dead space* is the portion of alveoli in the lungs in which there is no gas exchange. *Physiological dead space* is the combination of the anatomical and alveolar dead space, which is approximately 6 mL/kg in healthy cats. *Apparatus or mechanical dead space* is the part of the breathing circuit (e.g. endotracheal tube connector) from which carbon dioxide is not removed; rebreathing occurs

---

Anatomy

The glossoepiglottic frenulum runs from the dorsal surface of the tongue to the cranial aspect of the epiglottis. Pulling the tongue rostrally moves the tip of the epiglottis forward and down, exposing the laryngeal inlet and vocal cords.

Feline airways are small and more sensitive to trauma, spasm and edema than other species. The larynx may spasm during intubation. If this occurs, cyanosis and hypoxia develop and may be fatal. Laryngospasm is a well-known hazard for the anesthetist (*Box* 2.2; *Figure* 2.4). The use of a supraglottic airway device (e.g. v-gel) may circumvent

Table 2.1 Pharmacology and CV system.

	Increase	Decrease
Contractility	dissociative agents[a] (indirect), norepinephrine, epinephrine, ephedrine, dobutamine, dopamine	propofol, volatile anesthetics, barbiturates, lidocaine
Heart rate	dissociative agents[a] (indirect), norepinephrine, epinephrine, ephedrine, dobutamine, dopamine, anticholinergic drugs,[b] alfaxalone	opioids, agonists of α_2-adrenergic receptors
Blood pressure (BP = CO × SVR)	dissociative agents,[a] α_2 adrenergic agonists (transient), norepinephrine, epinephrine, ephedrine, dobutamine, dopamine, anticholinergic drugs,[b] vasopressin, phenylephrine	propofol, volatile anesthetics, alfaxalone, acepromazine, agonists of α_2-adrenergc receptors (late effect)
Cardiac output (CO = HR × SV)	dissociative agents,[a] norepinephrine, epinephrine, ephedrine, dobutamine, dopamine, anticholinergics drugs[b]	agonists of α_2-adrenergic receptors, volatile anesthetics, propofol, barbiturates, lidocaine, alfaxalone
Dysrhythmias	barbiturates, dissociative agents,[a] epinephrine,	lidocaine, acepromazine
Packed-cell volume	phenylephrine, epinephrine, agonists of α_2-adrenergic receptor	acepromazine

Notes:
a) Ketamine and tiletamine;
b) Atropine and glycopyrrolate.

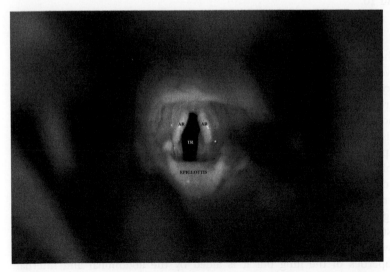

Figure 2.4 Feline larynx during intubation. Note the space between the arytenoid cartilages, necessary for the endotracheal tube to pass into the larynx and trachea. (AR) – Arytenoid cartilages; (TR) – opening into the trachea.

Box 2.2: The issue of laryngospasm in cats

- Cats are prone to laryngospasm, characterized by tight closure of the arytenoids in response to mechanical (during intubation) or chemical (detergent, disinfectants) stimulation
- Laryngospasm may occur both during intubation and as the endotracheal tube is removed and, less typically, later during recovery
- Laryngospasm can be blunted by application of 0.1 mL of lidocaine 2% onto the arytenoid cartilages before endotracheal intubation. Metered local anesthetic sprays at concentrations of 10% should be avoided due to the risk of toxicity. Additional excipients (e.g. methylparaben) found in some human products may cause fatal laryngeal cell damage and edema
- Local anesthetic spray should be allowed to take effect (30 seconds) and the glottis should reopen before intubation is attempted
- Laryngospasm is reduced, but not entirely prevented, by propofol, alfaxalone, and sedatives
- Laryngospasm can be prevented by IV administration of a neuromuscular blocking agent (e.g. atracurium) and this may be required in emergency. Cyanosis and hypoxemia develop rapidly when both laryngospasm and anesthetic-induced respiratory depression occur during induction of anesthesia; this can be ameliorated with preoxygenation
- Deep anesthesia enables intubation with less likelihood of laryngospasm but risks overdose

---

this problem. Potential complications associated with airway management are discussed in Chapters 1 and 10.

Physiology

Oxygen travels through the trachea, bronchi, and bronchioles into the alveolar sacs via bulk flow. The alveoli have a large surface area and pulmonary capillaries are intertwined around them. Oxygen tension in the alveolar capillaries is lower than in the alveoli. The oxygen tension gradient and large surface area enable rapid diffusion of oxygen from the alveoli into blood. Hemoglobin (Hb) is the major transport mechanism for oxygen. Oxygen binding is dependent on the affinity of Hb for oxygen molecules and is affected by temperature, pH, 2,3-diphosphoglycerate (DPG), and CO_2.

The feline diaphragm has more muscle fibers than the canine equivalent and motor function is controlled via the phrenic nerve, which arises from the ventral branches of cervical spinal nerves five, six, and seven. The diaphragm plays an important role during inspiration, along with the scalenus, serratus dorsalis cranialis, rectus thoracis, and external intercostal muscles. Inspiration is an active process and cats have a more compliant chest wall than other species. Expiration is mostly a passive process due to the elastic recoil properties of the lung but it is aided by the abdominal and internal intercostal muscles.

Table 2.2 Pharmacology and respiratory system

	Increase	Decrease
Minute ventilation (MV = TV × RR)	Agonists of β_2-adrenergic receptors (albuterol, terbutaline), doxapram	Opioids, propofol, barbiturates, dissociative anesthetics (apneustic pattern), alfaxalone, volatile anesthetics, agonists of α_2-adrenergic receptors
Bronchial tone	Chemicals, dust, smoke, desflurane	Sevoflurane, isoflurane, dissociative anesthetics, epinephrine, ephedrine, anticholinergic drugs

Overall, ventilation is dependent on feedback from the central nervous system (CNS) (brainstem, cortex, limbic system, and hypothalamus), central chemoreceptors (PaCO$_2$ – partial pressure of carbon dioxide in blood), peripheral chemoreceptors (pH, PaCO$_2$, PaO$_2$ – partial pressure of oxygen in blood), lung and peripheral receptors. Changes in PaCO$_2$ (< 35 mmHg or > 45 mmHg) are the major driving force for ventilation. Significant reductions in PaO$_2$ (< 60 mmHg) also cause increased ventilation ("hypoxic drive"). Feline pores of Kohn allow the passage of gas from poorly to highly ventilated areas of the lung, contributing to a high degree of collateral ventilation in this species.

Pharmacology

Table 2.2 describes the effects of sedatives and anesthetics on the respiratory system.

Nervous System

Central Nervous System (CNS) Anatomy

The CNS consists of the brain and the spinal cord. The brain is made up of the cerebrum, hypothalamus, thalamus, pons, cerebellum, and medulla oblongata. The primary energy sources for the brain are oxygen and glucose. Cerebrospinal fluid (CSF) plays an important role in protecting the CNS against trauma and in homeostasis of cerebral parenchymal interstitial fluid.

The blood-brain barrier is a permeable lipid barrier that separates the circulating blood from the brain's extracellular fluid. It restricts the movement of highly ionized, protein-bound, water-soluble, and large molecular weight substances into the brain. Penetrability of drugs through the barrier is dependent on molecular size, charge, lipid solubility and protein binding. Most anesthetic agents, oxygen, and CO$_2$ penetrate the blood-brain barrier readily. Permeability may increase with intracranial disease, neoplasia, inflammation, trauma, hypercapnia, sustained seizures, azotemia, and hypoxia.

The spinal cord is surrounded by three layers of meninges: dura mater, arachnoid membrane, and pia mater. The epidural space surrounds the dura mater and contains adipose tissue. The subarachnoid space is filled with CSF and is located between the arachnoid membrane and pia mater. The dorsal horn of the spinal cord is the primary site

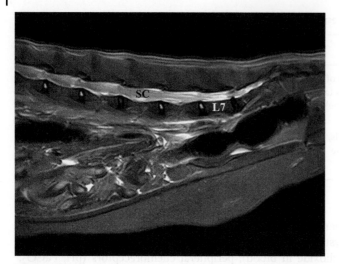

Figure 2.5 Magnetic resonance image of a feline lumbar and sacral spinal column. Note the spinal cord (SC) extending beyond the seventh lumbar (L7) vertebra.
Source: Courtesy of Mr. Wade Friedeck.

for sensory innervation and nociception. In cats, the arachnoid space extends beyond the lumbosacral junction (*Figure* 2.5), so epidural injections at this site are more likely to lead to accidental subarachnoid puncture (spinal or intrathecal) than in dogs (Chapter 5).

Peripheral Nervous System Anatomy

The peripheral nervous system is made up of sensory neurons that travel to the CNS (afferent) and motor fibers that travel from the CNS (efferent). The peripheral nervous system includes the autonomic nervous system, the parasympathetic and sympathetic nervous systems (PNS and SNS, respectively), and innervates vital organ systems including, but not limited to, the visual, cardiovascular, respiratory, reproductive, digestive, endocrine, and excretory systems.

Parasympathetic Nervous System (PNS)

- The cranial component is carried in cranial nerves II (oculomotor), VII (facial), IX (glossopharyngeal), and X (vagus). The vagus nerve carries parasympathetic nerve fibers to the heart, lungs, and abdominal organs, and accounts for 75% of the PNS
- The sacral component extends from three sacral spinal segments and supplies pelvic viscera
- The PNS contain two types of receptors: muscarinic and nicotinic. These receptors are activated by acetylcholine (ACh) both presynaptically and postsynaptically. Acetylcholinesterase degrades ACh into choline and acetate
  - Nicotinic receptors and ACh are responsible for skeletal muscle stimulation at the neuromuscular junction
  - Muscarinic receptors are found in secretory glands, smooth muscle, and the myocardium

- Clinical effects of parasympathetic stimulation include decreased heart rate, arteriolar vasodilation, bronchoconstriction, increased glandular secretions, miosis, and increased gastrointestinal motility

Sympathetic Nervous System (SNS)

- The SNS is located in the lateral horn of the spinal cord from the first thoracic to the fifth lumbar vertebra. It contains three major types of adrenergic receptors: dopaminergic, α (α_1 and α_2), and β (β_1, β_2 and β_3)
  - ACh is released from the preganglionic nerve ending whereas norepinephrine (NE) is released by most postganglionic nerve endings. Norepinephrine stimulates both α and β receptors within the splanchnic, cardiac, respiratory, and gastrointestinal systems
  - ACh is the main neurotransmitter activating muscarinic receptors on blood vessels in skeletal muscle producing vasodilation, and sweat glands. ACh also activates nicotinic receptors on the adrenal medulla
  - Dopamine and epinephrine are released from the adrenal gland(s) and stimulate dopamine and adrenergic receptors, respectively
- Clinical effects of the SNS include increased heart rate and contractility, bronchodilation, decreased intestinal activity, bladder relaxation, urinary sphincter constriction, decreased insulin secretion, glycogenolysis, gluconeogenesis, and lipolysis

Physiology

Autoregulation of cerebral blood flow (CBF) maintains constant cerebral perfusion during states of altered arterial blood pressure. This preserves perfusion when MAP is between approximately 60 mmHg and 160 mmHg. Mean blood pressure must be greater than 50 mmHg to prevent cerebral ischemia in cats. In cats with conditions that may induce systemic hypertension, for example cardiovascular and chronic kidney disease, the lower limits of cerebral autoregulation may shift upwards, closer to 80 mmHg. CBF is directly related to cerebral perfusion pressure (CPP) which in turn is directly related to MAP and indirectly related to intracranial pressure (ICP): CPP = MAP − ICP. Cats with increased ICP may have hypertension with reflex bradycardia (Cushing's reflex) (Chapter 9). Raised ICP associated with a space-occupying lesion may also cause changes in breathing pattern.

Pharmacology

Table 2.3 shows the effects of sedatives, anesthetics, and analgesics on the nervous system.

Urinary System

Anatomy

Feline kidneys are palpated with the right lying just ventral to the first-fourth lumbar vertebrae and the left just ventral to the second-fifth lumbar vertebrae. They have prominent capsular veins and are separated into two major areas; the cortex and medulla. Innervation of the kidneys is predominantly from sympathetic nerve fibers.

The nephron is the microscopic functional unit of the kidney. Feline kidneys contain fewer nephrons (approximately 200 000/kidney) when compared with the dog (approximately

Table 2.3 Pharmacology and neurological system.

	Increase	Decrease
Cerebral blood flow and intracranial pressure	Volatile anesthetics (> 1 × MAC*), dissociative anesthetics, hyperthermia, hypercapnia, hypoxemia, hypertension, vasodilators, vomiting	Volatile anesthetics (< 0.5 × MAC*), barbiturates, etomidate, propofol, midazolam, diazepam, alfaxalone
Sympathetic nervous system	Activation: inotropes, epinephrine, norepinephrine, dopamine, dobutamine, phenylephrine, ephedrine, albuterol, terbutaline	Local anesthetics via epidural or spinal route cause blunting of the SNS ("sympathetic blockade" results in vasodilation, venous pooling, and hypotension)
Parasympathetic nervous system	Anticholinergic agents (muscarinic receptors only)	Neuromuscular blocking agents (nicotinic receptors only)

*Minimum Alveolar Concentration

500 000/kidney). The nephron consists of the glomerulus, Bowman's capsule, proximal convoluted tubule, loop of Henle, distal convoluted tubule and the collecting ducts. The function of the nephron is to reabsorb water, electrolytes, and low molecular-weight proteins back into the circulation, and to eliminate unwanted solutes in urine.

Male cats have a long and narrow urethra. For anatomical reasons, urethral obstruction, caused by matrix plugs, is more likely to occur in male cats.

Renal Blood Flow and Autoregulation

The kidney receives 25% of the cardiac output via the renal artery, with the majority delivered to the renal cortex. The medulla receives a smaller portion, making it extremely sensitive to hypoxemia and hypotension.

Renal blood flow (RBF) is regulated both extrinsically and intrinsically, is dependent on adequate blood pressure, and is kept constant when MAP is within the range of approximately 75–160 mmHg (autoregulation). Extrinsically, angiotensin II, aldosterone, vasopressin, and atrial natriuretic peptides alter systemic blood pressure in response to changes in systemic blood volume to maintain RBF. Intrinsically, the renin-angiotensin-aldosterone system (RAAS) assists in regulating RBF and glomerular filtration rate (GFR). Both angiotensin II and aldosterone increase sodium and water retention promoting increases in intravascular volume and renal blood flow. Angiotensin II also increases prostaglandin production (PGE_2 and prostacyclin), which promotes renal arterial dilation protecting against ischemia. Decreased renal perfusion due to hypotension, hypovolemia or dehydration may exacerbate the renal toxicity of nonsteroidal anti-inflammatory drugs (NSAIDs) (Chapter 10 and 13).

Physiology

Blood filtration occurs in the glomerulus, a tuft of capillaries receiving blood from the afferent arteriole. Filtered blood exits the glomerulus via the efferent arteriole. The GFR is an important measure of renal function. Starling's forces are responsible for filtration of the solutes, small proteins, and water leaving the glomerulus (*Box* 2.3). Larger molecules and negatively charged ions (anions) do not readily cross the filtration barrier.

Box 2.3: Starling's forces and net filtration

- Starling's forces determine net filtration of a fluid across a capillary membrane.
- Net filtration is dependent on both hydrostatic and oncotic pressures within the intravascular and interstitial compartments:

$$\text{Net filtration} = K_f \left[(P_{cap} - P_{if}) - (\pi_P - \pi_{if}) \right]$$

K_f = filtration coefficient, P = hydrostatic pressure generated by the heart (P_{cap}) or tissues (P_{if}); π = oncotic pressure generated by plasma proteins (π_P) or filtered proteins and mucopolysaccharides in the interstitium (π_{if})

The proximal convoluted tubule reabsorbs 60% of the filtrate back into the systemic circulation. Glucose, sodium, chloride, potassium, calcium, insulin, glucagon, parathyroid hormone, and bicarbonate are reabsorbed here. Toxins, some drugs, hydrogen ions, creatinine, oxalates, prostaglandins, epinephrine, and endogenous waste products are not reabsorbed and are cleared from the systemic circulation:

- The descending loop of Henle aids in water reabsorption as well as some reabsorption of sodium, potassium, and chloride
- The ascending loop of Henle is primarily responsible for solute reabsorption. These cells are impermeable to water
- The distal convoluted tubule is the site for bicarbonate, sodium, and water reabsorption along with proton and potassium excretion. Since protons and potassium compete for excretion, hyperkalemic cats may develop concurrent acidemia because of the need to remove potassium (Chapter 9). The collecting tubule is primarily responsible for water regulation in response to arginine vasopressin (AVP)

The kidneys also play an important role in regulating systemic pH via reabsorption of bicarbonate in cases of chronic respiratory acidosis; this compensatory mechanism takes 24–36 hours to develop. In addition, erythropoietin is produced in the kidney and aids in red blood cell production; secondary anemia is common in chronic renal failure.

Pharmacology

Table 2.4 shows the effects of sedatives and anesthetic drugs on the urinary system.

- Nephrotoxic substances
  - Compound A: Sevoflurane at low flow rates in contact with dry older style CO_2 absorbents creates fluoride ions (Compound A). This is of negligible clinical significance when using nonrebreathing systems and fresh gas flows ≥ 200 mL/kg/hour
  - NSAIDs may decrease renal perfusion via their inhibition of vasodilatory prostaglandins and must be used with caution in patients with hypotension or hypovolemia
- Pharmacokinetics
  - Azotemia and renal dysfunction decrease anesthetic and sedative requirements by changing the blood-brain barrier permeability

Table 2.4 Pharmacology and urinary system.

	Increase	Decrease
Renal blood flow	Dopamine (controversial)	Volatile anesthetics, agonists of α_2- adrenergic receptors, hypotension
Urine output	Agonists of κ-opioid receptors (butorphanol), agonists of α_2- adrenergic receptors	Volatile anesthetics, pure agonists of μ-opioid receptor (parenteral or epidural)
Natriuresis	Dopamine (controversial)	Volatile anesthetics
Potentially nephrotoxicity (further description in the text)	Compound A, NSAIDs, aminoglycosides, vancomycin, polymyxin, ciprofloxacin, trimethoprim sulfamethoxazole, propylene glycol (some formulations of diazepam and etomidate), iodinated contrast media, gadolinium	

- Diazepam: hepatic metabolism of diazepam produces the active metabolite desmethyldiazepam and temazepam in cats (Chapter 3). Diazepam undergoes slow biotransformation in cats where there is inhibition of the bile acid efflux that results in accumulation of bile acid in the hepatocytes. These mechanisms can contribute to liver injury after repetitive administration of diazepam. Both the parent compound and its metabolites are eliminated via the kidney, and in cats with impaired renal clearance the clinical effects of diazepam may be prolonged (several days). Midazolam is the preferred benzodiazepine in cats
- Ketamine is metabolized in the liver to the active metabolite norketamine, which is renally excreted. In cats with significant renal impairment, the effect of both ketamine and norketamine may be prolonged

Hepatic System

Anatomy and Physiology

The liver is the largest endocrine organ in the body, located primarily in the thoracic part of the abdominal cavity. It is divided into six lobes by interlobar fissures: left and right lateral, left and right medial, quadrate, and caudate lobes. In cats, it may be difficult to distinguish between the quadrate and right medial lobes. The left lobes account for approximately 50% of the liver mass. The gall bladder resides between the right medial and quadrate lobe. In cats, the bile duct shares a common duct with the pancreas.

The hepatic portal system consists of the portal vein, hepatic artery, nerves, ducts, and lymphatics. The liver receives approximately 30% of the cardiac output. The portal vein delivers three-quarters of the liver's blood flow. The hepatic artery carries blood with higher oxygen content than the portal vein. Blood entering the portal vein comes from the abdominal organs and gastrointestinal tract. Hepatic innervation is from both the PNS and SNS, stimulating adrenergic, dopaminergic, and cholinergic receptors.

The major functions of the liver include production of albumin, coagulation, and clotting factors, acute phase proteins, urea, and plasma cholinesterases, as well as metabolism of carbohydrates, lipids, amino acids, ammonia, and drugs. The liver maintains oncotic pressure and stores glycogen. Hypoalbuminemia predisposes to ascites, and edema, and may affect the pharmacokinetics of drugs normally bound to albumin.

Hepatic Metabolism and Pharmacology of Anesthetics, Analgesics, and Sedatives

Some drugs that are administered via parenteral or rectal routes undergo the *first-pass effect*. In this case, metabolism by the liver decreases their bioavailability and systemic effects. This is particularly evident after oral (not buccal) administration of opioids: optimal analgesia does not occur.

- Phase I metabolism (oxidation, reduction, hydrolysis, deamination, sulfoxidation, and dealkylation or methylation) may produce inactive or active metabolites. The cytochrome P450 (CP450) and its subtypes are the most important hepatic enzymes in drug metabolism. They convert lipid-soluble anesthetics to more water-soluble compounds, which are eliminated via urine and bile. Some CP450 inducers (benzodiazepines, ketamine, and barbiturates) and inhibitors (cimetidine and chloramphenicol) have been identified. However, the clinical relevance of this in cats is unknown, especially with short-term administration
- Phase II metabolism (conjugation and glucuronidation) further increases water solubility and polarity, and enhances renal elimination. Some drugs are metabolized more slowly in cats when compared with dogs. Cats are deficient in glucuronyl transferases, which prolongs biotransformation of a number of drugs (propofol, carprofen, aspirin, acetaminophen) which may lead to toxicity of some such as acetaminophen (paracetamol) (e.g. methemoglobinemia) and salicylates. This issue appears to be most significant regarding the lack of metabolism of phenolic compounds. In cats, metabolism of acetaminophen produces reactive free radicals, which cause oxidative damage to erythrocytes and formation of methemoglobin and Heinz bodies. The metabolism of propofol in cats is unknown, but its slow clearance and prolonged elimination half life in this species may be associated with a deficiency in glucuronidation. Most anesthetic drugs require glucuronidation for metabolism, but cats may use alternative pathways. For example, morphine is metabolized via sulfate conjugation rather than glucuronidation in this species. Drugs that do not depend on glucuronidation include atracurium and remifentanil
- Benzyl alcohol, often used as a bacteriostatic preservative, requires glucuronidation for metabolism. Benzyl alcohol is used as a preservative in some formulations of propofol and carprofen. Excessive amounts (> 156 mg in 6.5 hours) may cause central nervous system toxicity (hyperesthesia, ataxia, depression, aggression, coma, death). The benzyl alcohol used in some formulations of propofol does not cause toxic effects in cats when used in normal clinical protocols

Endocrine System

- Exocrine pancreas:
  - Acini cells secrete digestive enzymes that contribute to gastrointestinal function, digestion, and motility

Table 2.5 Pharmacology and neuroendocrine system.

Anesthetic drug	Target endocrine organ	Pharmacological effect
Opioid agonists	Hypothalamus Adrenal gland	Alter thermoregulation usually resulting in hyperthermia (specifically in cats) Blunt the stress response
Acepromazine	Hypothalamus	Alters thermoregulation resulting in hypothermia
Agonists of α_2- adrenergic receptors	Adrenal gland Pancreas	Decrease stress response Hyperglycemia due to decreased insulin release from β cells
Etomidate	Adrenal gland	Reduction in cortisol and aldosterone production by inhibiting 11 β-hydroxylase for up to three hours in cats. Concern about repeat administration or infusion. Single-dose administration used with caution in adrenocortical disease (Addison's disease)

- Endocrine pancreas:
  - β cells: produce insulin which controls uptake, storage, and use of glucose by most body tissues; insulin enhances anabolism via glycogenesis, increased protein synthesis, glycolysis, and triglyceride storage; it inhibits catabolism
  - α cells: produce glucagon which increases blood glucose concentration. Glucagon decreases glycogen synthesis and increases both glycogenolysis and gluconeogenesis

Table 2.5 describes the effect of anesthetic agents on endocrine gland function.

Gastrointestinal System

Anatomy

The digestive tract includes the oropharynx, esophagus, stomach, intestines, and colon. The pancreas, liver, and biliary tract also play an important role in digestion. The tract contains smooth muscle with four major orientated layers: mucosa, submucosa, muscularis externa, and serosa. In cats, the first two-thirds of the esophagus have striated muscle.

The innervation of the gastrointestinal tract (GIT) contains both extrinsic (parasympathetic and sympathetic) and intrinsic (enteric nervous system (ENS)) components. Parasympathetic fibers to the upper tract are supplied via the vagus and pelvic nerves supply the lower tract. Sympathetic innervation is provided by spinal segments T1 to L3, and is typically inhibitory in the GIT. The ENS is located in the submucosal and myenteric plexus, receiving input from the PNS and SNS. Cats with GIT disease and undergoing abdominal laparotomy may have increased vagal tone with bradycardia.

Physiology

The major functions of the GIT, with aid from the neuroendocrine, pancreatic and hepatic systems, are to digest and absorb water, nutrients, electrolytes, minerals, vitamins, xenobiotics, proteins, lipids, carbohydrates, hormones, and bile secretions.

Total GIT transition time in cats is between 25 and 35 hours. Unlike other species, cats use a less intense system called a migrating spike complex to assist in emptying the stomach. Complete emptying of the stomach is less likely in this species. Gastric emptying time in conscious fed or unfed cats is approximately 9 hours and 1 hour, respectively. However, stress and fear may increase sympathetic tone, which decreases gastrointestinal transit time. Fasting times are often empirically suggested in cats and gastric emptying time in this species can be unpredictable (Chapter 10). Therefore, fasting period of more than 8 hours is most likely unnecessary. Water may be offered to cats up until an hour before surgery.

Pharmacology

Some drugs may cause emesis and nausea in cats. Vomiting is common after lower dosages and when the SC or IM route is used. Some opioid agonists (e.g. morphine and hydromorphone) stimulate the chemoreceptor trigger zone and dopamine receptors in the vomiting center to induce vomiting. Both neural and humoral pathways play an intricate role during emesis. Some other opioids such as buprenorphine and methadone do not cause vomiting. Agonists of α_2-adrenoceptors may also cause vomiting by stimulating the chemoreceptor trigger zone. Acepromazine has antiemetic properties, which may inhibit vomiting when administered 15 to 20 minutes before an opioid. However, this has not been demonstrated in cats.

Opioids are known to increase gastroesophageal reflux but this has not been thoroughly investigated in cats. Intestinal motility decreases after administration of opioids, agonists of α_2-adrenoceptors and volatile anesthetics. Appetite increases after propofol and diazepam administration. Life-threatening ulcers may be produced by NSAIDs when administered with corticosteroids, or when dosage intervals, data sheet dosing and contraindications are not observed. Chronic kidney disease leads to decreased appetite, weight loss and vomiting.

Maropitant (a neurokinin-1 receptor antagonist) is a very effective antiemetic in cats (e.g. for xylazine and uremia). Ondansetron (a serotonin 5-HT_3 receptor antagonist) prevents dexmedetomidine-induced vomiting in cats. This antiemetic drug is only effective when administered simultaneously with dexmedetomidine as it provides little benefit when administered 30 minutes before the sedative.

Further Reading

Apfel, C. C., Korttila, K., Abdalla, M., *et al.* (2004) A factorial trial of six interventions for the prevention of postoperative nausea and vomiting. *New England Journal of Medicine* **350**, 2441–2451.

Bodey, A. R., and Sansom, J. (1998) Epidemiological study of blood pressure in domestic cats. *Journal of Small Animal Practice* **39**, 567–573.

Brezis, M., and Rosen, S. (1995) Hypoxia of the renal medulla – its implications for disease. *New England Journal of Medicine* **332**, 647–655.

Castellanos, I., Couto, C. G., and Gray, T. L. (2004) Clinical use of blood products in cats: A retrospective study (1997–2000). *Journal of Veterinary Internal Medicine* **18**, 529–532.

Chandler, M. L., Guilford, G., and Lawoko, C. R. (1997) Radiopaque markers to evaluate gastric emptying and small intestinal transit time in healthy cats. *Journal of Veterinary Internal Medicine* **11**, 361–364.

Court, M. H. (2013) Feline drug metabolism and disposition: Pharmacokinetic evidence for species differences and molecular mechanisms. *Veterinary Clinics of North America: Small Animal Practice* **43**, 1039–1054.

Cowles, C. E. (2013) Neurophysiology and Anesthesia. In *Morgan and Mikhail's Clinical Anesthesiology*, 5th edn. (eds. J. Butterworth, D. Mackey, J. Wasnick). McGraw-Hill Education, New York, NY, pp. 575–592.

Cupples, W. A., and Braam, B. (2007) Assessment of renal autoregulation. *American Journal of Physiology* **292**, F1105–1123.

De Vos, W. C. (1993) Migrating spike complex in the small intestine of the fasting cat. *The American Journal of Physiology* **265**, G619–627.

Hanna, R. M., Borchard, R. E., and Schmidt, S. L. (1988a) Pharmacokinetics of ketamine HCl and metabolite I in the cat: A comparison of i.v., i.m., and rectal administration. *Journal of Veterinary Pharmacology and Therapeutics* **11**, 84–93.

Hanna, R. M., Borchard, R. E., and Schmidt, S. L. (1988b) Effect of diuretics on ketamine and sulfanilate elimination in cats. *Journal of Veterinary Pharmacology and Therapeutics* **11**, 121–129.

Kanda, T., and Hikasa, Y. (2008) Neurohormonal and metabolic effects of medetomidine compared with xylazine in healthy cats. *Canadian Journal of Veterinary Research* **72**, 278–286.

Maugeri, S., Ferrè, J. P., Intorre, L., *et al.* (1994) Effects of medetomidine on intestinal and colonic motility in the dog. *Journal of Veterinary Pharmacology and Therapeutics* **17**, 148–154.

Moon, P. F. (1997) Cortisol suppression in cats after induction of anesthesia with etomidate, compared with ketamine-diazepam combination. *American Journal of Veterinary Research* **58**, 868–871.

Nemoto, E. M., Hossmann, K. A., and Cooper, H. K. (1981) Post-ischemic hypermetabolism in cat brain. *Stroke* **12**, 666–676.

Papich, M. G. (2008) An update on nonsteroidal anti-inflammatory drugs (NSAIDs) in small animals. *Veterinary Clinics of North America: Small Animal Practice* **38**, 1243–1266.

Peachey, S. E., Dawson, J. M., and Harper, E. J. (2000) Gastrointestinal transit times in young and old cats. *Comparative Biochemistry and Physiology. Part A, Molecular and Integrative Physiology* **126**, 85–90.

Podell, M. (1998) Antiepileptic drug therapy. *Clinical Techniques in Small Animal Practice* **13**, 185–192.

Posner, L. P., Pavuk, A. A., Rokshar, J. L., *et al.* (2010) Effects of opioids and anesthetic drugs on body temperature in cats. *Veterinary Anaesthesia and Analgesia* **37**, 35–43.

Quimby, J. M., Brock, W. T., Moses, K., *et al.* (2015) Chronic use of maropitant for the management of vomiting and inappetence in cats with chronic kidney disease: A blinded, placebo-controlled clinical trial. *Journal of Feline Medicine and Surgery* **17**, 692–697.

Robinson, N. E. (1982) Some functional consequences of species differences in lung anatomy. *Advances in Veterinary Science and Comparative Medicine* **26**, 1–33.

van Beusekom, C. D., van den Heuvel, J. J., Koenderink, J. B., *et al.* (2015) Feline hepatic biotransformation of diazepam: Differences between cats and dogs. *Research in Veterinary Science* **103**, 119–125.

3

Sedation and Premedication

Paulo Steagall

Université de Montréal, Saint-Hyacinthe, Canada

Key Points

- Indications for sedation and premedication
- Definition of neuroleptanalgesia
- Drugs used for sedation including their clinical application, adverse effects and contraindications
- Practical tips on sedation and premedication

Introduction

Cats regularly require sedation to facilitate physical examination, handling, and diagnostic investigation. Premedication is the administration of sedatives or tranquilizers before general anesthesia. This is usually to render the cat cooperative, to reduce stress, and to provide analgesia in the preoperative period. A stress response leads to deleterious physiological effects through activation of the sympathetic nervous system. Analgesics (e.g. opioids) are administered as part of the premedication whenever pain is a concern or to reduce the dose of sedatives.

Sedation is commonly required in the following scenarios:

- To allow vascular access or venipuncture
- To allow minor noninvasive procedures such as urinary catheterization, bandage change, imaging, or other minor diagnostic procedures
- To provide anxyolisis, comfort, and perioperative analgesia
- To reduce the dose (requirements) of intravenous and inhalant anesthetics
- To smooth anesthetic induction and recovery
- To treat excitement and opioid-induced dysphoria without reversal of analgesia

There is a false impression that sedation is safer than general anesthesia. However, some sedatives may cause significant cardiorespiratory depression and potential hazards (e.g. regurgitation, hypoxemia) for the cat. This is particularly true for the critically ill, pediatric, or geriatric patient. In the latter cases, physiological systems

Feline Anesthesia and Pain Management, First Edition. Edited by Paulo Steagall,
Sheilah Robertson and Polly Taylor.

may already be compromised by an underlying disease, or may not yet be fully developed (as in pediatrics). In addition, general anesthesia allows airway control and ventilation with oxygen. It is recommended that vigilant monitoring is applied; the cat should be always under close supervision after administration of sedative drugs.

The choice of sedative for the procedure to be carried out and the required degree of sedation should be evaluated on a case-by-case basis (*Box* 3.1). A thorough physical examination is recommended to identify both minor and major pathology before selection of the appropriate sedative and analgesic therapy. Sedation of fractious cats can be challenging because the depth of sedation achieved with ketamine-based protocols is profound, with loss of protective reflexes. Patient history is often unknown.

The SC route of administration is often chosen for premedication because it is less painful. However, particularly with opioids (Chapter 13), this is *not* the best route as uptake is variable and unreliable. The IM route is preferred when an intravenous catheter is not in place. The buccal (oral transmucosal) route may be used to administer drugs in fractious patients or for analgesia.

Box 3.1: Neuroleptoanalgesia

Neuroleptanalgesia is a combination of a sedative or tranquilizer (i.e. acepromazine *or* an agonist of α_2-adrenergic receptors) with an analgesic, most commonly an opioid. The combination is synergistic, increasing the intensity of sedation and analgesia while decreasing the doses of each individual drug to be used. Opioids are included in the premedication for any procedure that may cause pain. This concept is widely used in feline practice.

Drugs used for Sedation in Cats

Some recommended drug combinations are given in *Table* 3.1.

Acepromazine

Mechanism of action: acepromazine decreases reaction to external stimuli (tranquilization with neuroleptic effects) by blocking central and peripheral dopaminergic receptors with variable sedative effects.

Key pharmacological features of acepromazine:

- Does *not* produce analgesia
- Produces minimal respiratory depression when administered alone to healthy cats
- Produces peripheral vasodilation (decreased systemic vascular resistance) by blockade of α_1-adrenergic receptors leading to hypothermia and hypotension especially in hypovolemic cats

- Hypothermia is also produced by depression of the hypothalamic thermoregulatory center
- There is *no* antagonist for acepromazine
- Undergoes hepatic metabolism and renal excretion (inactive metabolites)
- Produces an antiemetic effect by interacting with dopaminergic receptors in the chemoreceptor trigger zone
- Produces an antihistaminic effect by blocking histamine (H_1) receptors
- Recent retrospective studies have shown that acepromazine may be used in patients with history of seizures and epilepsy without reducing seizure threshold. This is still controversial, and acepromazine may be better avoided if other sedatives can be used. On the other hand, hospitalization can induce a stress response and evoke seizures in cats

Table 3.1 Drugs used for premedication and sedation in cats. These are commonly administered with opioids for neuroleptanalgesia.

Drug	Dosage regimens	Comments
Acepromazine	0.03–0.05 mg/kg IM, IV, SC	Mild sedation. Increasing doses do not always increase sedation in cats
Diazepam	0.2–0.5 mg/kg IV	Poor absorption after IM administration. Commonly used in combination with ketamine or propofol for anesthetic induction. Midazolam is the better alternative
Midazolam	0.2–0.5 mg/kg IM, IV	Commonly used in combination with ketamine or propofol for anesthetic induction
Xylazine	0.2–1 mg/kg IM, IV	Sedation when dexmedetomidine or medetomidine is not available. High prevalence of vomiting
Dexmedetomidine	3–20 μg/kg IM, IV	Lower doses are used for neuroleptanalgesia while high doses are administered for anesthesia in combination with ketamine and opioid (Chapter 4)
Medetomidine	6–40 μg/kg IM, IV	Same for dexmedetomidine with the exception that doses are doubled
Ketamine	3–10 mg/kg IM, PO	Chemical restraint. Ketamine may be used for sedation in cats when combined with midazolam and an opioid
Alfaxalone	2–3 mg/kg IM	Chemical restraint. Alfaxalone is administered in combination with midazolam and/or opioid for sedation of fractious cats
Atropine	0.02–0.04 mg/kg IV, IM	Does not produce sedation. Prevention or treatment of bradycardia
Glycopyrrolate	0.005–0.01 mg/kg IV, IM	Does not produce sedation. Prevention or treatment of bradycardia. Does not cross blood-brain barrier

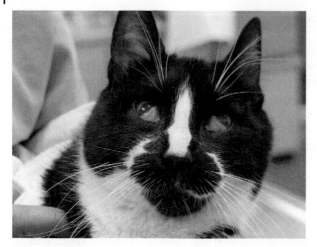

Figure 3.1 Protrusion of the third eyelid is commonly observed after administration of acepromazine and an opioid in cats.

Clinical Use

Acepromazine is commonly used as part of the premedication in combination with an opioid analgesic (e.g. morphine, methadone, hydromorphone, buprenorphine; Chapter 13) to facilitate catheterization. The onset and duration of action are approximately 15–20 minutes and 4 hours, respectively, but these effects can be variable. Acepromazine does not appear to reduce the prevalence of opioid-induced vomiting unless given 15 minutes before the opioid. However, these effects are not clearly established in cats. Protrusion of the third eyelid is commonly observed (*Figure* 3.1).

Acepromazine has been shown to decrease propofol requirements by 20–25% but this may not be observed in all cats. It is also administered to control postoperative agitation due to opioid-induced dysphoria or hyperthermia. In the latter case, its peripheral vasodilatory effects may help with cooling.

Acepromazine significantly decreases intraurethral pressure in preprostatic and prostatic regions of the urethra (smooth muscle) but not at the penile segment (striated muscles) so may not facilitate urethral catheterization. In addition, cats with urethral obstruction are often severely dehydrated and acepromazine may not be an option (see contraindications). A combination of acepromazine (0.1 mg/kg) and butorphanol (0.25 mg/kg), with or without ketamine (1.5 mg/kg) has been used for echocardiography without significantly changing the left atrial/ventricular size/function in cats. However, the study was performed in healthy patients and with high doses of acepromazine that are not commonly used in feline practice. Alternatively, low doses of acepromazine with butorphanol can be used to facilitate handling during echocardiography.

Contraindications

Because of its vasodilatory properties, acepromazine is contraindicated in cats at high risk of hypotension, hypovolemia, severe dehydration, or undergoing surgery with a high risk of bleeding (e.g. splenectomy, limb amputation). Animals treated with acepromazine may be more refractory to conventional treatment of hypotension, especially when it is used with

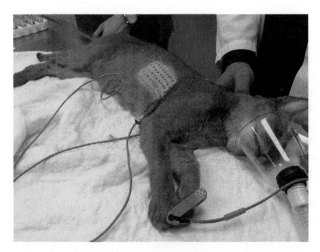

Figure 3.2 Intradermal skin testing in a cat. Acepromazine should be avoided due to its antihistaminic effects. The cat is commonly sedated with dexmedetomidine alone, or in combination with butorphanol. In cats undergoing heavy sedation, oxygen is administered using a face mask, and monitoring can be accomplished using "hands-on" techniques, pulse oximetry, and an electrocardiogram (Chapter 7).

volatile anesthetics. High doses of dopamine (up to 20 µg/kg/minute infusion IV) or ephedrine (0.1–0.2 mg/kg IV) may be required to treat hypotension in some instances. Acepromazine should be used with caution in critically ill cats or patients with hepatic and kidney disease. It has been shown to decrease platelet aggregation but the clinical significance of this finding is unknown. Anemic patients should not be given acepromazine as splenic sequestration of red blood cells will further decrease hematocrit. Acepromazine should be avoided in cats undergoing intradermal skin testing due to its antihistaminic effects (*Figure* 3.2).

Benzodiazepines

Mechanism of action: benzodiazepines act by facilitating the actions of gamma-amino-butyric acid (GABAa), the principal inhibitory neurotransmitter in the central nervous system. They do not activate GABAa but rather enhance the affinity of the neuro-transmitter for the receptor; the postsynaptic neurons are hyperpolarized and more resistant to excitation. Benzodiazepines have a synergistic effect when administered with barbiturates, alfaxalone, and propofol due to their similar mechanisms of action.

Key pharmacological features of benzodiazepines:

- Anticonvulsant activity
- No clinically relevant analgesia
- Minimal cardiorespiratory effects
- Extensive hepatic metabolism (low hepatic clearance); the metabolism is highly dependent on the intrinsic capacity of the cytochrome P450 enzymes
- Skeletal muscle relaxation
- Appetite stimulation
- Antagonism by benzodiazepine antagonists (e.g. flumazenil)
- High protein binding

Clinical Use

Benzodiazepines are never used for sedation and premedication in the young healthy adult because they may cause dysphoria, agitation, and disinhibition of aggressive behavior. However, midazolam may be administered in combination with an opioid (IV or IM) for sedation of geriatric or debilitated cats. However, excitement and aggression may be observed if the cat is not depressed or obtunded. More commonly, benzodiazepines are administered in combination with ketamine, propofol or alfaxalone for induction of general anesthesia. They counteract the muscular rigidity and seizure-like activity that may be observed after ketamine administration. Midazolam and diazepam both significantly decrease the dose of propofol required for tracheal intubation in healthy cats. Midazolam (0.25 mg/kg) and ketamine (3 mg/kg) given IM produce moderate sedation for noninvasive and nonpainful procedures. However, other protocols are better especially where agonists of α_2-adrenergic receptors are available.

Diazepam versus Midazolam

Diazepam is hydrophobic and not well absorbed IM, and midazolam is recommended for this route of administration. In addition, diazepam is less potent and may have long-term effects in cats due to slow elimination compared with midazolam as well as producing active metabolites via demethylation. Temazepam is the main metabolite that undergoes glucuronidation in cats. Diazepam undergoes slow biotransformation in cats where there is inhibition of the bile acid efflux that results in accumulation of bile acid in the hepatocytes. These mechanisms can contribute to liver injury after repetitive administration of diazepam.

Diazepam is commercially available in propylene glycol and may cause venoirritation and pain on injection because it is a hyperosmolar solution. Cardiac toxicity and cardiovascular depression due to propylene glycol administration is only a problem with repeated administration. Midazolam is water soluble, does not cause irritation or liver injury, and *it is the benzodiazepine of choice in cats.*

Zolazepam is commercially available in combination with tiletamine in many countries. It is used for induction and maintenance of general anesthesia. There are a number of injectable protocols using this combination (Chapter 4). Dosage regimens for flumazenil, a specific antagonist of benzodiazepine receptors, have not been reported in cats.

Contraindications

Benzodiazepines are not used for sedation of healthy cats, and they should be used cautiously in those with hepatic disease, if used at all. Acute hepatic necrosis has been reported after oral administration of diazepam but only following repeated administration.

Agonists of α_2-Adrenergic Receptors

Mechanism of action: agonists of α_2-adrenergic receptors (i.e. dexmedetomidine, medetomidine, and xylazine; others are rarely used in cats) bind to α_2-adrenergic receptors and produce reliable sedation in a dose-dependent manner. Sedation is produced by inhibition of the locus coeruleus, a vital modulator of vigilance in the brain as well as decreasing sympathetic nervous system outflow from the CNS to the periphery.

Key pharmacological features of agonists of α_2-adrenergic receptors:

- Peripheral vasoconstriction causing hypertension (increases in systemic vascular resistance) via binding to postsynaptic α_2-adrenergic receptor on the peripheral blood vessels. Reflex bradycardia, decreases in cardiac output, and coronary perfusion may result; Bradycardia and bradydysrhythmia (second-degree atrio-ventricular block) are also induced by increased vagal tone (first hemodynamic phase) (*Box 3.2*)
- Once vasoconstriction and hypertension subsides, bradycardia with hypotension may be observed (second hemodynamic phase)
- Respiratory depression when administered in combination with opioids *but not* when given alone
- Hypothermia is produced via depression of the hypothalamic thermoregulatory center
- Analgesia through decreased nociceptive input to the brain and inhibited release of excitatory neurotransmitters in the spinal cord
- Muscular relaxation
- Hepatic metabolism and renal excretion
- Inhibition of insulin release leading to hyperglycemia
- Inhibition of antidiuretic hormone (ADH) leading to increased urine production
- Direct stimulation of the chemoreceptor trigger zone inducing vomiting; higher prevalence of vomiting after xylazine than medetomidine
- Other effects include decreased gastrointestinal motility, suppression of the surgery-induced stress response, and decreased intraocular and intracranial pressure (as long as vomiting does not occur)

Box 3.2: To treat or not to treat α_2-agonist-induced bradycardia with anticholinergics?

Administration of anticholinergics (i.e. atropine or glycopyrrolate) to treat α_2-agonist-induced reflex bradycardia is controversial and often contraindicated. This is particularly true if the cat is hypertensive (blood pressure measured by Doppler ultrasound > 120 mmHg). Severe hypertension, tachycardia and impairment of cardiac function may be observed after administration of anticholinergics. Increases in heart rate may increase myocardial oxygen demand and reduce time for diastole. Tachycardia is not always associated with increases in cardiac output. Instead, the adverse effects of these drugs should be reversed with antagonists of α_2-adrenergic receptors such as atipamezole or yohimbine. However, if hypotension (decreased systemic vascular resistance) and bradycardia are observed, administration of anticholinergics might be acceptable.

Clinical Use

Agonists of α_2-adrenergic receptors are used for sedation to facilitate noninvasive procedures. The sedative, analgesic, and negative hemodynamic effects are dose dependent in cats so their use is limited to those that can tolerate such effects. They are used for

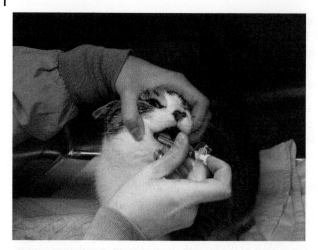

Figure 3.3 Dexmedetomidine can be administered by the buccal route for premedication in cats that do not tolerate needle injections. Sedation is less profound than when the same dose is administered IM.

premedication in combination with an opioid to reduce anesthetic requirements in a dose-dependent manner. Such premedication produces a substantial injectable and volatile anesthetic-sparing effect. Doses of injectable anesthetics and vaporizer concentrations should be reduced accordingly. The cornea should be lubricated in cases of profound sedation to avoid ulcers.

"Microdoses" (0.25–0.5 µg/kg of dexmedetomidine IV) are used to smooth anesthetic recovery and to treat dysphoria in healthy cats. The dose is diluted in saline 0.9% and given slowly to effect. High doses of agonists of α_2-adrenergic receptors (20–40 µg/kg of dexmedetomidine IM) are administered to facilitate handling of aggressive and feral cats. Dexmedetomidine can be administered by the buccal route (20 µg/kg) for "hands-off" premedication (*Figure* 3.3).

Dexmedetomidine and medetomidine are highly selective, specific, and potent agonists of α_2-adrenergic receptors when compared with xylazine. Dexmedetomidine is the pharmacologically active component of medetomidine. The former is twice as potent as the latter. Xylazine has a shorter duration of action and is often used when dexmedetomidine is not available. Some adverse effects observed after xylazine administration are most probably a result of their effects on α_1-adrenergic receptors. Agonists of α_2-adrenergic receptors are widely used as part of the "kitty magic" protocol for spay-neuter programs (Chapter 4).

Contraindications

Agonists of α_2-adrenergic receptors are best restricted to use in healthy adult cats, and should not be administered to patients that are hemodynamically compromised or unstable. Adverse effects as well as analgesia and sedation can be fully reversed with the competitive antagonist atipamezole given IM. Dexmedetomidine and medetomidine have been administered to cats with hypertrophic cardiomyopathy (HCM) and left-ventricular outflow tract (LVOT) obstruction in order to decrease LVOT velocity and pressure gradient, and eliminate outflow obstruction. This technique is particularly suited to sedation of aggressive cats with hyperthyroidism and HCM. In calm cats with HCM, appropriate sedation is often achieved with opioids alone. Agonists of α_2-adrenergic receptors are best avoided in cats with increased intraocular (e.g. glaucoma, open globe injuries) or intracranial pressure (e.g. head trauma, brain tumors) because of the risk of vomiting (Chapter 9).

If an antagonist is required, atipamezole is administered IM because tachycardia, hypotension, defecation and excitement may be observed after IV administration. Generally, the same original volume of standard dexmedetomidine or medetomidine preparations is administered when calculating the dose of atipamezole, however this may not be valid with new (i.e. more diluted) concentrations of dexmedetomidine. The IV route is only used in life-threatening conditions; in this case, it is diluted in saline 0.9% (up to 1 mL) and given slowly until the cardiovascular depression is reversed. Atipamezole has greater specificity for α_2-adrenergic receptors than yohimbine. Atipamezole is commonly administered to reverse the effects of dexmedetomidine and medetomidine whereas yohimbine is given when available to antagonize the effects of xylazine. Yohimbine is not available in the United Kingdom.

Anticholinergics

Mechanism of action: anticholinergics (atropine, glycopyrrolate and scopolamine) competitively and reversibly antagonize the effects of acetylcholine at cholinergic postganglionic sites (muscarinic but not nicotinic receptors). For this reason, they are called parasympatholytic (blockade of parasympathetic tone) agents. Muscarinic receptors are present in the heart, salivary glands, and smooth muscles of the gastro-intestinal and genitourinary tracts.

Key pharmacological features of anticholinergics:

- Increased heart rate. However, heart rate may decrease immediately after IV administration of small doses
- Mydriasis, with the exception of glycopyrrolate, which is a quaternary ammonium compound and does not cross the blood-brain barrier or the placenta. Mydriasis obstructs passage of intraocular fluid into the venous circulation thereby increasing intraocular pressure
- Inhibition of nasal, ocular, salivary, bronchial, gastrointestinal secretion
- Gastric pH and gastroesophageal sphincter tone are decreased, leading to an increased risk of gastroesophageal reflux and regurgitation during general anesthesia
- Decreased gastrointestinal motility
- Relaxation of bronchial smooth muscle and bronchodilation

Clinical Use

Anticholinergics are primarily used to prevent or treat bradycardia caused by increased vagal tone (drug-induced or from manipulation of head, neck or ophthalmic structures). They can decrease salivary and bronchial secretions in a clinically relevant manner.

Formation of mucus plugs is a concern due to the potential to reduce water content of salivary and airway secretions. Cats have small bronchi and bronchioles and even a small amount of bronchial secretion and plugs could cause airway obstruction and increased resistance to breathing.

Administration of anticholinergics is controversial. Some anesthesiologists give them routinely in the premedication to *prevent* bradycardia during anesthesia. Others administer anticholinergics only to *treat* bradycardia. It is of note that many cats will develop opioid-induced bradycardia during anesthesia, and increasing the heart rate will improve cardiac output and mean arterial pressure. However, in some instances, tachycardia will increase myocardial work and oxygen consumption and decrease coronary perfusion.

Glycopyrrolate is the common anticholinergic of choice as it is longer acting than atropine and does not cross the blood-brain/placental barriers. For this reason, if an anticholinergic is required, glycopyrrolate should be used in cesarean section. However, atropine has a shorter onset of action and is used for cardiopulmonary resuscitation (Chapter 10) or where glycopyrrolate is not available. Anticholinergics are also administered for counteracting the muscarinic effects of anticholinesterase drugs such as neostigmine, which is used to antagonize nondepolarizing neuromuscular blocking agents. In this situation, neostigmine and atropine are administered together at the end of surgery.

Contraindications

Anticholinergics are *not* routinely administered for the treatment of agonist of α_2-adrenergic receptor-induced bradycardia (*Box* 3.2) and they are contraindicated in cats with pulmonic or arterial stenosis, cardiomyopathy or pre-existing tachycardia. Atropine is contraindicated in cats with glaucoma.

Opioids

The pharmacological, analgesic, and adverse effects of opioids are discussed in detail in Chapter 13. However, opioids are commonly used for premedication and sedation as part of a neuroleptanalgesic or preventative analgesia protocol. Opioids produce adequate sedation in kittens (< 12 weeks) when administered alone. With appropriate doses and administration intervals, dysphoria and excitement (hyperactivity, agitation, difficult to handle and possible aggression) are rarely observed; euphoria is the typical behavioral effect induced by opioids, which will include kneading with the forepaws, rubbing on objects, purring, and rolling.

Opioids provide profound analgesia (agonists of μ-opioid receptors) with minimal effects on the cardiovascular system and without changes in myocardial contractility. They also have anesthetic-sparing effects (reduction in intravenous and inhalant anesthetic requirements). Opioid-induced bradycardia can easily be treated with anticholinergics. Dose-dependent respiratory depression becomes more evident when opioids are administered with other hypnotic anesthetics (propofol, alfaxalone, thiopental, inhalant anesthetics) or sedatives such as agonists of α_2-adrenergic receptors. Judicious monitoring of ventilation and oxygenation should be performed (Chapter 7) with the ability to provide oxygen during heavy sedation of ill cats if needed. Opioids should be used with caution in patients with elevated intracranial pressure because of the potential for hypoventilation and vomiting, which may further compromise their neurological status. Opioids may be reversed with the competitive antagonist naloxone, keeping in mind that the analgesic effects will also be terminated and that the duration of action of naloxone ($\approx$1 hour) may be shorter than the opioid, with the potential for renarcotization.

Ketamine and Alfaxalone

The pharmacological effects of ketamine and alfaxalone, together with their contra-indications and adverse effects, are discussed in Chapter 4. Ketamine (3–5 mg/kg) or alfaxalone (2–3 mg/kg) have been administered IM for premedication of the fractious or difficult cat. Ketamine is painful on injection due to it low pH. Alfaxalone is particularly useful for sedation of the geriatric but difficult cat. Both ketamine and alfaxalone may be combined with an opioid and midazolam (or acepromazine) to facilitate handling of these patients, however alfaxalone can be administered alone. At high doses (anesthesia for spay-neuter programs), both ketamine and alfaxalone given IM will induce general anesthesia. In the feral cat, ketamine (20 mg/kg) can be squirted into the mouth at the same time that the animal is hissing to facilitate handling. This approach produces excessive salivation and should only be considered as a last resort for chemical restraint.

Trazodone

Trazodone is an antagonist of serotonin receptors with anxiolytic, mild sedative, and antidepressant effects. It is administered to control anxiety related to car rides and veterinary visits, as difficulty with transport is the main cause of limited feline veterinary care compared with dogs. Adverse effects have not been clearly reported but decreased activity is observed after administration of 50, 75, and 100 mg/cat of trazodone PO without affecting behavior during patient examination. Trazodone should be given 2 hours before transportation. Trazodone interferes with central serotonin receptors and there may be potential for the serotonin syndrome (Chapter 15).

Other Drugs

Gabapentin (25 mg/kg PO) and amitriptyline (10 mg/cat PO) appear to produce sedation in cats and have been used as alternatives to trazodone for feline transportation; however little is known about their clinical value in this respect, nor their potential adverse effects.

Several protocols have been described for sedation or premedication of cats using a range of drug combinations (*Table* 3.2). Each has its own advantages and disadvantages to be considered.

Table 3.2 Examples of drug combinations for sedation or premedication in cats. Each protocol has its own advantages and disadvantages to be considered.

Drug combination	Dosage regimens (mg/kg and route of administration)	Comments
Examples of acepromazine combinations[a]		
Acepromazine + butorphanol	0.05 + 0.2 mg/kg IM, respectively	Mild sedation. Short-acting analgesic effects. Noninvasive procedures
Acepromazine + buprenorphine	0.03 + 0.02 mg/kg IM, respectively	Good analgesia for moderate pain (e.g. ovariohysterectomy) when combined with NSAIDs. Euphoric behavior. In the United States, buprenorphine should be administered at 0.24 mg/kg SC (Simbadol®) (Chapter 13)
Acepromazine + hydromorphone OR methadone	0.03 + 0.1 OR 0.4 mg/kg IM, respectively	Good analgesia for severe pain (e.g. fracture) especially when combined with NSAIDs and local anesthetics. Other full agonists of μ-opioid receptors can be used
Examples of dexmedetomidine combinations[b]		
Dexmedetomidine + butorphanol	0.01 + 0.2 mg/kg IM, respectively	Good sedation for radiographs, noninvasive diagnostic and minor surgical procedures or premedication of a healthy cat
Dexmedetomidine + hydromorphone OR methadone	0.01 + 0.1 OR 0.4 mg/kg IM, respectively	Excellent sedation and premedication before surgery. Good analgesia and commonly used for painful (moderate or severe pain) procedures. Other full agonists of μ-opioid receptors can be used
Other examples		
Ketamine + midazolam + butorphanol	5 + 0.25 + 0.2 mg/kg IM, respectively	Chemical restraint of the fractious cat. Doses of ketamine can be increased for more reliable sedation. Alfaxalone (2–3 mg/kg) can replace ketamine
Midazolam + hydromorphone or methadone	0.25 + 0.1 OR 0.4 mg/kg IM, respectively.	Sedation and premedication of debilitated or geriatric cats. Butorphanol can replace hydromorphone or methadone if nonpainful

Notes:
a) These protocols can be administered by the IV route. However, acepromazine may not be needed if a catheter is already in place. In this case, opioids are administered alone.
b) Other drug protocols using dexmedetomidine are provided in Chapter 4 for spay-neuter programs. In addition, lower doses of dexmedetomidine can be administered after preanesthetic assessment and on a case-by-case basis.

Further Reading

Bortolami, E., and Love, E. J. (2015) Practical use of opioids in cats: A state-of-the-art, evidence-based review. *Journal of Feline Medicine and Surgery* **17**, 283–311.

Center, S. A., Elston, T. H., Rowland, P. H., et al. (1996) Fulminant hepatic failure associated with oral administration of diazepam in 11 cats. *Journal of the American Veterinary Medical Association* **209**, 618–625.

Deutsch, J., Jolliffe, C., Archer E., *et al.* (in press) Intramuscular injection of alfaxalone in combination with butorphanol for sedation in cats. *Veterinary Anaesthesia and Analgesia.* doi.org/10.1016/j.vaa.2016.05.014

Escobar, A., Pypendop, B. H., Siao, K. T., *et al.* (2012) Effect of dexmedetomidine on the minimum alveolar concentration of isoflurane in cats. *Journal of Veterinary Pharmacology and Therapeutics* **35**, 163–168.

Hall, T. L., Duke, T., Townsend, H. G., *et al.* (1999) The effect of opioid and acepromazine premedication on the anesthetic induction dose of propofol in cats. *Canadian Veterinary Journal* **40**, 867–870.

Indrawirawan, Y., and McAlees, T. (2014) Tramadol toxicity in a cat: Case report and literature review of serotonin syndrome. *Journal of Feline Medicine and Surgery* **16**, 572–578.

Lamont, L. A., Bulmer, B. J., Sisson, D. D., *et al.* (2002) Doppler echocardiographic effects of medetomidine on dynamic left ventricular outflow tract obstruction in cats. *Journal of the American Veterinary Medical Association* **221**, 1276–1281.

Marks, S. L., Straeter-Knowlen, I. M., Moore, M., *et al.* (1996) Effects of acepromazine maleate and phenoxybenzamine on urethral pressure profiles of anesthetized, healthy, sexually intact male cats. *American Journal of Veterinary Research* **57**, 1497–1500.

Orlando, J. M., Case, B. C., Thomson, A. E., *et al.* (2016) Use of oral trazodone for sedation in cats: A pilot study. *Journal of Feline Medicine and Surgery* **18**, 476–482.

Park, F. M. (2012) Successful treatment of hepatic failure secondary to diazepam administration in a cat. *Journal of Feline Medicine and Surgery* **14**, 158–160.

Pascoe, P. J., Ilkiw, J. E., and Pypendop, B. H. (2006) Effects of increasing infusion rates of dopamine, dobutamine, epinephrine, and phenylephrine in healthy anesthetized cats. *American Journal of Veterinary Research* **67**, 1491–1499.

Pypendop, B. H., Barter, L. S., Stanley, S. D., *et al.* (2011) Hemodynamic effects of dexmedetomidine in isoflurane-anesthetized cats. *Veterinary Anaesthesia and Analgesia* **38**, 555–567.

Pypendop, B. H., and Ilkiw, J. E. (2014) Relationship between plasma dexmedetomidine concentration and sedation score and thermal threshold in cats. *American Journal of Veterinary Research* **75**, 446–452.

Robinson, R., and Borer-Weir, K. (2015) The effects of diazepam or midazolam on the dose of propofol required to induce anaesthesia in cats. *Veterinary Anaesthesia and Analgesia* **42**, 493–501.

Santos, L. C., Ludders, J. W., Erb, H. N., *et al.* (2010) Sedative and cardiorespiratory effects of dexmedetomidine and buprenorphine administered to cats via oral transmucosal or intramuscular routes. *Veterinary Anaesthesia and Analgesia* **37**, 417–424.

Slingsby, L. S., Taylor, P. M., and Monroe, T. (2009) Thermal antinociception after dexmedetomidine administration in cats: A comparison between intramuscular and oral transmucosal administration. *Journal of Feline Medicine and Surgery* **11**, 829–834.

Steagall, P. V., Taylor, P. M., Brondani, J. T., *et al.* (2008) Antinociceptive effects of tramadol and acepromazine in cats. *Journal of Feline Medicine and Surgery* **10**, 24–31.

Stevens, B. J., Frantz, E. M., Orlando, J. M., *et al.* (2016) Efficacy of a single dose of trazodone hydrochloride given to cats prior to veterinary visits to reduce signs of transport- and examination-related anxiety. *Journal of the American Veterinary Medical Association* **249**, 202–207.

Tamura, J., Ishizuka, T., Fukui, S., *et al.* (2015) Sedative effects of intramuscular alfaxalone administered to cats. *Journal of Veterinary Medical Sciences* **77**, 897–904.

van Beusekom, C. D., van den Heuvel, J. J., Koenderink, J. B., *et al.* (2015) Feline hepatic biotransformation of diazepam: Differences between cats and dogs. *Research in Veterinary Science* **103**, 119–125.

Ward, J. L., Schober, K. E., Fuentes, V. L., *et al.* (2012) Effects of sedation on echocardiographic variables of left atrial and left ventricular function in healthy cats. *Journal of Feline Medicine and Surgery* **14**, 678–685.

4

Injectable Anesthetics and Induction of Anesthesia

Paulo Steagall

Université de Montréal, Saint-Hyacinthe, Canada

Key Points

- Choosing the appropriate anesthetic regimen on a case-by-case basis
- Considerations for injectable-only protocols versus volatile anesthesia
- Anesthetics and their pharmacology, clinical application, adverse effects, and contraindications
- Considerations for induction using volatile anesthetics, including their advantages and disadvantages
- Use of total intravenous anesthesia (TIVA) and injectable-only protocols

Introduction

Injectable anesthetics, given by the IV route, are used most commonly for induction of general anesthesia for short procedures, or are followed by maintenance with volatile anesthetics. An injectable-only protocol may be selected for maintenance of anesthesia when volatile anesthesia is not available, or for technical reasons such as airway procedures. Injectable-only protocols, often administered IM are widely used for neutering procedures. They may be more practical and cost effective than volatile anesthesia but should be managed and chosen judiciously.

Considerations for injectable-only protocols include:

- Repeated injections may result in drug accumulation and slow anesthetic recovery
- Drugs administered by the IM route cannot be titrated or adjusted to effect, and may result in profound effects or failure to achieve anesthesia
- Endotracheal intubation is not always performed and airways are not protected. There is a risk of regurgitation and aspiration. In this case, means of securing an airway and providing oxygenation are important and should be available (Chapter 1)
- Equipment for gaining IV access should be available (Chapter 1)
- Fluid therapy is indicated in most cases (Chapter 8) but routine feline neutering does not always require it
- Anesthesia for complex surgical procedures is best maintained using volatile anesthetics and balanced anesthesia

Feline Anesthesia and Pain Management, First Edition. Edited by Paulo Steagall, Sheilah Robertson and Polly Taylor.
© 2018 John Wiley & Sons, Inc. Published 2018 by John Wiley & Sons, Inc.

- Anesthetic monitoring is strongly recommended with any anesthetic technique; it decreases morbidity and mortality

General Considerations for Induction of Anesthesia

The choice of anesthetic drug for induction of anesthesia should be evaluated on a case-by-case basis. A thorough physical examination is essential before selection of the appropriate anesthetic and analgesic therapy (Chapter 1); however, this may not be possible in fractious or feral cats. Patient status, presence of disease (type, duration, organ system), type of procedure (surgery, diagnostic examination), availability of drugs, and the experience of the anesthetist will ultimately determine the anesthetic protocol.

Venous access can be achieved in cats using a variety of intravenous catheters (Chapter 1). The IV route allows the anesthetic dose to be administered "to effect". Transition from an injectable induction to volatile anesthesia is generally smooth. "Off-needle" injections are not best practice for induction of anesthesia; this technique is often used, but it does carry the risk of perivascular injection. An IV catheter should be placed for long procedures and when intravenous fluids and additional drugs will be administered. The buccal (oral transmucosal) route of administration is reserved for ketamine squirted into the mouth of fractious cats that do not tolerate physical restraint. Some drugs such as ketamine or alfaxalone can be administered IM for chemical restraint (Chapter 3), which will facilitate handling and IV catheterization and decrease the anesthetic induction dose.

Induction of anesthesia is one of the most critical events for the cat since most anesthetics cause a degree of cardiorespiratory depression. Apnea, hypoxemia, hypotension, and hypoventilation may all occur. The clinician should be ready to intervene, and a checklist is recommended before anesthesia (Chapter 1).

Critically ill patients should be stabilized before general anesthesia (Chapter 9). In such cases, preoxygenation for 3 minutes and continuous ECG monitoring during anesthetic induction is recommended (*Figure* 4.1).

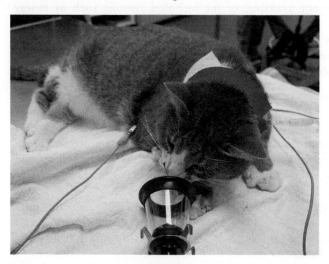

Figure 4.1 A cat is preoxygenated before induction of anesthesia. An ECG is monitored continuously during the perioperative period.

Drugs used for Induction of Anesthesia

Table 4.1 shows recommended doses for injectable agents. The veterinarian should be aware of the current national scheduling and regulation control of these medicines in whichever country they practice.

Propofol

Mechanism of action: GABA is the main inhibitory neurotransmitter in the central nervous system (CNS) and binds to gamma aminobutyric acid (GABA$_A$) receptors. Propofol exerts its effect at GABA$_A$ receptors. It hyperpolarizes the postsynaptic cell membrane causing functional inhibition of the postsynaptic neuron by increasing chloride conductance. Propofol also decreases the rate of dissociation of GABA from the receptor leading to increased GABA activity and depression of the CNS.

Commercial Preparations

Propofol is not soluble in water and is prepared commercially as a lipid emulsion containing soybean oil, glycerol, and egg lecithin. This formulation will promote rapid bacterial growth and the solution should be discarded 6–8 hours after the vial is opened. Mixing of propofol with other drugs using the same syringe is not recommended. Current formulations do not normally cause pain or tissue damage after perivascular injection.

Table 4.1 Suggested doses for induction and maintenance of anesthesia with injectable agents.

Drug[a]	Doses for induction[b]	Infusion rates	Comments
Alfaxalone	3–5 mg/kg IV	0.2–0.3 mg/ kg/minute	Cardiorespiratory depression. Greater margin of safety versus propofol.
Propofol	4–8 mg/kg IV	0.2–0.4 mg/ kg/minute	Cardiorespiratory depression. Smooth induction and recovery.
Ketamine[c]	5 mg/kg IV 10–15 mg/kg IM	0.01–0.04 mg/ kg/minute	Infusion rates used for antihyperalgesia. High doses will contribute to anesthesia. Excreted mostly unchanged in cats.
Tiletamine-zolazepam	1–2 mg/kg IV 3–6 mg/kg IM		Chemical restraint or injectable-only anesthesia. Apneustic breathing in spay-neuter programs.
Thiopental	5–10 mg/kg IV		Cardiorespiratory depression. Neuroprotection.
Etomidate	2 mg/kg IV		Minimal cardiovascular effects. Adrenal suppression.

Notes:
a) Doses are commonly reduced when propofol, alfaxalone, thiopental, and etomidate are administered with midazolam.
b) Lower doses are used after premedication.
c) Rarely administered alone. For IM administration, ketamine is commonly combined with an opioid and midazolam or dexmedetomidine.

A formulation of propofol ("Propofol 28" or "PropoFloPlus"), containing the preservative benzyl alcohol, is designed to reduce anesthetic waste. This product can be used for up to 28 days after broaching without refrigeration. Propofol 28 is not approved for use in cats in all countries but it is widely used in cats in Europe.

A number of clear preparations of propofol have become available globally but should be used with extreme caution as the vehicle may cause serious irritation or even cardiovascular collapse.

Pharmacology

Key pharmacological features of propofol:

- Does not produce antinociception
- Decreases cerebral metabolic oxygen consumption, cerebral blood flow, and intracranial pressure
- Has antiepileptic activity but myoclonus or excitatory movements may occasionally be seen at a light depth of anesthesia
- Produces significant cardiovascular depression by decreasing systemic vascular resistance (vasodilation), mean arterial blood pressure, cardiac output, myocardial contractility, and depression of sympathetic nervous system activity
- Produces dose-dependent respiratory depression including apnea. Hypoventilation and decreased tidal volume result in hypercapnia
- Blunts the ventilatory response to increases in carbon dioxide (CO_2) and hypoxemia. These effects can be observed even at low doses
- Has high metabolic clearance and is rapidly redistributed after administration. Propofol can be used in cats with hepatic or renal disease since rapid tissue uptake occurs. It is primarily metabolized by the liver but there is also extrahepatic uptake in the lungs
- It is not clear whether propofol increases intraocular pressure in cats. Propofol has been used successfully in cats with glaucoma as long as the cough reflex is minimized during intubation (Chapter 1)
- Reduces gastroesophageal sphincter pressure and gastric pressure, predisposing the cat to gastroesophageal reflux during anesthesia
- May cause oxidative injury of red blood cells with Heinz body formation and repeated exposure can result in inappetence and prolonged recovery. However, this effect appears to be dose related
- Is a phenolic compound, and cats have reduced ability to conjugate it. Delayed anesthetic recovery may occur in cats after prolonged infusions or repeated exposures due to slow clearance of propofol

Clinical Use

Propofol is only effective when administered IV and is widely used for induction of anesthesia. It has a short duration of action after a single injection (3–5 minutes), and produces smooth induction and recovery from anesthesia. Premedication reduces propofol requirements; this is especially obvious after use of agonists of α_2-adrenergic receptors. Propofol is commonly given in combination with other agents such as benzodiazepines (diazepam or midazolam) or ketamine (so-called "ketofol") (*Box* 4.1).

In general, cats will require higher doses on a mg/kg basis compared with dogs. The goal of using propofol in combination with other drugs is to reduce the dose and cardiovascular depression. This is particularly important in geriatric and compromised cats. Lower doses of propofol (1–2 mg/kg) may be administered to healthy cats after premedication with acepromazine or dexmedetomidine and an opioid. Midazolam, diazepam or ketamine is then injected and finally, propofol injected again, if needed. Propofol should always be administered slowly (over at least 30–60 seconds) to reduce the likelihood of apnea and cardiorespiratory depression. Smaller doses of propofol are required for supraglottic airway device placement when compared with endotracheal intubation (Chapter 1).

Box 4.1: The use of "ketofol" in feline anesthesia

The combination of propofol and ketamine has been used with the goal of maximizing the benefits while minimizing the adverse effects of each drug alone. For example, a calm and smooth recovery is produced by propofol, but not ketamine. On the other hand, sympathetic stimulation with increases in heart rate and blood pressure and minimal respiratory depression are produced by ketamine. The latter effects can override the cardiorespiratory depression produced by propofol alone. This protocol is an attempt to use the "best of both worlds" in terms of anesthetic effects of propofol and ketamine. After premedication, propofol (2 mg/kg) is administered before ketamine (2 mg/kg) to avoid muscle rigidity.

Propofol can be used for induction of anesthesia in cats with head trauma or space-occupying lesions, especially when barbiturates are not available. In these cases, a secure airway is required so that eucapnia can be maintained to avoid increases in intracranial pressure (Chapter 9).

The cardiovascular depressant effects of propofol may be severe in some cats; for example, those that are volume depleted or have hypertrophic cardiomyopathy (HCM). Respiratory depression is less of a concern if an airway can be readily secured and respiratory support provided. These depressant effects are likely to be exacerbated by co-administration of volatile anesthetics. However, the effect is short lived and the patient normally starts to breathe spontaneously a few minutes after drug administration. Propofol is an appropriate choice for cesarean section, when there is increased intracranial pressure and in the face of hepatic (e.g. lipidosis) or renal disease (Chapter 9).

Cats may sneeze during recovery from propofol anesthesia. They will often paw at their nose and mouth. These effects are self-limiting and do not require treatment. In addition, opisthotonus and spontaneous muscle activity can occur during induction and do not require any treatment. Repeated injections of propofol may cause delayed recovery. In cats undergoing daily general anesthesia, propofol should alternate with other drugs (alfaxalone or ketamine/benzodiazepine) or be coadministered with benzodiazepines to reduce the dose and therefore daily exposure.

Contraindications

Propofol should be used judiciously in cats with cardiovascular disease and hypovolemia. Cats with respiratory disease and brachycephalic breeds should be closely monitored after administration of propofol and provided with oxygen.

Alfaxalone

Mechanism of action: alfaxalone is a synthetic neurosteroid with a similar mechanism of action to propofol and barbiturates, modulating the $GABA_A$ receptor, producing anesthesia and muscle relaxation. Alfaxalone is devoid of steroid activity despite its similarities to the progesterone molecule.

Commercial Preparations

Alfaxalone has low solubility in water and was first manufactured in combination with alfadalone (alphadolone) and dissolved in a castor-oil-based surfactant called Cremophor EL (commercially marketed as Saffan for cats and Althesin for humans). This formulation caused anaphylactic reactions manifesting as edema of the pinna and forepaws and occasionally bronchoconstriction; pulmonary edema and death were also reported. It was a remarkably successful anesthetic with a good safety record in cats but was withdrawn because of the adverse effects produced by the solvent. The current formulation of alfaxalone is water soluble with cyclodextrin (Alfaxan® or Alfaxan-HPCD), and does not produce the adverse effects mentioned above. Alfaxalone does not contain a microbiocidal preservative and labeled recommendations vary between "discard within a few hours of broaching the vial" to "keep refrigerated for up to 7 days," depending on the country.

Pharmacology

Key pharmacological features of alfaxalone:

- Does *not* produce antinociception
- Decreases cerebral metabolic oxygen consumption, cerebral blood flow, and intracranial pressure
- Produces dose-dependent cardiovascular depression by decreasing systemic vascular resistance (vasodilation), cardiac output and mean arterial blood pressure. Increases in heart rate are often observed
- Produces dose-dependent respiratory depression including decreases in respiratory rate and tidal volume leading to hypoventilation and hypercapnia. As with propofol, apnea may be observed but is less common than after propofol. Slow administration reduces the prevalence of apnea
- Does not accumulate at clinical doses and can be used as a bolus, by "top-up" doses or by infusion for TIVA. It has high clearance with primary hepatic metabolism and renal elimination
- Reduces gastroesophageal sphincter pressure and gastric pressure, predisposing the cat to reflux during anesthesia
- Does not cause oxidative injury of red blood cells with Heinz body formation

Clinical Use

Alfaxalone is approved for IV administration. However, IM injection has been used for chemical restraint (Chapter 3). The dose for induction of anesthesia in nonpremedicated cats is 5 mg/kg, but is reduced after premedication (1–3 mg/kg). Alfaxalone has a short duration of action (3–5 minutes but up to 10 minutes after a second bolus), and produces a smooth induction. However agitation and dysphoria may be seen during recovery especially if premedication was not used. These effects can be decreased by leaving the cat undisturbed in a quiet cage and ensuring good postoperative pain management (Chapter 13).

Cardiorespiratory depression is short lived. These effects can be minimized by slow (over 60 seconds) administration. Alfaxalone can be used in cats with head trauma or space-occupying lesions since it decreases intracranial pressure. In these cases, securing an airway is important so that ventilation can be supported (Chapter 9). Alfaxalone has been used in compromised cats for induction of anesthesia in combination with benzodiazepines and opioids (Chapter 3, Chapter 9).

Alfaxalone has been used for cesarean section in dogs without negative impact on Apgar scores; it should be a reasonable choice for induction of anesthesia in cats undergoing this procedure. Alfaxalone is a good choice of anesthetic for examination of laryngeal function in cats as it does not affect arytenoid cartilage motion. It is also an option when TIVA is required, although long-term anesthesia with alfaxalone has not yet been evaluated in cats. Anesthesia was uneventful when alfaxalone was used for induction in juvenile cats (< 12 weeks of age) undergoing neutering procedures.

Box 4.2 compares and contrasts propofol and alfaxalone.

Box 4.2: The advantages and disadvantages of propofol and alfaxalone

Cardiorespiratory depression, quality of induction and recovery from propofol and alfaxalone are similar, with both anesthetics increasing the risk of gastroesophageal reflux. However, apnea is less common and recovery may sometimes be agitated with paddling and trembling after alfaxalone. In cats with hepatic or renal disease, propofol is the anesthetic of choice. The cost differential between the two agents varies from one country to another. Alfaxalone can be administered by the IM or SC route for chemical restraint, an important advantage over propofol. However, high volumes of injection will be required, and prolonged and poor recoveries can be observed when high doses are used. Alfaxalone has greater margin of safety when compared with propofol.

Contraindications

No studies have been published on the impact of impaired hepatic or renal function on pharmacokinetic variables or recovery duration after the administration of alfaxalone. It is not clear whether accumulation occurs or if recovery from anesthesia is delayed.

Dissociative Anesthetics (Ketamine and Tiletamine)

Most of our knowledge of dissociative anesthetics is based on studies using ketamine. Tiletamine has not been widely studied but it is believed that its mechanism of action and general pharmacology are similar to ketamine.

Mechanism of action: ketamine and tiletamine cause *dissociation* between the thalamus and the limbic system, and amnesia, but *not* muscle relaxation. They bind to a number of receptors throughout the body but most notably they are noncompetitive antagonists at N-methyl D-aspartate (NMDA) receptors. Ketamine is considered to be an antihyperalgesic agent. Suppression of neutrophil production and inflammation may result in some analgesic effect.

Commercial Preparations

Ketamine is commercially available as a racemic mixture in an acidic solution (pH 3.5–5.5). This solution causes pain on IM injection. Ketamine S (+) is available in many countries. Theoretically, this is twice as potent as racemic ketamine with a better antihyperalgesic effect and fewer adverse effects. However, to date, there is no clear evidence for these advantages in the cat. Benzethonium chloride is the preservative used in most ketamine preparations.

Tiletamine is commercially available only in combination with zolazepam, a benzodiazepine, and is marketed for IM administration in cats. The powder is reconstituted with sterile water for injection to produce a solution that contains 50 mg/mL of each drug or 100 mg/mL of the combination. The dose is usually expressed in terms of the combined drugs. Tiletamine and zolazepam have plasma half lives between 2 and 4 hours, and 4.5 hours, respectively.

Pharmacology

Key pharmacological features of dissociative anesthetics:

- Produce antinociception by antagonism of NMDA receptors (*Box* 4.3). However, these drugs are not sufficient for painful procedures when used alone
- Increase cerebral oxygen consumption, cerebral blood flow, and intracranial pressure. The latter is exacerbated by hypercapnia
- Cause direct myocardial depression (*in vitro* ketamine studies). However, dissociative anesthetics inhibit uptake of catecholamines back into postganglionic sympathetic nerve endings, producing an indirect sympathetic effect
- Exert some anticholinergic effects. Administration of these agents in healthy cats usually increases heart rate, cardiac output, myocardial contractility, and blood pressure
- Produce minimal respiratory depression. The ventilatory response to increased $PaCO_2$ (partial pressure of carbon dioxide in the blood) is maintained. However, a decrease in respiratory rate and tidal volume may be seen, particularly during deep anesthesia, or when used in combination with other anesthetic/sedative drugs. Irregular respiratory patterns (apneustic ventilation) may be seen
- Ketamine is rapidly distributed after injection and has a short elimination half life. Ketamine is partially metabolized by the liver into an active metabolite (norketamine), which has an anesthetic effect. *In contrast to other species, ketamine is primarily excreted unchanged via the kidney in cats*
- Increase intraocular pressure
- Risk of corneal abrasion since eyes remain open and tear formation is reduced.
- Do *not* significantly change gastroesophageal sphincter pressure and gastric pressure

---

Box 4.3: NMDA receptor and ketamine as an adjuvant analgesic

The NMDA receptor is activated by glutamate and glycine, which are excitatory neuro-transmitters in the dorsal horn of the spinal cord (increased nociception). This receptor is involved with pain processing, central sensitization with consequent hyperalgesia and allodynia (Chapter 11). Ketamine is used *at subanesthetic doses* in the prevention and treatment of central sensitization, neuropathic, and cancer pain. The drug is combined with opioids, local anesthetics, and NSAIDS in the treatment of pain (Chapter 13).

Clinical Use

Dissociative anesthetics produce a cataleptic state, which is characterized by open eyes, mydriasis, muscle rigidity, and increased lacrimation and salivation. Tiletamine is only available in combination with zolazepam, and ketamine is usually administered in combination with a benzodiazepine or an agonist of α-2 adrenergic receptors for induction of anesthesia (*Table* 4.1) or as part of TIVA. Dissociative anesthetics produce rapid onset of anesthesia. Muscle rigidity, agitation, salivation, and hyperexcitability may be observed after ketamine or tiletamine/zolazepam administration when used alone. The quality of recovery from anesthesia is suboptimal. On the other hand, protective laryngeal reflexes are maintained. Ketamine is a good choice for induction of anesthesia in sick cats with hypovolemia, dehydration, and sepsis because of its sympathomimetic effects. In addition, ketamine can be administered at low doses in combination with midazolam and butorphanol for nonpainful diagnostic procedures or for chemical restraint in cats that are difficult to handle (Chapter 3). Ketamine is also used as an infusion and as part of balanced anesthesia (Chapter 6).

Ketamine can confound the psychomotor subscale of the UNESP-Botucatu multi-dimensional composite pain scale. Cats may show behaviors that can be confused with pain after ketamine administration even if they have not had surgery (Chapter 12).

Ketamine and tiletamine/zolazepam combinations are widely used for spay-neuter programs (see below). Duration of anesthesia with tiletamine/zolazepam is longer (30–40 minutes) when compared with ketamine (10–15 minutes); however, this will vary according to the protocol.

Contraindications

Alternatives to the dissociative agents are best chosen for cats with the following conditions: head trauma or space-occupying lesions, increased intraocular pressure, HCM, pregnancy, lower urinary tract obstruction, renal or hepatic disease, and cesarean section (Chapter 9).

Barbiturates

Mechanism of action: barbiturates interact with the $GABA_A$ receptor in the CNS and have a similar mechanism of action to propofol and alfaxalone. They can also mimic the action of GABA by directly activating $GABA_A$ receptors.

Commercial Preparations

Barbiturates are prepared commercially from highly alkaline solutions (sodium salts), and are dissolved in water for injection or saline 0.9% to make an appropriate concentration for administration. They should not be mixed with other drugs, which are acidic in solution. Thiopental is commercially available as a powder, which has a long shelf life; however, once reconstituted, the solution should be used within 6 days if stored at room temperature and 2 weeks when refrigerated. Thiopental solutions cause tissue necrosis and pain if injected perivascularly. If this happens, saline 0.9% should be injected into SC tissues as a diluent with or without local anesthetic. A local anesthetic cream can also be applied for pain relief.

Pharmacology

Key pharmacological features of thiopental

- Does *not* produce antinociception
- Produces rapid onset of anesthesia. Awakening from anesthesia is largely attributed to redistribution of the drug from the brain to skeletal muscles
- Decreases cerebral metabolic oxygen consumption, cerebral blood flow, and intra-cranial pressure, and has antiepileptic activity
- Produces significant cardiovascular depression by decreasing systemic vascular resistance (vasodilation), cardiac output, myocardial contractility, and mean arterial blood pressure. These effects are dose dependent
- Produces dose-dependent respiratory depression including decreases in respiratory rate and tidal volume leading to hypoventilation and hypercapnia. Apnea may be observed but is less likely with slow (over at least 60 seconds) administration
- Decreases intraocular pressure
- Is metabolized in the liver and excreted by the kidneys. Recovery from anesthesia is significantly prolonged if incremental doses are used to maintain anesthesia
- Thiopental is highly bound to proteins. This may potentially lead to an enhanced anesthetic effect in cases of hypoalbuminemia, or, at least theoretically, when other protein-bound drugs are used
- It reduces hematocrit and total protein concentration due to splenic sequestration

Clinical Use

Thiopental and pentobarbital were commonly used for induction of anesthesia in cats, but are now almost universally replaced by alfaxalone and propofol. Pentobarbital is commonly administered for euthanasia.

Thiopental produces rapid onset and short duration of anesthesia (5–10 minutes); however, recovery may be very prolonged if it is used to maintain anesthesia. The main use of thiopental would be for induction of anesthesia in cats with head trauma or space-occupying lesions, because of its neuroprotective effects, which are also observed with alfaxalone and propofol.

Contraindications

Barbiturates are not recommended for cats in the following circumstances: cardiomyopathy, respiratory disease, pregnancy, lower urinary tract obstruction, anemia, renal or hepatic disease, and cesarean section (Chapter 9).

Etomidate

Mechanism of action: etomidate is an imidazole compound that binds to specific sites at the $GABA_A$ receptors, enhancing GABA activity and producing anesthesia.

Commercial Preparation

Etomidate is a nonveterinary product containing propylene glycol, which causes pain and vascular irritation during injection, and may result in hemolysis due to its high osmolality (4640 mOsm/L). Lipid emulsion formulations cause fewer adverse effects.

Pharmacology

Key pharmacological features of etomidate:

- Does *not* produce antinociception
- Produces rapid onset of anesthesia
- Decreases cerebral metabolic oxygen consumption, cerebral blood flow, and intracranial pressure via cerebral vasoconstriction. It has antiepileptic activity. Myoclonus or excitatory ("paddling") movements are often seen if cats are not heavily sedated before administration of etomidate or if low doses are given. These side effects are reduced by benzodiazepines
- Suppresses adrenocortical function by inhibiting the conversion of cholesterol to cortisol. This effect lasts between 2 and 4 hours after administration. Maintenance of anesthesia with etomidate has been associated with higher mortality rates in humans, especially in the face of sepsis, which may be a consequence of suppressed adrenocortical function
- Produces minimal cardiovascular depression; a unique feature of etomidate
- Produces minimal respiratory depression and does not blunt the ventilatory response to increases in CO_2
- Decreases intraocular pressure
- Is metabolized in the liver and excreted by the kidneys
- Reduces gastroesophageal sphincter pressure and gastric pressure, predisposing the cat to gastroesophageal reflux during anesthesia

Clinical Use

There is a lack of studies on the use of etomidate in cats. It produces rapid onset and short duration of anesthesia after IV administration. Etomidate is not widely used in cats because it is expensive, it causes retching and adrenocortical suppression, and may cause hemolysis. Myoclonia may be seen during induction or recovery, but this is minimized by coadministration of a benzodiazepine. Etomidate is suitable for cats with cardiorespiratory disease, or those with hypovolemia or severe dehydration (Chapter 9). It can be also used for cats with ocular or cardiac disease, or those with head trauma.

Contraindications

Etomidate is not recommended for cats with hepatic or renal disease, sepsis, adrenal suppression, or anemia. Judicious use is recommended in hypo or hyperadrenocorticism.

Fentanyl plus Midazolam

Anesthesia can often be induced with a combination of IV fentanyl (2–5 µg/kg) and midazolam (0.25–0.5 mg/kg) in critically ill, debilitated, injured cats (Chapter 9). This protocol produces minimal cardiorespiratory depression and is a good choice for cats whose cardiovascular function is not stable. A small IV dose of propofol or alfaxalone (0.5 mg/kg) may be required if the desired end point is not reached (e.g. intubation).

Induction with Volatile Anesthetics

Induction of anesthesia using a "cat chamber" or a "cat bag" is discussed in Chapter 1. This technique should not be used on a routine basis but may be chosen when injectable methods are not possible or have failed, or may be chosen to minimize handling. Environmental pollution must be considered (Chapter 6). Some cats become excited and upset during the process (*Figure* 4.2). Mask techniques should also not be a routine technique but may be chosen when intravenous access is difficult, or has failed, or the cat

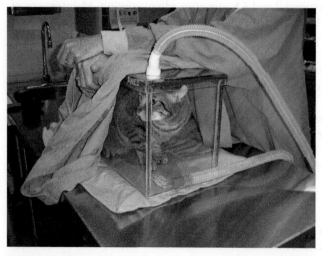

Figure 4.2 A cat is anesthetized in a chamber with appropriate scavenging of gases. Sevoflurane is the preferred volatile agent.

is to be anesthetized on a daily basis. Maintenance for short procedures such as blood donation can continue using a tight fitting mask (*Figure* 10.2). Sedation will decrease the "dose" of inhalant required and time to loss of consciousness. Low-stress handling is essential to ensure a calm and cooperative cat (e.g. towel wraps or "cat bags"), and to prevent injury to personnel. The mask alone is introduced to the cat to test its reaction before proceeding. Oxygen alone is turned on first, then the vaporizer setting is increased in 0.5 % increments – either every five breaths or every 15–30 seconds; if the cat becomes excited the vaporizer is increased to the maximum setting until the cat ceases struggling. Respiratory rate and mucus membrane color can be monitored by observation and heart rate palpated through the towel or bag. If available, sevoflurane is preferred for mask and chamber induction. Higher concentrations can be administered from the outset because it is nonirritant, making time to unconsciousness shorter and less stressful.

Total Intravenous Anesthesia (TIVA)

Volatile anesthesia is commonly used for maintenance of anesthesia in clinical practice (Chapter 6). However, it produces dose-dependent cardiorespiratory depression. Inhalation anesthesia is also unsuitable for some procedures, such as airway examination, bronchoalveolar lavage, and bronchoscopy. Cats that are mechanically ventilated for nonanesthetic-related treatment (including but not limited to head trauma, aspiration pneumonia, severe pulmonary contusions) are usually heavily sedated or anesthetized using injectable intravenous drugs. TIVA is a technique for providing general anesthesia using a single or a combination of injectable agents. With the correct choice of drugs TIVA may offer some benefits compared with inhalant anesthesia; these primarily relate to better cardiovascular stability, and calm and predictable recovery from anesthesia. TIVA has been administered using alfaxalone or propofol alone, or by combining propofol or alfaxalone with ketamine or short-acting opioids (e.g. fentanyl, alfentanil or remifentanil) (*Table* 4.1). Anesthesia is induced using a bolus of the chosen agent, then maintained with the same drug with or without additional agents given by infusion (*Box* 4.4). Cats developed less respiratory depression using TIVA with alfaxalone when compared with propofol for ovariohysterectomy. An analgesic drug is always administered with propofol or alfaxalone when using TIVA for painful procedures. Anesthetic recoveries may be prolonged when using propofol for TIVA.

Box 4.4: Administration of drug infusions in anesthesia

Constant rate infusion (CRI) is defined as a continuous administration of a set dose regimen through an electronic delivery device to maintain constant plasma levels. *Target-controlled infusion* (TCI) is based on complex algorithms and PK values, and infusion rates are administered by a delivery device to obtain a specific plasma (effect site) concentration to produce a desired effect. Analgesic and anesthetic CRI and TCI are used both for TIVA and for balanced anesthesia during inhalant anesthesia in cats (Chapter 6).

Infusion Devices

There are two types of infusion device for clinical use: *volumetric infusion pumps* may use peristaltic, piston or shuttle delivery systems to supply high volumes with low accuracy (± 10%). *Syringe drivers* use a stepper motor with a drive screw, and are more suitable for administering drugs when high accuracy (± 5%) is required. A calculator feature allows the user to enter body weight, drug concentration, and the desired infusion rate. As with vaporizers, the anesthetist will alter the setting based on depth of anesthesia. This equipment is illustrated in *Figure* 8.1.

Injectable-only Protocols

Feline population control has become extremely important in our society. Injectable-only anesthesia with appropriate analgesia has become a crucial component of humane spay-neuter programs. The Association of Shelter Veterinarians has published guide-lines for spay-neuter programs and how they are best implemented and performed. Some considerations for anesthetic protocols are:

- The need for analgesia, muscle relaxation, immobility, and loss of consciousness
- Low-volume injections with a wide margin of safety and possible reversibility (especially for agonists of α_2-adrenergic receptors)
- Rapid and smooth recovery from anesthesia
- Protocol will ultimately be dictated by the number and type of cats (e.g. feral or community cats), the skill and efficiency of technical assistance, timing and surgical competence, financial constraints of the program, drug availability, equipment, and facilities

The anesthetic management should take into consideration that kittens represent a large part of the population in these programs.

- Kittens (6–12 weeks) are usually fasted for no more than 2 hours to avoid hypo-glycemia. Fasting times are controversial and it is now accepted that adult cats do not require prolonged fasting (8–12 hours). Fasting for approximately 4 hours should be sufficient
- Hypothermia must be prevented by avoiding conductive heat loss, limiting body cavity exposure, and keeping hair removal and wetting with cleansing and antiseptic solutions to a minimum
- Intubation is not always practical in spay-neuter programs but may be required for treatment of hypoventilation, hypoxemia and respiratory arrest, and the appropriate equipment should be available. A supraglottic airway devices is an excellent option for rapid and nontraumatic intubation in these cases (Chapter 1)
- IV catheterization is usually not practical, and is often not performed in spay-neuter programs. This is particularly true when experienced personnel are involved and surgery times are short. However, it may be important for administration of "top ups" during anesthesia, or for emergency drugs. Even if not routinely used, equipment for IV catheterization should be available

- Incisional, intraperitoneal, and intratesticular blocks are highly recommended as part of the multimodal protocol for postoperative analgesia (Chapter 5). Local anesthetics are cost effective, widely available, and will reduce injectable anesthetic requirements
- Administration of nonsteroidal anti-inflammatory drugs (NSAIDs) is controversial because patient history is often unknown, and preanesthetic blood work is not routinely performed. They should be administered according to the veterinarian's

Table 4.2 Suggested anesthetic protocols for spay-neuter programs.

Anesthetic protocol[a]	Comments
Buprenorphine Dexmedetomidine Ketamine	Add equal volumes of buprenorphine (0.3 mg/mL), dexmedetomidine (0.05 mg/mL) and ketamine (100 mg/mL) into a sterile vial. The dose is 0.1 mL/kg of the mixture IM.
"Kitten Quad" Buprenorphine Midazolam Ketamine Medetomidine	60 mg/m^2 ketamine $+ 180 \text{ µg/m}^2$ buprenorphine $+ 3 \text{ mg/m}^2$ midazolam and either 600 µg/m^2 medetomidine or 300 µg/m^2 dexmedetomidine. An excellent chart can be found online at http://www.cats.org.uk/uploads/documents/Earlier_neutering_priciples-Dosage_Chart.pdf (accessed July 4, 2017) Equal volumes of medetomidine (1 mg/mL), ketamine (100 mg/mL), midazolam (5 mg/mL) and buprenorphine (0.3 mg/mL) are mixed in the same syringe and administered at the same time. Examples: 1 kg = 0.06 mL of each agent; 2 kg = 0.1 mL; 3 kg = 0.13 mL; 4 kg = 0.16 mL; 5 kg = 0.18 mL. Note that dosing is nonlinear, and the use of an application is recommended. The Kitten Quad App is available on Android, iPhone, and Windows.
"TKX" Tiletamine/Zolazepam Ketamine Xylazine[b]	In one bottle of tiletamine/zolazepam, add 4 mL of ketamine (100 mg/mL) and 1 mL (100 mg/mL) of xylazine. Each mL contains 80 mg of ketamine, 20 mg of xylazine, 50 mg tiletamine and 50 mg zolazepam. The dose is 0.25 mL for a 3 kg cat IM. The addition of an opioid such as buprenorphine (0.02 mg/kg) IM is recommended. Supplemental doses of 0.05–0.1 mL IV or IM (total) may be required.
"TTDex" Tiletamine/Zolazepam Butorphanol Dexmedetomidine	In one bottle of tiletamine/diazepam, add 2.5 mL of dexmedetomidine and 2.5 mL of butorphanol. Each mL contains 50 mg tiletamine, 50 mg zolazepam, 0.25 mg dexmedetomidine, and 5 mg butorphanol. The dose is 0.03–0.04 mL/kg IM for surgical anesthesia.

Notes:
a) Monitoring and oxygen supplementation are recommended. If needed and if the equipment is available, maintenance of anesthesia in female cats can be performed with isoflurane administered by mask or following placement of a supraglottic airway device or intubation. Atipamezole (0.2 mg/kg, IM) or yohimbine (0.4 mg/kg) can be given to shorten anesthetic recovery times when dexmedetomidine or xylazine has been used, respectively. Administration of NSAIDs is recommended if there are no contraindications. Intraperitoneal and intratesticular blocks will provide additional analgesia.
b) When dexmedetomidine is not available or when cost is prohibitive.

discretion, the patient's health status and the exclusion of any contraindications. Nonsteroidal anti-inflammatory drugs play a major role in postoperative pain relief
- Monitoring is commonly performed manually and by auscultation. This includes assessment of anesthetic depth (pulse palpation, heart rate, respiratory rate, mucous membrane color, and neurological reflexes). Pulse oximetry is practical and useful with protocols where oxygen is not routinely administered (Chapter 7)
- A protocol for anesthetic emergencies should be in place with standard kits and equipment readily available (Chapter 10). Personnel should be trained for emergency procedures
- Adjustments to the range of recommended dosages, regimens, and techniques to suit the conditions of each center are to be expected
- A successful program includes necropsy and tentative diagnosis of any deaths. Case-based discussions ("rounds") are important to review anesthetic records and communication of all parties involved
- Anesthetic recovery should be monitored until the cats are at least in sternal recumbency. Hypothermia is a common complication and warming methods should be employed (*Figure* 10.8)
- Transportation to the operating facility should be by trained personnel and in suitable vehicles and traps or carriers. Patient identification and space allocation are important to organize in advance to avoid stress and accidents
- Free-roaming cats and cats from shelters may have upper respiratory disease, and the attending veterinarian will be required to make decisions on whether or not these patients undergo anesthesia and surgery

Some injectable-only anesthetic protocols are suggested in *Table* 4.2.

Further Reading

Bley, C. R., Roos, M., and Price, J. (2007) Clinical assessment of repeated propofol-associated anesthesia in cats. *Journal of the American Veterinary Medical Association* **231**, 1347–1353.

Boudreau, A. E., Bersenas, A. M., Kerr, C. L., *et al.* (2012) A comparison of three anesthetic protocols for 24 hours of mechanical ventilation in cats. *Journal of Veterinary Emergency and Critical Care* **22**, 239–252.

Buisman, M., Wagner, M. C., Hasiuk, M. M., *et al.* (2016) Effects of ketamine and alfaxalone on application of a feline pain assessment scale. *Journal of Feline Medicine and Surgery* **18**, 643–651.

Campagna, I., Schwarz, A., Keller, S., *et al.* (2015) Comparison of the effects of propofol or alfaxalone for anaesthesia induction and maintenance on respiration in cats. *Veterinary Anaesthesia and Analgesia* **42**, 484–492.

Hall, T. L., Duke, T., Townsend, H. G., *et al.* (1999) The effect of opioid and acepromazine premedication on the anesthetic induction dose of propofol in cats. *Canadian Veterinary Journal* **40**, 867–870.

Ko, J., and Berman, A. (2010) Anesthesia in shelter medicine. *Topics in Companion Animal Medicine* **25**, 92–97.

Griffin, B., Bushby, P. A., McCobb, E., *et al.* (2016) The association of shelter veterinarians' 2016 veterinary medical care guidelines for spay-neuter programs. *Journal of the American Veterinary Medical Association* **249**, 165–188.

Mathis, A., Pinelas, R., Brodbelt, D. C., *et al.* (2012) Comparison of quality of recovery from anaesthesia in cats induced with propofol or alfaxalone. *Veterinary Anaesthesia and Analgesia* **39**, 282–290.

Mosing, M., Reich, H., and Moens, Y. (2010) Clinical evaluation of the anaesthetic sparing effect of brachial plexus block in cats. *Veterinary Anaesthesia and Analgesia* **37**, 154–161.

O'Hagan, B. J., Pasloske, K., McKinnon, C., *et al.* (2012) Clinical evaluation of alfaxalone as an anaesthetic induction agent in cats less than 12 weeks of age. *Australian Veterinary Journal* **90**, 395–401.

Posner, L. P., Asakawa, M., and Erb, H. N. (2008) Use of propofol for anesthesia in cats with primary hepatic lipidosis: 44 cases (1995–2004). *Journal of the American Veterinary Medical Association* **232**, 1841–1843.

Ravasio, G., Gallo, M., Beccaglia, M., *et al.* (2012) Evaluation of a ketamine-propofol drug combination with or without dexmedetomidine for intravenous anesthesia in cats undergoing ovariectomy. *Journal of the American Veterinary Medical Association* **241**, 1307–1313.

Schwarz, A., Kalchofner, K., Palm, J., *et al.* (2014) Minimum infusion rate of alfaxalone for total intravenous anaesthesia after sedation with acepromazine or medetomidine in cats undergoing ovariohysterectomy. *Veterinary Anaesthesia and Analgesia* **41**, 480–490.

Steagall, P. V., Aucoin, M., Monteiro, B. P., *et al.* (2015) Clinical effects of a constant rate infusion of remifentanil, alone or in combination with ketamine, in cats anesthetized with isoflurane. *Journal of the American Veterinary Medical Association* **246**, 976–981.

Taboada, F. M., and Murison, P. J. (2010) Induction of anaesthesia with alfaxalone or propofol before isoflurane maintenance in cats. *Veterinary Record* **167**, 85–89.

Tamura, J., Ishizuka, T., Fukui, S., *et al.* (2015) Sedative effects of intramuscular alfaxalone administered to cats. *Journal of Veterinary Medical Sciences* **77**, 897–904.

Tzannes, S., Govendir, M., Zaki, S., *et al.* (2000) The use of sevoflurane in a 2:1 mixture of nitrous oxide and oxygen for rapid mask induction of anaesthesia in the cat. *Journal of Feline Medicine and Surgery* **2**, 83–90.

Warne, L. N., Beths, T., Whittem, T., *et al.* (2015) A review of the pharmacology and clinical application of alfaxalone in cats. *Veterinary Journal* **203**, 141–148.

Whittem, T., Pasloske, K. S., Heit, M. C., *et al.* (2008) The pharmacokinetics and pharmacodynamics of alfaxalone in cats after single and multiple intravenous administration of Alfaxan at clinical and supraclinical doses. *Journal of Veterinary Pharmacology Therapeutics* **31**, 571–579.

Williams, L. S., Levy, J. K., Robertson, S. A., *et al.* (2002) Use of the anesthetic combination of tiletamine, zolazepam, ketamine, and xylazine for neutering feral cats. *Journal of the American Veterinary Medical Association* **220**, 1491–1495.

Zonca, A., Ravasio, G., Gallo, M., *et al.* (2012) Pharmacokinetics of ketamine and propofol combination administered as ketofol via continuous infusion in cats. *Journal of Veterinary Pharmacology and Therapeutics* **35**, 580–587.

5

Local Anesthetics and Loco-regional Techniques

Francesco Staffieri[1] and Paulo Steagall[2]

[1]*University of Bari, Bari, Italy*
[2]*Université de Montréal, Saint-Hyacinthe, Canada*

Key Points

- Basic pharmacology of local anesthetics
- Factors influencing onset and duration of action of local anesthetics
- Local anesthetic-induced toxicity
- Local anesthetics used in clinical practice
- Basic principles of electrical nerve location
- Description of loco-regional anesthetic techniques suitable for clinical practice

Introduction

Local anesthetics block neuronal voltage-gated Na^+ channels and voltage-dependent K^+ and Ca^{2+}. By doing so, they block the generation and propagation of electrical impulses in a reversible manner. These mechanisms produce loss of *sensory, motor, and autonomic* function. Loco-regional anesthetic techniques are widely used in the management of perioperative pain (*Box 5.1*).

Box 5.1: Advantages of using perioperative local anesthetic techniques

- They provide preventive and multimodal perioperative analgesia. Local anesthetics can be administered in combination with opioids, agonists of α_2-adrenergic receptors, ketamine, and NSAIDs (Chapter 13)
- They decrease/blunt the stress response to surgical trauma: local anesthetic techniques used before surgery reduce the neuroendocrine response to surgery
- They prevent the development of central sensitization: local anesthetics are the only drugs that completely block peripheral nociceptive input
- They reduce volatile and injectable anesthetic requirements (anesthetic "sparing effect"). They diminish autonomic responses to surgical stimuli, which improves intraoperative cardiopulmonary function, and facilitate a rapid and smooth recovery

---

Feline Anesthesia and Pain Management, First Edition. Edited by Paulo Steagall, Sheilah Robertson and Polly Taylor.

Nerve branches of the maxillary, inferior alveolar (mandibular), intercostal, and those innervating the thoracic and pelvic limbs are commonly blocked as part of loco-regional anesthetic techniques in cats. Knowledge of anatomy and clinical pharmacology of local anesthetics is required to ensure these techniques are safe and effective.

Physicochemical and Pharmacodynamic Properties of Local Anesthetics

Local anesthetics have a lipophilic aromatic unsaturated ring linked to a hydrophilic amino group by an intermediate hydrocarbon chain. The latter contains either an ester or an amide group, which defines the type of metabolism, and serves as the basis for classification (esters vs amide local anesthetics). The amino group is usually a tertiary amine and determines the degree of water solubility (molecular dissociation and combination with sodium channels).

- Most of these drugs are formulated as a racemic mixture (1:1). Ropivacaine and levobupivacaine are exceptions
- Local anesthetics have a *nonionized*, lipid-soluble form (base) and an *ionized* water-soluble form (conjugated acid). The dissociation constant (pKa) corresponds to the pH at which the acid and base forms exist in equal amounts. This is calculated using the Henderson–Hasselbalch equation:

  $$pKa = pH - \log[\text{base}]/[\text{acid}]; \text{where the pH is that of the solution or tissue.}$$

- Local anesthetics have a pKa between 7.5 and 9 and are formulated as acid solutions of hydrochloride salts (pH 3.5–5.0). This formulation gives a net prevalence of the ionized form, and is therefore water soluble
- When a local anesthetic solution is injected into body tissues with a physiological pH (7.4), the nonionized lipid-soluble form will prevail. This is critical for the drug effect since the nonionized form crosses biological membranes. In inflamed tissues, the ionized form prevails, explaining why local anesthetics are usually ineffective in these conditions (acidic pH)
- Protein binding influences the drug activity because only the unbound free fraction is pharmacologically active. Higher protein binding is associated with a longer duration but slow onset of action. Protein binding is pH-dependent, and is reduced in pathological conditions such as acidemia
- Lipid solubility promotes sequestration of the local anesthetic into lipophilic compartments (i.e. myelin) from where the drug is slowly released. Lipid solubility is directly correlated with potency (*Box* 5.2). It also contributes to the slower onset and longer duration of action of the highly lipid-soluble drugs
- Potency can be defined as the minimum concentration of a local anesthetic required to block nerve conduction
- Increased protein binding, potency, and the effect of the local anesthetic on vascular tone (i.e. vasoconstriction), correlate with increased duration of action
- The concentration of a local anesthetic required to block nerve conduction is *inversely* related to the *length of the nerve* in contact with the anesthetic solution

---

Box 5.2: Potency and lipid solubility of local anesthetics: Practical implications

- Potency and lipid solubility (octanol: buffer partition coefficient) are positively correlated
- Bupivacaine is almost ten times more lipid soluble (partition coefficient of 3440) than lidocaine (partition coefficient of 366). *In vivo* potency of bupivacaine is four times that of lidocaine
- The higher lipid solubility of bupivacaine accounts for the lower concentrations (0.125 – 0.75%) required to produce nerve block when compared with lidocaine (1–2%)
- The high lipid solubility of bupivacaine accounts for the slower onset (20–30 minutes) and longer duration of action (3–6 hours) when compared with lidocaine (5–10 minutes and 1–2 hours, respectively)

Axons and Nerve Fibers

Axons may be classified on their structure (myelinated and unmyelinated), diameter, and function (*Table* 5.1). The small unmyelinated axons (C fibers) are more susceptible to local anesthetics followed by small myelinated axons (B fibers), and large myelinated (Aα and Aβ) fibers. Clinical experience shows that autonomic responses are inhibited before sensory (pain, loss of sensation, and light touch), and motor blockade. The resolution of nerve block follows the reverse order. This phenomenon is known as *differential block,* and is influenced by many other factors (i.e. characteristics of the local anesthetic, length of nerve in contact with the anesthetic solution, position of the single axon in the nerve bundle, frequency of discharge of the nerve). Some local anesthetics may cause sensory

Table 5.1 Classification of nerve fibers with regard to structure (myelinated and unmyelinated), diameter and function.

Type of fiber	Structure	Diameter (μm)	Function	Conduction (m/s)	Susceptibility to local anesthetics (*in vitro*)	Order of blockade (*in vivo*)
Aα	Myelinated	12–20	Motor and proprioception	30–120	++	5
Aβ	Myelinated	5–12	Sensory (touch and pressure)	30–70	++	4
Aγ	Myelinated	3–6	Muscle tone to the muscle spindle	15–35	+++	3
Aδ	Myelinated	2–5	Pain (fast), touch, temperature	5–25	++	2
B	Unmyelinated	< 3	Autonomic function	3–15	++	1
C	Unmyelinated	0.3–1.4	Pain (slow), autonomic function, temperature	0.7–1.3	+	2

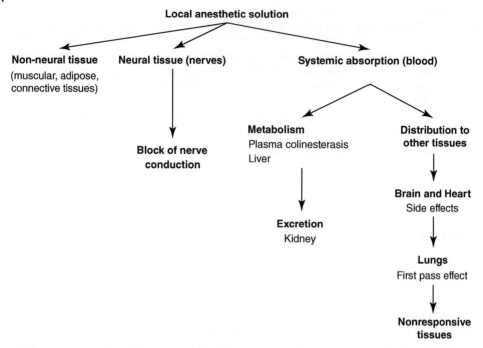

Figure 5.1 Absorption, distribution, metabolism, and excretion of local anesthetics.

blockade with apparent sparing of motor blockade (e.g. ropivacaine), and this is known as *sensitive-motor dissociation*. For example, if ropivacaine is used, a cat may be able to walk postoperatively (lack of motor impairment) while sensory block is still present after epidural administration or a sciatic-femoral nerve block.

Pharmacokinetics

Figure 5.1 shows the classic absorption, distribution, metabolism, and excretion after the administration of local anesthetics.

Factors Influencing Onset and Duration of Action

- *Site of injection* is the most important factor influencing the onset of local anesthetic block. The anesthetic solution should be injected as close as possible, but not into, the nerve for the most rapid onset of anesthesia
- *Dose, volume, and concentration* of the local anesthetic solution influence onset, magnitude, and duration of anesthesia. Higher concentrations are normally preferred. If the local anesthetic is diluted this reduces concentration, and might affect duration of anesthesia. On the other hand, in small animals such as the cat it may be necessary to use dilute solutions so that an adequate volume can be used without giving a toxic dose

- *Physical and chemical characteristics* of the local anesthetic solution influence the onset of anesthesia (see lipid solubility, potency above). This may explain the slow onset of action of the lipophilic drugs (such as bupivacaine, ropivacaine), despite their greater potency
- Duration of anesthesia depends on clearance of the local anesthetic solution from the site of action, which, in turn, will depend on the dose, blood flow, and lipophilicity of the drug

Metabolism

Amino-esters such as tetracaine, procaine, and benzocaine are *not* recommended in feline anesthesia. They are hydrolyzed into para-aminobenzoic acid (PABA), which may cause an allergic reaction and methemoglobinemia (Chapter 2).

Amino-amide local anesthetics include lidocaine, mepivacaine, prilocaine, bupivacaine, ropivacaine, and levobupivacaine. These drugs are largely metabolized by cytochrome P450 enzymes in the liver. Conjugation and glucuronidation (phase II of hepatic metabolism) increase water solubility and polarity, thereby facilitating renal elimination. Cats are deficient in glucuronyl transferases; this impairs biotransformation of local anesthetics and makes this species more prone to toxicity (Chapter 2). Prilocaine undergoes hydrolysis to o-toluidine, a compound capable of oxidizing hemoglobin to methemoglobin, which does not bind to oxygen and leads to cyanosis. Clearance of amide local anesthetics may be reduced or prolonged by decreased hepatic blood flow (e.g. decreased cardiac output and hypotension).

Adjuvants

Local anesthetics are commonly administered with adjuvant drugs to modify their onset and duration of action. The advantages and disadvantages of these adjuvants are described in *Table* 5.2.

Local Anesthetics

The most common local anesthetics used in feline practice are presented in *Table* 5.3.

Lidocaine

Lidocaine is the most popular local anesthetic in veterinary practice, and is considered to be the prototype of the amino-amide group. It is available in concentrations of 0.5%, 1%, and 2% with or without epinephrine (adrenaline), and in a gel preparation in concentrations of 2.5% to 5%. Doses should not exceed 10 mg/kg.

Lidocaine is administered as part of topical or infiltration anesthesia, peripheral nerve (brachial plexus, sciatic, and femoral nerve, "ring block" e.g. for onychectomy), and neuraxial (epidural and spinal) blocks. Lidocaine is routinely applied to the larynx before intubation to avoid laryngospasm (Chapter 1 and 2).

Table 5.2 Adjuvant drugs administered with local anesthetics.

Adjuvant	Advantages	Disadvantages	Mechanism of action	Comments
Vasoconstrictors (epinephrine 1:200 000 (5 µg/mL))	Prolong the duration of the block; increase the intensity of the block; reduce the systemic absorption of local anesthetics	Potential ischemic nerve injury; accidental intravascular and high doses cause systemic effects	Reduction of local blood flow and clearance of the drug; direct stimulation of the α_2-adrenergic receptors	1:200 000 concentrations can be obtained by adding 0.1 mL of 1:1000 epinephrine (0.1 mg) to 20 ml of local anesthetic solution
Agonists of α_2-adrenergic receptors (dexmedetomidine)	Shorten onset of the block; longer duration of sensory and motor block; enhance the quality of block	Accidental intravascular and high doses cause systemic effects	Direct supraspinal and spinal mechanisms; local effect mediated by hyperpolarization of C fibers; local vasoconstriction	Clinical experience suggests that a solution of local anesthetic containing 0.5–1 µg/mL of dexmedetomidine is effective in small animal patients
Sodium bicarbonate	Reduce pain of injection of local anesthetic solution; shorten the onset of the block	Excessive alkalinization (pH > 7) may cause precipitation of local anesthetic solutions	Raises the pH of the local anesthetic solution (alkalinization) increasing the amount of nonionized lipid soluble form of the local anesthetic	The recommended dose of sodium bicarbonate solution is 0.1 mEq per mL of local anesthetic solution
Hyaluronidase	Improves the diffusion of local anesthetic into the tissues	Allergic reactions have been reported in humans	The enzyme breaks down hyaluronic acid, which is a constitutive component of the connective tissue in the extracellular matrix	The efficacy of this technique is unproven
Opioids	Potentiation of sensory block without impairing motor function; prolonged duration of action	Epidural morphine may result in urine retention and pruritus	Opioids exert their analgesic action through a variety of supraspinal and spinal mechanisms, including attenuation of C fiber-mediated nociception	Morphine is the most widely used epidural opioid in veterinary medicine (alone or in combination with local anesthetic)

Lidocaine (1 mg/kg IV) is a class Ib antiarrhythmic drug that can be used to treat cardiac ventricular dysrhythmias. When administered intravenously either as a bolus or as a constant rate infusion it can provide prokinetic, anti-dysrhythmic, inhalant-anesthetic sparing, anti-inflammatory and analgesic effects. In cats, intravenous infusions of lidocaine (25–50 µg/kg/minute) reduce isoflurane requirements but cause cardiovascular

Table 5.3 Common local anesthetics used in feline practice.

Local anesthetic	pK$_a$	Protein binding (%)	Onset (minutes)	Duration of the block (hours)	Relative potency (lidocaine = 1)
Lidocaine	7.7	55–65	5–15	1–2	1
Mepivacaine	7.6	75–80	5–15	1.5–2.5	1
Bupivacaine	8.1	85–95	10–20	4–6	4
Ropivacaine	8.1	94	10–20	3–5	3
Levobupivacaine	8.1	97	10–20	4–6	4

depression which is greater than an equipotent dose of isoflurane alone. Thus, in cats, lidocaine infusion is not recommended to reduce inhalant agent requirements or as a component of a multimodal analgesic plan (Chapter 6).

Lidocaine Patch

Lidocaine can be administered by the transdermal route (*Figure* 13.5). Lidocaine adhesive patches provide pain relief in a safe manner with minimal systemic absorption and poor bioavailability (6%). The 700 mg patch (50 mg/g of adhesive) is applied over the area of need, and measurable concentrations can be detected in plasma after 12 hours. However, an analgesic effect is observed at the site earlier due to a local effect. This formulation should be used as part of multimodal analgesia, but is not available in all countries.

Eutectic Mixture of Lidocaine and Prilocaine

This is a commercial mixture of lidocaine 2.5%, and prilocaine 2.5% (1:1) for topical anesthesia. Application of the cream does not result in significant systemic absorption or adverse effects in healthy cats. It has been shown to be efficacious for venipuncture and intravenous catheter placement (*Figure* 5.2).

Bupivacaine and Levobupivacaine

Bupivacaine is a highly lipophilic amino-amide local anesthetic. It is significantly more cardiotoxic than other local anesthetics and must *never* be administered by the IV route. Doses should not be greater than 2 mg/kg. Concentrations of 0.25%, 0.5%, and 0.75% are available commercially with or without epinephrine.

Levobupivacaine is an isomer (S-enantiomer) of bupivacaine, and produces less cardiotoxicity than the racemic mixture. The physicochemical properties and clinical uses are similar to bupivacaine but the drug is more expensive in most countries. Adverse effects were not reported when levobupivacaine (2 mg/kg) was used for feline femoral and sciatic nerve block.

Ropivacaine

Ropivacaine is an amino-amide local anesthetic with intermediate potency and long duration of action. It is marketed as a pure S-enantiomer. It produces less cardiovascular

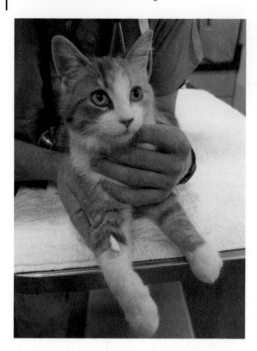

Figure 5.2 A eutectic mixture of lidocaine and prilocaine cream is used to desensitize the skin before venous catheterization and venipuncture. The area should be covered by an occlusive bandage for 20–30 minutes before puncture. Blanching or hyperemia may be noted in the area of application after removal of the occlusive bandage. Adverse reactions have not been reported in cats.

and central nervous system (CNS) adverse effects compared with bupivacaine. It is available in concentrations up to 1%. Ropivacaine causes sensory block but limited motor blockade which is often beneficial in clinical cases. However, its use in cats is not well documented.

Mixing Local Anesthetics

Historically, lidocaine 2% and bupivacaine 0.5% have been mixed together to decrease the onset of action of bupivacaine while increasing the duration of action of lidocaine. However, these drugs have different pKa and percentage protein binding, and there is little evidence that this combination is better than bupivacaine alone. The results may be unpredictable and the duration of action actually decreased. For example, epidural administration of lidocaine and bupivacaine produced a similar onset of sensory block to either drug alone. When anesthetics are combined, the total dose should be calculated as a fraction of each anesthetic's maximum dose to avoid toxicity.

Adverse Effects

Neurotoxicity
Local anesthetics can produce irreversible or reversible nerve damage. Local neurotoxicity is directly related to the potency of a local anesthetic. However, adverse effects are rare if normal clinical precautions are taken (*Box* 5.3).

Box 5.3: Risk factors associated with toxicity of local anesthetics

- Excessive doses or concentration of the local anesthetic solution; this is not a problem when recommended doses and concentrations are used
- Addition of epinephrine to the local anesthetic solution (especially if administered for limb block) carries a risk of central or peripheral ischemic tissue injury
- Use of spinal or epidural catheters (increases the risk of inflammation and spinal cord damage)
- Contamination of the local anesthetic solution
- Use of preservatives; this is particularly important with repeated epidural injections of solutions containing preservatives that are neurotoxic to the spinal cord

---

Neurotrauma can be caused by direct nerve damage or intraneural injection. *A local anesthetic solution should never be injected if resistance to injection is experienced.* Recent studies using ultrasound-guided techniques showed that intraneural injection is common but often occurs without causing neurologic lesions. Use of electrical peripheral nerve stimulators and ultrasonography should reduce the incidence of such complications.

Systemic Toxicity
Systemic toxicity is usually produced by accidental intravascular injection of the local anesthetic solution. It results from high plasma concentrations affecting the central nervous system followed by respiratory and cardiovascular depression, and death (*Figure* 5.3). Bupivacaine is the exception to this rule; it causes immediate cardiovascular toxicity.

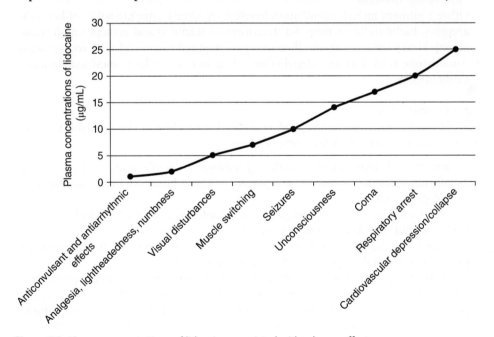

Figure 5.3 Plasma concentrations of lidocaine associated with adverse effects.

Systemic toxicity can be prevented by

- Using recommended doses and concentrations
- Confirming negative aspiration of blood before injection (risk of intravascular injection)
- Using an ECG or Doppler ultrasound to monitor cardiovascular function and for rapid recognition of dysrhythmias. Bupivacaine is injected slowly
- Appropriate knowledge of anatomical landmarks and the risks associated with each technique

Signs of central nervous toxicity include agitation, muscle twitching, seizures, stupor, and coma. Some of these signs are not observed if the cat is anesthetized. In this case, apnea and cardiovascular collapse (decreased cardiac contractility, bradycardia, hypotension, and dysrhythmias) will result. Severe cardiovascular depression (bradycardia, sinus arrest, and severe hypotension) has been reported in a cat after receiving bupivacaine (1.6 mg/kg) for an inferior mandibular block. Accidental IV injection may have occurred.

Treatment of Systemic Toxicity

- Administration or infusion of local anesthetics should be stopped immediately
- Anticholinergics and positive inotropes are recommended for treatment of bradycardia and hypotension
- If signs do not resolve within minutes, an intravenous lipid emulsion (Intralipid®, 4 mL/kg bolus, followed by 0.5 mL/kg/minute for 10 minutes) is administered. This will also increase the chance of successful resuscitation after cardiac arrest following bupivacaine overdose
- Other treatment includes ventilation (respiratory arrest), administration of benzodiazepines, barbiturates or propofol (treatment of seizures) and epinephrine (cardiac arrest). Heavy sedation or anesthesia may be required to control neurological signs
- Amiodarone is used as an antiarrhythmic drug in cases of local anesthetic-induced cardiotoxicity

Other Complications
Knowledge of feline anatomy and good local anesthetic technique should enable effective blocks to be produced with few complications.

- Hematoma and bleeding can occur during administration of a local anesthetic. This is usually not a problem; however, an epidural or spinal hematoma may cause serious neurologic deficit
- Aseptic techniques prevent development of infection; a block should never be performed through known infected tissue
- Penetration of the globe has been reported in a cat following an intraoral maxillary nerve block for oral surgery. Enucleation was required
- Suspected brainstem anesthesia following a retrobulbar block has been reported in a cat: the patient became apneic and ventilation was required in the intra- and early postoperative period. Postoperative neurological signs included nystagmus, absent menace response, mydriasis, and lack of dazzle and direct pupillary light reflex. All neurological signs resolved within 3 hours of extubation

Techniques for Nerve Location

Some peripheral nerve blocks may be guided using electrical nerve stimulator (ENS) or ultrasonography. Methods employing ENS are convenient, safe, and affordable for administration of local anesthetics. The ENS is attached to an insulated needle (*Box* 5.4) generating an electrical field in the tissues surrounding a target nerve. This results in depolarization and muscle contractions that are used to confirm correct needle placement (*Figure* 5.4). Most cats will require heavy sedation or general anesthesia for this procedure.

Box 5.4: The insulated needle

An insulated needle is electrically isolated with the exception of its tip. In cats, a 23 or 22-G needle with a length of 25–50 mm (1–2 inches) is most commonly used. The needle is equipped with a luer lock (with or without a short extension line) to connect the syringe and avoid excessive movements. The dead space of the extension line and needle should be taken into account when calculating the volume to be injected.

Ultrasonography allows direct visualization of nerves, vessels, and surrounding structures during application of peripheral nerve block. This may reduce complications such as nerve damage, bleeding, and hematoma; however, it requires training and the equipment is expensive. Use of ENS and ultrasonography reduces the dose of local anesthetic required to produce effective nerve block and increases the rate of success.

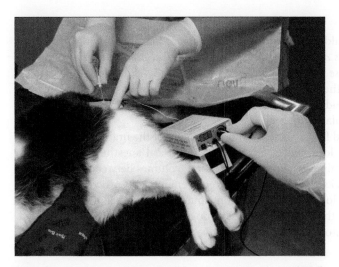

Figure 5.4 Sciatic nerve block. An electrical nerve stimulator (ENS) is used to locate the sciatic nerve for administration of the local anesthetic. A typical nerve stimulator delivers currents at a variable frequency (1–4 Hz) and intensity (0 and 4–5 mA). There are two electrical cables (not shown); one (negative charge, cathode, black color) is connected to the insulated needle while the second (positive charge, anode, red color) is attached to the skin of the cat and distal to the needle (*Box* 5.4). Muscle contraction usually disappears after injection. This is due to the solution deposited between the needle and the nerve and should not be considered a sign of onset of the block.

These advantages are particularly important in cats because of the increased risk of toxicity resulting from their poor hepatic glucuronidation.

Local Anesthetic Techniques

Some basic principles are employed before application of all local anesthetic techniques (*Box* 5.5). Local anesthetic techniques should not be used in proximity to any cancerous tumors since neoplastic cells may be disseminated. This section briefly describes common local anesthetic techniques used in feline practice.

Box 5.5: Basic principles that are applied with local anesthetic techniques

- Aseptic technique is always employed. Chlorhexidine ($\leq$ 0.12% solution to avoid swelling and irritation) can be applied before local anesthetic techniques in the oral cavity
- Careful calculation of local anesthetic dose is essential to avoid toxicity. Cats are relatively small and possess poor metabolic capabilities (i.e. glucuronidation) (Chapter 2)
- Negative aspiration of blood should be confirmed before injection. This is particularly important when bupivacaine is administered because of its cardiotoxicity
- Lack of resistance to injection; intraneural injection followed by nerve damage has been associated with high resistance during injection

---

Head

All dental procedures should be performed under general anesthesia with a properly secured airway. *Mouth gags are no longer applied for surgical procedures involving the head and oral cavity because they are associated with postanesthetic blindness* (Chapter 1 and 10). Oral local anesthetic techniques require simple, low-cost material such as disposable 1 mL syringes and 23 or 25-G 25-30 mm (1.2 inch) needles. Larger needles may cause nerve and vascular damage.

Dental blocks can be used for extractions and for surgery of the oral cavity, including maxillectomy and mandibulectomy. A small quantity of local anesthetic (most commonly lidocaine or bupivacaine) is required. In general, volumes between 0.1–0.25 mL are appropriate. These blocks reduce anesthetic requirements and procedure-induced increases in heart rate and blood pressure, and contribute to the control of postoperative pain. It is important to note that techniques used in dogs cannot be directly extrapolated to the cat due to some anatomical differences between species.

Infraorbital Nerve Block (*Figure* 5.5.1)
The infraorbital foramen is located just ventral to the orbit, and a bony ridge can be palpated in cats. The infraorbital canal is much shorter in the cat than in dogs. It is only a few millimeters in length. The needle is introduced ventrally and advanced approximately 2 mm since eye penetration may occur. Both the intraoral (or subgingival) and extraoral approaches are acceptable.

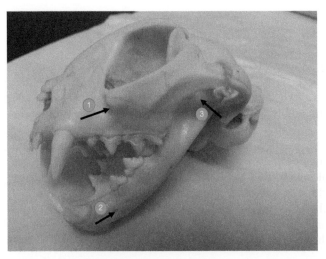

Figure 5.5 Common local anesthetic blocks of the oral cavity. Anatomical location of the infraorbital nerve block (1), mental nerve block (2) and inferior alveolar (mandibular) nerve block (3).

Anesthesia of the infraorbital nerve as it leaves the canal will produce ipsilateral anesthesia of the nasal, labial, and rostral soft tissue. *A maxillary block is required to desensitize the incisor teeth.*

Mental Nerve Block (*Figure* 5.5.2)
In cats, the middle mental foramen can be located between the third premolar and the canine tooth. However, it is difficult to palpate because it is located medial to the lip frenulum. The foramen is small and to avoid nerve damage it should not be penetrated. The needle is gently inserted rostro-caudally at the lateral aspect of the mandible, and local anesthetic is injected over the foramen.

This block desensitizes the rostral lower lip and mandible, and the canine and incisor teeth. It is commonly performed for mandibular symphysis repair or extraction of the ipsilateral lower incisor teeth.

Inferior Alveolar (Mandibular) Nerve Block (*Figure* 5.5.3)
The inferior alveolar foramen is located on the medial side of the mandible approximately halfway between the angular process of the mandible and the last molar tooth. This foramen may be difficult to palpate in cats but the block can still be performed successfully. Some cats do not have the concavity of the ventral margin of the mandibular ramus, which can be easily located in dogs. An extraoral approach is commonly used for this block; however, an intraoral technique is also acceptable.

Two imaginary lines are used to locate the mandibular foramen. One is perpendicular to the lateral canthus of the eye and ventral portion of the mandible, which crosses with another line dividing the dorsal and ventral teeth arcade, and parallel to the ventral portion of the mandible. Where these lines intersect indicates the injection point.

A mandibular nerve block produces sensory and motor block of the mandible including teeth, lower lip, part of the tongue, and hard and soft tissues.

Maxillary Nerve Block

The percutaneous approach for the maxillary nerve block involves desensitizing the maxillary nerve as it enters the pterygopalatine fossa. The nerve is located ventral to the rostral aspect of the zygomatic arch and caudal to the vertical aspect of the maxillary bone. The needle is inserted in a rostro-medial direction just below the ventral border of the zygomatic arch, and between the caudal aspect of the maxilla, and the vertical ramus of the mandible. The needle should be directed towards the pterygopalatine fossa.

For the intraoral approach, the needle is bent to a 45° angle and advanced dorsally, and caudal to the molar tooth. The needle is pointed towards the maxillary foramen in the pterygopalatine fossa. Global penetration has been reported in cats after a maxillary block using the intraoral technique (see other complications above).

This block produces anesthesia of the ipsilateral maxilla including teeth, palate, and the skin of the nose, cheek, and upper lip, as the infraorbital nerve and branches of the pterygopalatine nerve branches are also blocked.

Peribulbar and Retrobulbar Blocks

Anesthesia of the eye and the orbit is achieved by blocking the ophthalmic branch of the trigeminal nerve. Advantages include excellent analgesia, reduction of analgesic and anesthetic requirements, akinesia, and blunting of the oculocardiac reflex.

Retrobulbar anesthesia is achieved by injecting a small volume of local anesthetic solution intraconally (i.e. inside the extraocular muscle cone). A 38 mm (1.5 inch), 22-G needle is bent at the midpoint by approximately 20°. The needle is inserted through the superior eyelid of the medial region of the orbit and advanced approximately 30 mm (1.2 inches) towards the caudal pole of the globe but in close proximity to the orbital wall. Intraconal placement of the needle can be performed under ultrasound guidance. One mL of the local anesthetic solution is injected once the needle tip is in the intraconal space.

A 15 mm (5/8th inch), 25-G needle is used for the *peribulbar* block. The needle is inserted through the superior eyelid in the medial region of the orbit and advanced to its full length in close proximity to the orbital wall, and 2–3 mL of local anesthetic is injected. Peribulbar injection relies on the distribution of local anesthetic rather than direct retrobulbar anesthesia.

Possible complications of retrobulbar anesthesia include an oculocardiac response, retrobulbar hemorrhage, intravenous injection of anesthetic, globe perforation, extra-ocular muscle damage, and intrathecal injection which can induce seizures or cardio-respiratory arrest.

Thoracic Limbs

Intravenous regional anesthesia ("Bier" block) is rarely performed in cats. Application of a tourniquet has been shown to carry a significant risk of nerve damage and paralysis in cats.

Brachial Plexus (using ENS)

This block is indicated for anesthesia of structures distal to the middle third of the humerus. The goal is to anesthetize the axillary, musculocutaneous, radial, median, and

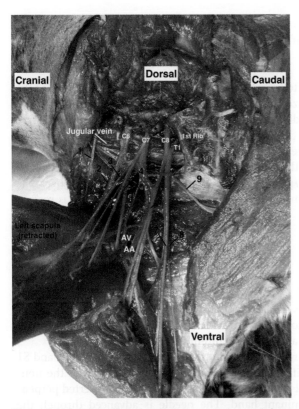

Figure 5.6 Anatomy of the brachial plexus in the cat (left lateral view). The cervical (C6, C7, C8) and thoracic (T1) nerve roots and their branches form the brachial plexus. *Transverse processes of the fifth, sixth and seventh cervical vertebrae. AA: Axillary artery; AV: Axillary vein; 1. Nerve to the muscle brachiocephalicus; 2. Suprascapular nerve; 3. Subscapular nerve; 4. Axillary nerve; 5. Musculocutaneous nerve; 6. Radial nerve; 7. Median nerve; 8. Ulnar nerve; 9. Thoracodorsal nerve. *Source*: Courtesy of Dr. Marina Evangelista.

ulnar nerves (*Figure* 5.6). The brachial plexus comprises a number of different nerves and there is a higher prevalence of "patchy anesthesia" (i.e. some nerves are anesthetized but not all of them) when compared with other loco-regional anesthetic techniques.

The scapulo-humeral joint, acromion, the jugular vein, greater tubercle, and the first rib are identified. The needle is introduced in a cranio-caudal direction, medial to the scapulohumeral joint, cranial to the acromion, and dorsal to the jugular vein. It is directed perpendicular to a line between the acromion and the cranial border of the greater tubercle of the humerus, and advanced towards the first rib at the ventral border of the scalenus muscle. The ENS is set to deliver a 0.6–0.8 mA current output at 2 Hz. The needle is slowly advanced towards the nerve until flexion of the elbow and contraction of the biceps brachii muscle is observed. Correct needle placement is confirmed when the response is observed at 0.4 mA, but not at 0.2 mA (risk of intra-neural injection). Local anesthetic is injected at 0.3 mL/kg. The axillary artery and vein are located within the axillary space and there is a risk of inadvertent intravascular injection if negative aspiration is not performed and repeated during the injection procedure.

When a peripheral nerve stimulator is not available, the same technique is applied using the aforementioned landmarks and the blind technique.

Metacarpal/Metatarsal "Ring" Block

These blocks are used for onychectomy, where this procedure is still performed. For the thoracic limbs, this block desensitizes the dorsal and palmar branches of the ulnar nerve, the superficial branches of the radial nerve, and the median nerve. The injections are performed close to the carpus. For the pelvic limbs, this block desensitizes the superficial and deep peroneal nerve and the tibial nerve, and lateral and plantar nerves. The injections are performed close to the metatarsal joint. Local anesthetic is administered subcutaneously over the palmar/plantar aspect of the limbs and anesthetizes the superficial nerves. A 25- or 27-G needle is used. Bupivacaine or ropivacaine is recommended for prolonged anesthesia.

Pelvic Limbs

Lumbosacral Epidural

Lumbosacral epidural anesthesia is indicated for surgery caudal to the diaphragm. This block blunts the stress response to surgery, provides intraoperative and postoperative analgesia, and decreases inhalant anesthetic requirements during surgery.

The cat is positioned in sternal recumbency and the spinous processes of L7 and S1 and the iliac tuberosity are identified with the middle finger and thumb of the non-dominant hand. A 22-G, 25 mm (1 inch) Tuohy (preferably) needle is inserted perpendicular to the skin with the dominant hand. The needle is advanced through the subcutaneous tissues, and the needle stylet is removed with the nondominant hand. The needle hub is filled with local anesthetic for the hanging drop technique. The needle is further advanced until the *ligamentum flavum* is punctured and loss of resistance is felt while the local anesthetic is aspirated due to negative pressure within the epidural space. Puncture of the *ligamentum flavum* will produce a "pop" sensation although this may be quite subtle in cats. Additionally, the hanging drop with aspiration of local anesthetic is not always reliable in cats.

Lidocaine or bupivacaine is injected in combination with preservative-free morphine (0.1 mg/kg) (total volume of injection is 0.2 mL/kg) (Chapter 13). Slow injection is important to achieve a homogenous distribution of the drug within the epidural space, and prevent "patchy" anesthesia, which occurs when some spinal nerves are left unaffected.

In cats, the dural sac extends further caudally than in other species and penetration of the duramater can occur with consequent leakage of cerebrospinal fluid into the needle hub (Chapter 2). In this case, the needle should be pulled back a little before injection. If this does occur, use of preservative free drugs is essential.

Epidural injection should not be performed if there is skin infection at the puncture site. Other contraindications for this technique include coagulation disorders, spinal cord trauma, hypovolemia, and septicemia.

Sacrococcygeal Epidural

This is a simple, easy, and readily applicable technique for catheterization of male cats with urethral obstruction (*Figure 9.2*). The cat is sedated, if not depressed, and positioned in sternal recumbency. The sacrococcygeal area is prepared aseptically. The space between the sacrum and first coccygeal vertebra is identified. Lidocaine 2% is injected (0.1–0.2 mL/kg) using a 25-G, 25 mm (1 inch) needle at a 30–45° angle and advanced through the interacuate ligament and *ligamentum flavum*. The needle is repositioned if bone is encountered, or if blood is aspirated. The technique produces anesthesia of the perineal area, penis, urethra, colon, and anus.

Sciatic and Femoral Nerve Block (using the ENS Technique)

Sciatic and femoral nerve blocks provide analgesia and probably fewer complications than epidural anesthesia for pelvic limb surgery in dogs, and may equally be applied in cats. These blocks are usually combined and should result in anesthesia of the femur, stifle, tibia, tarsus, metatarsus, digits, as well as other pelvic structures.

The *sciatic nerve block* is performed with the cat in lateral recumbency (*Figure 5.4*). The greater trochanter and the ischiatic tuberosity are palpated and the insulated needle is inserted at the midpoint between these landmarks. Initially, the ENS is set to deliver a 0.5–0.6 mA current output at 2 Hz. The needle is slowly advanced towards the nerve until dorsiflexion or plantar extension of the foot is observed. Correct needle placement is confirmed when the response is observed at 0.4 mA, but not at 0.2 mA (risk of intraneural injection).

A *femoral nerve block* is performed using a ventral (inguinal) approach with the cat in dorsal recumbency (*Figure 5.7*). The pelvic limb to be injected is abducted at 90° and extended caudally. The femoral triangle (delineated by the pectineus muscle caudally, the sartorius muscle cranially and the iliopsoas laterally) is identified. The puncture site is located cranial to the femoral artery. The insulated needle is advanced towards the iliopsoas muscle until contraction of the quadriceps muscle results in stifle extension. Negative aspiration is essential prior to injection in this area due to the proximity of the femoral artery.

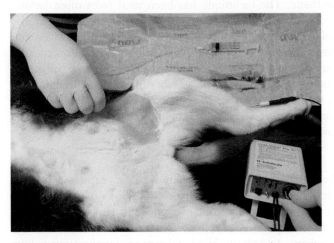

Figure 5.7 Femoral nerve block. An electrical nerve stimulator (ENS) is used to locate the femoral nerve for administration of the local anesthetic.

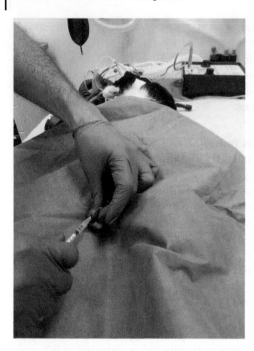

Figure 5.8 Intratesticular anesthesia. This block blunts stress response to castration, decreases intraoperative and postoperative pain and incidence of rescue analgesia. Inhalant anesthetic requirements during surgery are reduced. Under general anesthesia and aseptic conditions, a 23-G or 25-G needle is inserted into the testicular parenchyma and approximately 0.25–0.5 mL of lidocaine per testis is injected after aspiration to prevent intravascular injection.

Other Techniques

Intratesticular Block
The intratesticular block is indicated for anesthesia of the testicles in cats undergoing castration. The technique is shown in *Figure* 5.8.

Intraperitoneal and Incisional Anesthesia
Incisional anesthesia is accomplished by infiltrating the skin in the surroundings of the surgical field with local anesthetic. The technique has been used most often before laparotomy, and as part of a multimodal analgesic protocol. Doses of local anesthetic are calculated (*Figure* 5.9), and additional loco-regional blocks should be taken into account. For example, half of the dose should be used for each block if both incisional and intraperitoneal techniques are employed. For laparotomy, local anesthetic is injected into the subcutaneous tissues along the linea alba, just before final aseptic preparation.

Intraperitoneal anesthesia with bupivacaine provides postoperative analgesia in cats undergoing ovariohysterectomy; plasma concentrations of bupivacaine were below toxic levels. The technique is shown in *Figure* 5.9.

Wound "Soaker" Catheters
Local anesthetics can be delivered through diffusion ("wound soaker") catheters that are embedded near or in surgical sites and used to deliver continuous or intermittent infusions of local anesthetic for postoperative pain management. However, "patchy" distribution can occur and the technique is best applied as part of a multimodal protocol, and not as a "stand-alone" analgesic technique. The incidence of complications is low and the need for rescue analgesics is commonly reduced in the postoperative period.

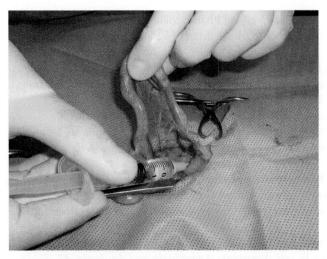

Figure 5.9 Intraperitoneal anesthesia. Bupivacaine 0.5% (2 mg/kg) is diluted with an equal volume of saline 0.9% resulting in a final concentration of 0.25%. This is equally divided into three parts and instilled into the peritoneal space, specifically over the right and left ovarian pedicles and caudal uterus before ovariohysterectomy, using a 3 mL syringe attached to a 22-G × 30 mm (1.2 inches) catheter.

Further Reading

Abelson, A. L., McCobb, E. C., Shaw, S., *et al.* (2009) Use of wound soaker catheters for the administration of local anesthetic for post-operative analgesia: 56 cases. *Veterinary Anaesthesia and Analgesia*, **36**, 597–602.

Aguiar, J., Chebroux, A., Martinez-Taboada, F., *et al.* (2015) Analgesic effects of maxillary and inferior alveolar nerve blocks in cats undergoing dental extractions. *Journal of Feline Medicine and Surgery*, **17**, 110–116.

Aprea, F., Vettorato, E., and Corletto, F. (2011) Severe cardiovascular depression in a cat following a mandibular nerve block with bupivacaine. *Veterinary Anaesthesia and Analgesia*, **38**, 614–618.

Bauquier, S. H. (2012) Hypotension and pruritus induced by neuraxial anaesthesia in a cat. *Australian Veterinary Journal*, **90**, 402–403.

Benito, J., Monteiro, B., Lavoie, A. M., *et al.* (2016) Analgesic efficacy of intraperitoneal administration of bupivacaine in cats. *Journal of Feline Medicine and Surgery*, **18** (11), 906–912.

de Vries, M., and Putter, G. (2015) Perioperative anaesthetic care of the cat undergoing dental and oral procedures: Key considerations. *Journal of Feline Medicine and Surgery*, **17**, 23–36.

Enomoto, M., Lascelles, B. D., and Gerard, M. P. (2016) Defining the local nerve blocks for feline distal thoracic limb surgery: A cadaveric study. *Journal of Feline Medicine and Surgery*, **18**, 838–845.

Holmstrom, S. E., Bellows, J., Colmery, B., *et al.* (2005) AAHA dental care guidelines for dogs and cats. *Journal of the American Animal Hospital Association*, **41**, 277–283.

Ko, J. C., Maxwell, L. K., Abbo, L. A., *et al.* (2008) Pharmacokinetics of lidocaine following the application of 5% lidocaine patches to cats. *Journal of Veterinary Pharmacology and Therapeutics*, **31**, 359–367.

Lawal, F. M., and Adetunji, A. (2009) A comparison of epidural anaesthesia with lignocaine, bupivacaine and a lignocaine-bupivacaine mixture in cats. *Journal of the South African Veterinary Association*, **80**, 243–246.

Moldal, E. R., Eriksen, T., Kirpensteijn, J., *et al.* (2013) Intratesticular and subcutaneous lidocaine alters the intraoperative haemodynamic responses and heart rate variability in male cats undergoing castration. *Veterinary Anaesthesia and Analgesia*, **40**, 63–73.

Moldal, E. R., Kirpensteijn, J., Kristensen, A. T., *et al.* (2012) Evaluation of inflammatory and hemostatic surgical stress responses in male cats after castration under general anesthesia with or without local anesthesia. *American Journal of Veterinary Research*, **73**, 1824–1831.

Mosing, M., Reich, H., and Moens, Y. (2010) Clinical evaluation of the anaesthetic sparing effect of brachial plexus block in cats. *Veterinary Anaesthesia and Analgesia*, **37**, 154–161.

O'Hearn, A. K., and Wright, B. D. (2011) Coccygeal epidural with local anesthetic for catheterization and pain management in the treatment of feline urethral obstruction. *Journal of Veterinary Emergency and Critical Care*, **21**, 50–52.

Oliver, J. A., and Bradbrook, C. A. (2013) Suspected brainstem anesthesia following retrobulbar block in a cat. *Veterinary Ophthalmology*, **16**, 225–228.

Perry, R., Moore, D., and Scurrell, E. (2015) Globe penetration in a cat following maxillary nerve block for dental surgery. *Journal of Feline Medicine and Surgery*, **17**, 66–72.

Pypendop, B. H., and Ilkiw, J. E. (2005a) Assessment of the hemodynamic effects of lidocaine administered IV in isoflurane-anesthetized cats. *American Journal of Veterinary Research*, **66**, 661–668.

Pypendop, B. H., and Ilkiw, J. E. (2005b) The effects of intravenous lidocaine administration on the minimum alveolar concentration of isoflurane in cats. *Anesthesia and Analgesia*, **100**, 97–101.

Shilo-Benjamini, Y., Pascoe, P. J., Maggs, D. J., *et al.* (2013) Retrobulbar and peribulbar regional techniques in cats: A preliminary study in cadavers. *Veterinary Anaesthesia and Analgesia*, **40**, 623–631.

Shilo-Benjamini, Y,. Pascoe, P. J., Maggs, D. J., *et al.* (2014) Comparison of peribulbar and retrobulbar regional anesthesia with bupivacaine in cats. *American Journal of Veterinary Research*, **75**, 1029–1039.

Smith, M. M., Smith, E. M., La Croix, N., *et al.* (2003) Orbital penetration associated with tooth extraction. *Journal of Veterinary Dentistry*, **20**, 8–17.

Souza, S. S., Intelisano, T. R., De Biaggi, C. P., *et al.* (2010) Cardiopulmonary and isoflurane-sparing effects of epidural or intravenous infusion of dexmedetomidine in cats undergoing surgery with epidural lidocaine. *Veterinary Anaesthesia and Analgesia*, **37**, 106–115.

Stevens-Sparks, C. K., and Strain, G. M. (2010) Post-anesthesia deafness in dogs and cats following dental and ear cleaning procedures. *Veterinary Anaesthesia and Analgesia*, **37**, 347–351.

Thomasy, S. M., Pypendop, B. H., Ilkiw, J. E., *et al.* (2005) Pharmacokinetics of lidocaine and its active metabolite, monoethylglycinexylidide, after intravenous administration of lidocaine to awake and isoflurane-anesthetized cats. *American Journal of Veterinary Research,* **66,** 1162–1166.

Weil, A. B., Ko, J., and Inoue, T. (2007) The use of lidocaine patches. *Compendium: Continuing Education for Veterinarians,* **29,** 208–210.

Woodward, T. M. (2008) Pain management and regional anesthesia for the dental patient. *Topics in Companion Animal Medicine,* **23,** 106–114.

6

Inhalation and Balanced Anesthesia

Bruno Pypendop

University of California, Davis, CA, United States

Key Points

- Inhalant anesthetics are most commonly used for maintenance of anesthesia. However they may result in hypotension and low cardiac output
- Dexmedetomidine or lidocaine decreases inhalant requirements and improves blood pressure but reduces cardiac output more than an equipotent concentration of the inhalant drug alone
- Opioids provide good analgesia and exert a variable effect on inhalant requirements. At high doses, they cause tachycardia, hypertension, and hyperthermia
- Ketamine decreases volatile anesthetic requirements, but its hemodynamic effects in combination with these drugs have not been well characterized in cats
- Nonrebreathing circuits are typically used in feline anesthesia and require the use of high fresh gas flow

Volatile Anesthetics

Volatile anesthetic agents are widely used for maintenance of anesthesia in cats. Some advantages include predictable and rapid adjustment of anesthetic depth and fast recovery. These drugs are not dependent on liver metabolism or renal excretion. The mechanism of action of inhalant anesthetics has not been elucidated but it may involve nonspecific effects on lipid membranes, interactions with ion channels or receptors, or both.

Intubation of the airways (e.g. endotracheal tube or supraglottic airway device, Chapter 1) is most commonly used to deliver these anesthetics to the patient. Oxygen is administered along with the inhalant anesthetic (volatile anesthetics and nitrous oxide), and ventilation is easily controlled if needed. Both these features may decrease morbidity and mortality, although endotracheal intubation in cats has been reported to increase the risk of death (Chapter 1). A well-fitting mask is acceptable for short periods of anesthesia.

Four volatile anesthetics have been widely used in cats: halothane, isoflurane, sevo-flurane, and desflurane; only the three latter agents are currently available in the United

Feline Anesthesia and Pain Management, First Edition. Edited by Paulo Steagall, Sheilah Robertson and Polly Taylor.

States and Europe. In addition, desflurane does not appear to be commonly used in current veterinary practice. While nitrous oxide is still available, it does not induce unconsciousness alone in cats and therefore is used as part of a balanced anesthetic technique. The following section discusses the main features of these anesthetics.

Halothane

- Halothane is a halogenated hydrocarbon discovered in the early 1950s and introduced in veterinary anesthesia in the late 1950s
- Its vapor pressure is 244 mm Hg at 20 °C, and it is usually delivered via a precision, out-of-circuit vaporizer
- Its chemical structure lacks the ether group found in isoflurane, sevoflurane, and desflurane; this feature has been implicated in the higher dysrhythmogenic potential of halothane
- Thymol is added to its preparation; it can damage the anesthetic vaporizer, which therefore requires regular service and calibration
- Its blood:gas partition coefficient is 2.4, which makes it the volatile anesthetic with the highest solubility in blood among the ones in current use; therefore it has a slower onset and offset of action than other volatile anesthetics
- Its MAC (minimum alveolar concentration required to prevent a response in 50% of the population) is 1.14% in cats. Halothane is the most potent of the volatile anesthetics in current use
- Halothane has the potential to cause hepatitis, although this has not been reported in cats. In contrast to other inhalant anesthetics in current use, halothane sensitizes the myocardium to catecholamine-induced dysrhythmias, and should be used with caution in patients at risk for dysrhythmias, or in combination with other dysrhythmogenic agents
- Halothane depresses myocardial contractility in a concentration-dependent manner, and to a larger extent than isoflurane

Isoflurane

- Isoflurane is a fluorinated ether released for veterinary use in the late 1980s. Commercially available products are stable and do not require a preservative
- Its vapor pressure is 240 mmHg at 20 °C, and it is usually delivered via a precision, out-of-circuit vaporizer
- It has a low blood:gas partition coefficient (1.46). This results in rapid anesthetic induction and recovery. Isoflurane undergoes minimal hepatic metabolism (0.2%)
- Its MAC is between 1.63 and 2.21% in cats. Cardiopulmonary studies at 1.3 MAC in cats reported minimal cardiopulmonary depression, especially in cats breathing spontaneously. At 2.0 MAC (deep anesthesia), isoflurane caused hypotension and hypercapnia; however, cardiac index was maintained. On the other hand, cardiac index decreased when the hypercapnia was corrected by controlled ventilation. In the cat, respiratory rate tends to be maintained as dose is increased whereas tidal volume decreases. The alveolar concentration that causes apnea is 2.4 MAC

- Mean arterial blood pressure decreased from 95 ± 5 mmHg in the conscious cat to 60 ± 7 mmHg at 1.5% inspired concentration and 40 ± 2 mmHg at 2.5% inspired concentration. Isoflurane does not sensitize the heart to catecholamines
- It has a strong pungent odor and cats may resist its administration via a facemask

Sevoflurane

- Sevoflurane is also a fluorinated ether, it was released for veterinary use in the late 1990s
- Its vapor pressure is 160 mmHg at 20 °C, and it is usually delivered via a precision, out-of-circuit vaporizer
- It has a lower blood:gas partition coefficient (0.68) than isoflurane; induction and recovery from anesthesia should be more rapid with sevoflurane than isoflurane. It undergoes minimal hepatic metabolism (2–5%)
- Its MAC is between 2.58 and 3.41% in cats. The cardiopulmonary effects at 1.25, 1.5, and 1.75 MAC of sevoflurane have been reported in cats. Sevoflurane-induced dose-dependent cardiovascular depression characterized by decreases in arterial blood pressure, cardiac index, and stroke index. Arterial blood pressure was better maintained with sevoflurane than isoflurane, thus limiting hypotension despite substantial myocardial depression
- Sevoflurane causes dose-dependent respiratory depression, although it appears less severe than reported in other species. Like isoflurane, sevoflurane does not sensitize the heart to catecholamines
- It has a more pleasant odor than isoflurane and it is better tolerated for mask induction than isoflurane. It is currently more expensive than isoflurane, particularly when the difference in potency is taken into account

Desflurane

- Desflurane is also a fluorinated ether, currently approved only for use in humans
- Its vapor pressure is 700 mmHg at 20 °C. The boiling point is close to room temperature, so all changes in temperature result in large changes in vapor pressure. Desflurane requires a unique and expensive precision, out-of-circuit vaporizer that heats the agent in order to deliver accurate concentrations. The vaporizer therefore requires an electrical source and warming up before use. These features and the high cost, especially considering its potency, limit the use of desflurane in veterinary anesthesia
- Desflurane has the lowest blood:gas partition coefficient (0.42) among volatile anesthetics. It results in very rapid anesthetic induction and recovery. Desflurane undergoes minimal hepatic metabolism (0.02%)
- It is the least potent volatile anesthetic with a MAC of approximately 10% (9.79–10.27%) in cats. The cardiopulmonary effects of 1.3 and 1.7 MAC of desflurane have been reported in cats. Desflurane at 1.7 MAC decreased mean arterial pressure and induced marked hypercapnia, although cardiac index was not affected. However, cardiac index was decreased when hypercapnia was corrected by mechanical

ventilation. In the cat, respiratory rate tends to be maintained as dose is increased whereas tidal volume decreases
- Like isoflurane and sevoflurane, desflurane does not sensitize the heart to catecholamines; however, it appears to be irritant to airways

Balanced Anesthetic Techniques

Balanced anesthesia relies on combining drugs to produce anesthesia so that the dose of each drug can be reduced, in an attempt to decrease the adverse effects produced. Specific drugs are often administered for specific effects such as analgesia.

Volatile anesthetics result in poor hemodynamics (low blood pressure and cardiac output) when administered at concentrations that produce a surgical depth of anesthesia. Balanced anesthesia is often advocated to decrease volatile anesthetic requirements, and improve cardiovascular performance and analgesia. Techniques include the administration of opioids (following parenteral, transdermal, and epidural administration), ketamine, nitrous oxide, lidocaine (following intravenous administration), gabapentin, and dexmedetomidine in combination with volatile anesthetics (Table 6.1).

Table 6.1 Drugs that are administered for balanced anesthesia in cats.

Agent	Dose	Comments
Fentanyl	LD: 5 µg/kg IV slow bolus CRI: 0.1–0.4 µg/kg/minute	May or may not reduce inhalant requirements; good analgesia; requires mechanical ventilation; low to moderate doses may cause bradycardia; high doses may cause hypertension, tachycardia, and hyperthermia.
Ketamine	LD: 0.5–1 mg/kg IV bolus CRI: 20–30 µg/kg/minute	Decreases inhalant requirements by approximately 50%. Cardiovascular effects in combination with inhalants have not been studied in detail.
Nitrous oxide	50–70% inspired concentration	May or may not reduce inhalant requirements; may provide analgesia; sympathetic stimulant; increases blood pressure but not cardiac output.
Lidocaine	LD: 1 mg/kg IV bolus CRI: 50–80 µg/kg/minute	Decreases inhalant requirements by approximately 20%. Increases blood pressure but decreases cardiac output. Used for prevention or treatment of ventricular dysrhythmias.
Dexmedetomidine	LD: 0.5 µg/kg IV bolus CRI: 0.5 µg/kg/hour	Decreases inhalant requirements by approximately 50%. Decreases heart rate by approximately 19% and cardiac output by approximately 34%; increases mean arterial pressure by approximately 61% and systemic vascular resistance by approximately 181%. Worsens cardiovascular performance compared to inhalant alone. May be useful to provide analgesia or sympatholysis.

Notes: LD – loading dose; CRI – constant-rate infusion.

Opioids

Intravenous Administration

In human anesthesia, administration of high doses of opioids has become popular during general anesthesia. Opioids decrease volatile requirements in a dose-dependent manner, and produce or promote stable hemodynamics in both the presence and absence of noxious stimuli. In cats, the magnitude of decreases in these requirements (i.e. decrease in MAC) appears to be significantly smaller than in other species. Large doses of opioids stimulate the sympathetic nervous system and result in tachycardia, hypertension, and hyperthermia. In addition, the effects of opioids on the MAC may be highly variable. In some studies, a clinically relevant effect (i.e. decrease in MAC) was demonstrated while others failed to do so (see below). Nevertheless, IV administration of moderate to high doses of opioids during volatile anesthesia are expected to *result in good to excellent analgesia and blunting of autonomic responses to noxious stimulation (while directly increasing blood pressure and heart rate).*

Maximal reduction in the MAC of a volatile anesthetic by a specific drug is defined as the reduction achieved when further increases in plasma drug concentration do not result in a further reduction in MAC. The effects of high and low doses of different opioids on the MAC of isoflurane have been studied in cats and are summarized below.

- Low and high doses of morphine, butorphanol, buprenorphine, and U50488H (an experimental kappa agonist) decreased MAC by 12 and 28%, 18 and 19%, 11 and 14%, and 4 and 11%, respectively
- Maximal MAC reduction during administration of alfentanil was up to 35% in a later study using target-controlled infusions (Chapter 4) in cats
- Agonists of μ-opioid receptors such as morphine and alfentanil appear to have the potential to reduce MAC to a larger extent than agonists of κ-opioid receptor and antagonists of μ-opioid receptors such as butorphanol, or pure κ-opioid receptor agonists such as U50488H
- In a different study, with the exception of alfentanil, high plasma concentrations of fentanyl, sufentanil, and remifentanil did not significantly reduce the MAC of inhalant anesthetics in cats; MAC reduction during administration of alfentanil was 16.2%
- Remifentanil decreased the MAC of isoflurane between 23–30% in a further study, whereas it did not influence MAC in a different study. A ceiling effect was reported where high doses of remifentanil did not further decrease MAC
- These studies highlight the large individual variability with opioid-induced MAC sparing in cats. *Opioids will decrease volatile anesthetic requirements in some cats but this effect may not be observed in others*

Better cardiovascular performance was reported in cats when alfentanil/isoflurane was compared with an equipotent isoflurane alone MAC multiple. Alfentanil was found to attenuate most of the hemodynamic and metabolic responses to noxious stimulation. However, increases in plasma concentrations of epinephrine and norepinephrine were reported resulting in tachycardia and hypertension (*Figure* 6.1). These effects could be detrimental in some cats where balanced anesthesia would be considered desirable (e.g. cats with hypertrophic cardiomyopathy, the most common type of cardiac disease in cats, Chapter 9). In summary, sympathetic stimulation may be observed during general anesthesia when high dose opioid infusions are used.

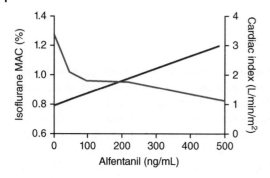

Figure 6.1 Effect of alfentanil on the MAC of isoflurane (red line) and effect of equipotent concentrations of isoflurane and alfentanil combined on cardiac index (blue line). This figure shows that alfentanil causes a moderate decrease in MAC, and a large increase in cardiac index (only one alfentanil concentration studied). The increase in cardiac index was due to increases in heart rate and stroke volume presumably caused by sympathetic stimulation. Alfentanil is uncommonly used in veterinary medicine, but fentanyl may have similar effects. Note that 500 ng/mL is a very high plasma alfentanil concentration; based on pharmacokinetic data, an equipotent plasma fentanyl concentration (50 ng/mL) would be achieved by administering a loading dose of 12 µg/kg, followed by a constant rate infusion of 1 µg/kg/minute (60 µg/kg/hour).

Fentanyl is more commonly used for balanced anesthesia in cats than other opioids. Based on published pharmacokinetic data in isoflurane-anesthetized cats, a loading dose of 0.2 µg/kg, and a constant rate infusion (CRI) of 0.02 µg/kg/minute (1.2 µg/kg/hour) of fentanyl would be required to maintain plasma concentrations of 1 ng/mL (lower analgesic concentration) at steady state. A loading dose of 12 µg/kg followed by a CRI of 1 µg/kg/minute (60 µg/kg/hour) would be required to maintain plasma concentrations of 50 ng/mL (maximal MAC reduction) at steady state (*Box 6.1*).

Box 6.1: Balanced anesthesia with fentanyl

In clinical practice, when using fentanyl for balanced anesthesia in cats, a loading dose of 5 µg/kg is administered followed by an infusion of 0.4 µg/kg/minute. This would be expected to result in good analgesia, and possibly some, but not maximal, MAC reduction. Isoflurane, sevoflurane or desflurane is administered concurrently, at the lowest concentration necessary to achieve surgical depth of anesthesia. Doses are reduced to avoid dysphoria approximately 30 minutes prior to the end of surgery. In cats, unlike in dogs, heart rate does not decrease and administration of an anticholinergic agent is usually not required.

Opioid infusion techniques induce less respiratory depression in cats when compared with dogs; however, assisted or mechanical ventilation may be still required. Cats may become hypersensitive to touch and sound during recovery of anesthesia after prolonged opioid infusions. This can be minimized with a quiet environment and minimal handling.

Epidural Administration

Opioids may be administered by the epidural or subarachnoid (spinal, intrathecal) route to provide analgesia, and possibly reduce the MAC of volatile anesthetics (Chapter 5 and

Chapter 13). Opioids produce analgesia without interfering with motor function. While opioids are generally administered by this route to provide postoperative analgesia, their effects are also observed intraoperatively if administered early enough in the pre-operative period.

Epidural administration of morphine (0.1 mg/kg) decreased the MAC of isoflurane by 31%. However, in another study, significant decreases in the MAC of isoflurane were not recorded after epidural administration of morphine (0.1 mg/kg) or buprenorphine (12.5 µg/kg) in cats. The latter study suggested important individual variability. In any case, lack of MAC reduction should not be interpreted as lack of antinociception; the same dose of morphine produced significant thermal antinociception from 1 to 24 hours. The potential of epidural opioids to improve hemodynamics when combined with volatile anesthetics for balanced anesthesia appears limited.

Transdermal Administration

Administration of fentanyl by the transdermal route using a human patch may provide postoperative analgesia. This is not to be confused with a veterinary licensed transdermal solution of fentanyl in dogs (Recuvyra®), which should not be administered to cats (Chapter 13) and is no longer available.

The fentanyl patch must be placed before surgery in order to be effective in the postoperative period. Thus, plasma fentanyl concentrations within the analgesic range may be present during surgery and contribute to balanced anesthesia. Transdermal fentanyl (25 and 50 µg/hour patches) was reported to reduce the MAC of isoflurane by 17 and 18%, respectively. Possible hemodynamic benefits of this technique in combination with volatile anesthetics have not been evaluated.

Ketamine

Ketamine has been reported to decrease the MAC of isoflurane in cats by 45, 63, and 75% when administered by CRI at 23, 46, and 115 µg/kg/minute. Corresponding plasma ketamine concentrations were 1.8, 2.7, and 5.4 µg/mL; for comparison, a study in isoflurane-anesthetized dogs reported that plasma concentrations of ketamine between 2–3 µg/mL would provide maximum benefits for balanced anesthesia (improved hemo-dynamics and ventilation compared with volatile anesthetic alone). Administration of approximately 50 µg/kg/minute of ketamine in cats appears to produce plasma concen-trations in that range; however, these doses are higher than those used in clinical practice (10–20 µg/kg/minute). In-depth studies on the cardiovascular effects of ketamine in combination with volatile anesthesia have not been reported in cats; however, both arterial blood pressure and heart rate increase during ketamine administration. Recovery may be prolonged when using high ketamine doses for long periods of infusion. Further work is needed to define infusion doses before this can be recommended in cats. Some studies are summarized below:

- A recent study reported the effects of ketamine in combination with remifentanil in isoflurane-anesthetized cats. Ketamine increased the MAC-reducing effect of remi-fentanil but there was no difference in heart rate or blood pressure in cats anesthetized

with isoflurane alone, isoflurane with remifentanil, and isoflurane with remifentanil and ketamine
- The effects of ketamine in combination with morphine and lidocaine (MLK) or fentanyl and lidocaine (FLK) have been studied in dogs. At the doses used, morphine (0.2–0.24 mg/kg/hour), lidocaine (3 mg/kg/hour), ketamine (0.6 mg/kg/hour), and MLK significantly reduced the MAC of isoflurane by 48, 29, 25, and 45%, respectively. These reductions were not significantly different between morphine and MLK but the percent MAC reduction of both treatments was significantly greater than lidocaine and ketamine infusions
- In dogs, FLK (fentanyl 0.0036 mg/kg/hour, lidocaine 3 mg/kg/hour, ketamine 0.6 mg/kg/hour) was reported to reduce the MAC of isoflurane by approximately 100% (e.g. produce immobility in response to noxious stimulation without addition of an inhalant anesthetic)
- These drug combinations are commonly administered as balanced anesthetic techniques in veterinary practice. In some cases, these protocols have been administered to cats; however, some practitioners do not include lidocaine. It should be stressed that the cardiovascular effects of ketamine during inhalant anesthesia have not been determined in cats, and those of fentanyl and lidocaine appear to be different between dogs and cats (see below)
- Further studies are needed to evaluate the potential benefits of such combinations in cats and until adequate information is available these combinations should be used with caution in cats

Nitrous Oxide

Nitrous oxide has been a common component of general anesthetic techniques in human anesthesia; however, its use in veterinary anesthesia has been less widespread. Nitrous oxide has low solubility in blood, and results in rapid onset and offset of effect with limited cardiorespiratory depression. In veterinary anesthesia some have reported minimal advantages in supplementing more potent volatile anesthetics while others have concluded that its analgesic properties reduce the need for high concentrations of volatile anesthetics, which ultimately minimizes cardiopulmonary depression.

In cats, nitrous oxide decreased the MAC of halothane in a concentration-dependent manner (e.g. by 19% with 50% nitrous oxide and by 31% with 75% nitrous oxide). On the other hand, consistent reduction in the MAC of isoflurane was not observed in a similar study. This may suggest that the effects of nitrous oxide on the MAC of isoflurane are highly variable. Interestingly, interaction of nitrous oxide and halothane, and with isoflurane, was reported to be additive and antagonistic, respectively. The cardiovascular effects of isoflurane alone versus isoflurane (at the same concentration) and 70% nitrous oxide showed that in cats the combination improved arterial pressure due to vaso-constriction. Overall, beneficial effects (e.g. increased cardiac output) were not reported; however, clinical impression is that addition of nitrous oxide to isoflurane will often stabilize mean arterial blood pressure within a normal range despite changes in surgical stimulation, especially in critically ill cats.

Potential delivery of a hypoxic mixture is of great concern (Chapter 10) when using nitrous oxide since a high concentration of the gas is administered with oxygen and a volatile anesthetic. Because of an increase in the alveolar to arterial oxygen tension difference in cats under general anesthesia, an inspired oxygen concentration of at least 33% is recommended; this concentration should be measured (Chapter 7) rather than assumed based on relative flows of oxygen and nitrous oxide. When inspired oxygen concentration cannot be measured, target nitrous oxide concentration (based on relative oxygen and nitrous oxide flows) should not exceed 50%. It has been argued that due to its low potency, nitrous oxide produces minimal benefits when administered at concentrations lower than 50%.

Precautions should be taken when nitrous oxide is used:

- Because of the decrease in inspired oxygen fraction inherent to the use of nitrous oxide, it should not be administered to cats with respiratory dysfunction unless the arterial oxygen tension can be measured
- Potential problems associated with *gas spaces* can arise when an animal previously breathing air is given a gas mixture containing nitrous oxide. Since nitrous oxide moves into gas spaces more rapidly than nitrogen moves out, an increase in volume in compliant spaces, or an increase in pressure in noncompliant spaces may occur. Thus nitrous oxide should not be administered to cats with pneumothorax or in situations where air embolus could occur (e.g. spinal surgery)
- At the end of anesthesia, the rapid transfer of nitrous oxide from the blood into the lung, related to the large partial pressure gradient, results in a transient but marked decrease in alveolar and therefore arterial oxygen tensions. For this reason, it is recommended to administer 100% oxygen for a minimum of 10 minutes following discontinuation of nitrous oxide administration
- As nitrous oxide is not absorbed by activated charcoal canisters, active scavenging is necessary to prevent contamination of the environment and personnel exposure (*Box 6.2*). These factors have reinforced the opinion of some authors that the cost:benefit ratio does not justify the use of nitrous oxide in veterinary patients

---

Box 6.2: Environmental effects of nitrous oxide

Nitrous oxide contributes to the greenhouse effect and global warming, and to ozone depletion. These effects, combined with its low anesthetic potency in dogs and cats, potential for abuse, potential for affecting human health through chronic exposure to low concentrations, and cost, have led some authors to claim that it should not be used in veterinary practice

---

Lidocaine

Lidocaine is a local anesthetic agent (Chapter 5); its IV administration has been reported to provide perioperative analgesia in humans. In addition, it reduces the requirement for both volatile and injectable anesthetics. In cats, lidocaine decreases the MAC of isoflurane in a plasma concentration-dependent manner: MAC was reduced by 3 to 52% with plasma concentrations ranging from 1 to 10 µg/mL (*Figure 6.2*). The decrease in MAC was linear within that range. However, administration of lidocaine was associated with *greater cardiovascular depression than an equipotent concentration of*

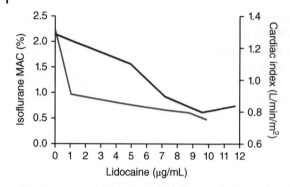

Figure 6.2 Effect of lidocaine on the MAC of isoflurane (red line), and effect of equipotent concentrations of isoflurane and lidocaine combined on cardiac index (blue line). This figure shows that while lidocaine decreases MAC in a plasma concentration-dependent manner, the combination of lidocaine and isoflurane results in lower cardiac index than an equipotent (higher) concentration of isoflurane alone.

isoflurane alone. Oxygen delivery decreased and it could result in poor tissue oxygenation. Therefore administration of lidocaine is not recommended for balanced anesthesia in cats if the goal is to improve hemodynamics; IV lidocaine is used for other reasons such as the treatment of ventricular dysrhythmias.

Dexmedetomidine

Dexmedetomidine is an agonist of α_2-adrenergic receptors with sedative, analgesic, and anesthetic-sparing effects. It causes cardiovascular depression characterized by bradycardia, decreased cardiac output and increased systemic vascular resistance (Chapter 3).

In dogs, IV dexmedetomidine (0.5 µg/kg loading dose followed by 0.5 µg/kg/hour) decreased the MAC of isoflurane by approximately 20% without producing significant cardiovascular depression. In cats, it decreased the MAC of isoflurane in a plasma concentration-dependent manner by up to 85%. In a follow-up study, dexmedetomidine produced cardiovascular depression (decrease in cardiac output and oxygen delivery, and increase in systemic vascular resistance) in a plasma concentration-dependent manner. This cardiovascular depression resulted in lower cardiovascular performance than isoflurane alone within the range of plasma dexmedetomidine concentrations studied, despite the decrease in MAC (see *Figure* 6.3). Administration of dexmedetomidine is not recommended for balanced feline anesthesia if the goal is to improve hemodynamics; dexmedetomidine may provide other benefits (e.g. analgesia, muscle relaxation).

Gabapentin

Gabapentin is an anticonvulsant drug. It produces sedation and possibly analgesia in various species including cats (Chapter 13 and Chapter 15). In humans, it is widely used in the treatment of a variety of painful conditions. Some studies have suggested benefits

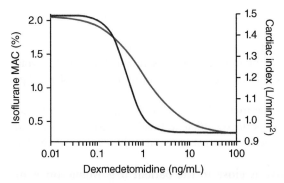

Figure 6.3 Effect of dexmedetomidine on the MAC of isoflurane (red line) and effect of equipotent concentrations of isoflurane and dexmedetomidine combined on cardiac index (blue line). The lines represent the modeled concentration-effect relationship. This figure shows that while dexmedetomidine decreases MAC in a plasma concentration-dependent manner, the combination of dexmedetomidine and isoflurane results in lower cardiac index than an equipotent (higher) concentration of isoflurane alone.

when gabapentin is combined with other analgesic drugs to treat perioperative pain. In cats, gabapentin did not change the MAC of isoflurane over a wide range of plasma drug concentrations (1–20 μg/mL), and it does not appear to be suitable for balanced anesthetic techniques in cats.

Balanced Anesthesia Summary

Some agents (lidocaine, dexmedetomidine) have been shown to decrease the MAC of volatile anesthetics while worsening cardiovascular performance when compared with a higher, equipotent dose of the anesthetic alone. Some agents (nitrous oxide, opioids) may or may not decrease MAC, and may or may not improve hemodynamics; ketamine appears to decrease MAC but its cardiovascular effects in combination with volatile anesthetics have not been studied in cats. If the goal of balanced anesthesia is to improve hemodynamics, the quest continues for the ideal agent in cats. However, some of these drugs are useful for balanced anesthesia if the goal is to improve analgesia.

Breathing Systems

Breathing systems are required to deliver inhalant anesthetics to a cat. Minute ventilation is a combination of a small tidal volume with a high respiratory rate in cats (Chapter 2). Some basic information about breathing systems are included below:

- The anesthetic circuit must be small and light to allow easy access to the patient, have minimal dead space, offer little resistance to respiration, and provide a method of controlling ventilation when necessary
- Nonrebreathing systems are commonly used in cats. Ayre's T-piece, Jackson-Rees, Lack, and Bain circuits are among the most popular systems in feline anesthesia (*Box* 6.3). The Bain and Jackson-Rees circuits are commonly used in North America

(*Figure* 6.4). A "mini Lack" specially sized for cats has become popular in the United Kingdom (*Figure* 6.5a)

- High fresh gas flows are necessary to prevent rebreathing of expired gas when using nonrebreathing systems. The lowest theoretical fresh gas flow achievable to avoid rebreathing of expired gas equals minute ventilation: approximately 150 mL/kg/minute in anesthetized cats
- High-fresh gas flows may induce hypothermia and increase costs with volatile anesthesia
- Most nonrebreathing systems are not perfectly efficient; this is at least in part related to the distance between the patient and the exhaust (pop-off) valve or equivalent (e.g. open reservoir bag)
- Systems in which the exhaust valve is close to the patient (e.g. Mapleson A or Magill, Lack) are highly efficient during spontaneous ventilation; fresh gas flows that are similar to minute ventilation may be sufficient to prevent rebreathing of expired gas
- Systems in which the exhaust valve is farther away from the patient (e.g. Mapleson D, Bain) are less efficient; a fresh gas flow higher than minute ventilation is required to prevent rebreathing of expired gas; for the Bain circuit, a minimum of 200 mL/kg/minute has been recommended, and this may be insufficient in some conditions (e.g. rapid shallow breathing)
- Although rebreathing systems are not commonly used in cats, modern technology, and light materials have enabled the design of circle systems suitable for very small animals (*Figure* 6.5b). These enable low flows to be used in the same way as in larger animals

Mechanical (or intermittent positive pressure) ventilation is sometimes necessary in anesthetized cats, for example to avoid excessive hypercapnia, during the use of neuromuscular blocking agents, or during thoracic surgery. During positive pressure ventilation, Mapleson A systems are inefficient; higher fresh gas flows are required to prevent rebreathing of expired gas than during spontaneous ventilation. In addition, the location of the exhaust valve (close to the patient) may make mechanical ventilation difficult using this system. These factors have led some authors to conclude that Mapleson A systems should not be used for mechanical ventilation. Mapleson D (e.g. Bain) and F (e.g. Jackson-Rees) are as efficient during spontaneous and mechanical ventilation, and similar fresh gas flows can be used in both conditions without causing rebreathing of expired gas. Rebreathing systems are also suitable for mechanical ventilation.

One study compared the cardiopulmonary effects of a pediatric circle system with an oxygen flow of 0.5 L/minute, an adult circle with an oxygen flow of 0.5 L/minute, and an Ayre's T-piece with an oxygen flow of 3 L/minute during halothane anesthesia in cats. Variables (heart rate, cardiac output, stroke volume, arterial pressure, venous pressure, systemic vascular resistance, respiratory rate, end-tidal concentrations of carbon dioxide, end-tidal concentrations of halothane, arterial blood gas and pH, temperature and ECG) were not statistically or clinically different among groups during 135 minutes of anesthesia. It was concluded that none of the systems was superior to the others. However, this study was conducted in healthy cats, and the conclusions may not apply to sick patients that may not tolerate increases in the work of breathing.

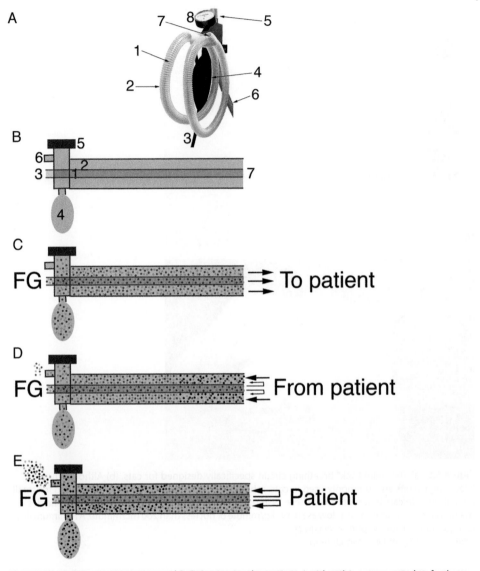

Figure 6.4 A: Bain circuit picture and B: Bain circuit schematic. 1: inside tubing, connected to fresh gas flow line; 2: outside tubing, connected to reservoir bag and exhaust system; 3: fresh gas flow line; 4: reservoir bag; 5: adjustable pressure limiting (pop-off) valve; 6: exhaust tubing; 7: patient connection; 8: circuit manometer (low pressure gauge). C: movement of gas during inspiration; D: movement of gas during expiration; E: movement of gas during expiratory pause. The green dots represent oxygen, the purple dots represents inhalant anesthetic, and the black dots represent carbon dioxide. During inspiration, gas devoid of carbon dioxide flows from the inside and outside tubing towards the patient. During expiration, gas containing carbon dioxide flows from the patient to the outside tubing; continuous flow in the inside tubing prevents expiratory gas to flow in it. During the pause between expiration and inspiration, continuous flow of fresh gas in the inside tubing "flushes" gas in the outside tubing towards the exhaust, resulting in accumulation of fresh gas in the outside tubing prior to the next inspiration.

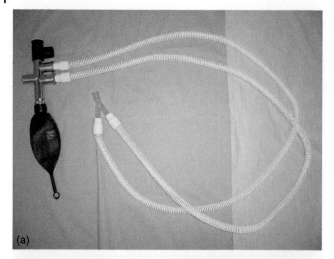

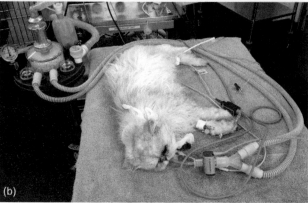

Figure 6.5 (a) The "mini-Lack" breathing circuit specifically designed for cats. (b) Although nonre-breathing circuits are commonly used in cats, rebreathing circle circuits specifically designed for small animals enable cats to benefit from these systems as much as larger animals. This system enables maintenance flow rates to be as low as 30 mL/kg/minute or not less than 200 mL/minute. A minimum flow is required to ensure vaporizer accuracy.
Source: Courtesy of Dr. Colin Dunlop.

Box 6.3: Advantages and disadvantages of nonrebreathing systems

Advantages of nonrebreathing systems include small dead space, minimal resistance to breathing, minimal drag on the endotracheal tube due to the light weight, no dilution of fresh gas with expired gas (the inhalant concentration dialed on the vaporizer is the inspired inhalant concentration), rapid changes in anesthetic concentration, and low cost of purchase. Disadvantages include potential for rebreathing of expired gas if fresh gas flow is not high enough, loss of heat and moisture related to the use of high fresh gas flow, waste of inhalant anesthetic and oxygen due to the high fresh gas flow, atmospheric pollution related to the use of high fresh gas flow, and inefficiency of some systems during intermittent positive pressure ventilation

---

Further Reading

Aguado, D., Benito, J., and Gomez de Segura, I. A. (2011) Reduction of the minimum alveolar concentration of isoflurane in dogs using a constant rate of infusion of lidocaine-ketamine in combination with either morphine or fentanyl. *Veterinary Journal* **189**, 63–66.

Brosnan, R. J., Pypendop, B. H., Siao, K. T., *et al.* (2009) Effects of remifentanil on measures of anesthetic immobility and analgesia in cats. *American Journal of Veterinary Research* **70**, 1065–1071.

Escobar, A., Pypendop, B. H., Siao, K. T., *et al.* (2012) Effect of dexmedetomidine on the minimum alveolar concentration of isoflurane in cats. *Journal of Veterinary Pharmacology and Therapeutics* **35**, 163–168.

Ferreira, T. H., Aguiar, A. J., Valverde, A., *et al.* (2009) Effect of remifentanil hydrochloride administered via constant rate infusion on the minimum alveolar concentration of isoflurane in cats. *American Journal of Veterinary Research* **70**, 581–588.

Golder, F. J., Pascoe, P. J., Bailey, C. S., *et al.* (1998) The effect of epidural morphine on the minimum alveolar concentration of isoflurane in cats. *Journal of Veterinary Anaesthesia* **25**, 52–56.

Hartsfield, S. M., and Sawyer, D. C. (1976) Cardiopulmonary effects of rebreathing and nonrebreathing systems during halothane anesthesia in the cat. *American Journal of Veterinary Research* **37**, 1461–1466.

Ilkiw, J. E., Pascoe, P. J., and Fisher, L. D. (1997) Effect of alfentanil on the minimum alveolar concentration of isoflurane in cats. *American Journal of Veterinary Research* **58**, 1274–1279.

Imai, A., Ilkiw, J. E., Pypendop, B. H., *et al.* (2002) Nitrous oxide does not consistently reduce isoflurane requirements in cats. *Veterinary Anaesthesia and Analgesia* **29**, 98.

Lerche, P., Muir, W. W., 3rd, and Bednarski, R. M. (2000) Nonrebreathing anesthetic systems in small animal practice. *Journal of the American Veterinary Medical Association* **217**, 493–497.

Muir, W. W., 3rd, Wiese, A. J., and March, P. A. (2003) Effects of morphine, lidocaine, ketamine, and morphine-lidocaine-ketamine drug combination on minimum alveolar concentration in dogs anesthetized with isoflurane. *American Journal of Veterinary Research*, **64**, 1155–1160.

Pascoe, P. J., Ilkiw, J. E., Craig, C., *et al.* (2007) The effects of ketamine on the minimum alveolar concentration of isoflurane in cats. *Veterinary Anaesthesia and Analgesia* **34**, 31–39.

Pascoe, P. J., Ilkiw, J. E., and Fisher, L. D. (1997) Cardiovascular effects of equipotent isoflurane and alfentanil/isoflurane minimum alveolar concentration multiple in cats. *American Journal of Veterinary Research* **58**, 1267–1273.

Pypendop, B. H., Barter, L. S., Stanley, S. D., *et al.* (2011) Hemodynamic effects of dexmedetomidine in isoflurane-anesthetized cats. *Veterinary Anaesthesia and Analgesia* **38**, 555–567.

Pypendop, B. H., and Ilkiw, J. E. (2005a) Assessment of the hemodynamic effects of lidocaine administered IV in isoflurane-anesthetized cats. *American Journal of Veterinary Research* **66**, 661–668.

Pypendop, B. H., and Ilkiw, J. E. (2005b) The effects of intravenous lidocaine administration on the minimum alveolar concentration of isoflurane in cats. *Anesthesia and Analgesia* **100**, 97–101.

Pypendop, B. H., Ilkiw, J. E., Imai, A., *et al.* (2003) Hemodynamic effects of nitrous oxide in isoflurane-anesthetized cats. *American Journal of Veterinary Research* **64**, 273–278.

Pypendop, B. H., Pascoe, P. J., and Ilkiw, J. E. (2006) Effects of epidural administration of morphine and buprenorphine on the minimum alveolar concentration of isoflurane in cats. *American Journal of Veterinary Research*, **67**, 1471–1475.

Reid, P., Pypendop, B. H., and Ilkiw, J. E. (2010) The effects of intravenous gabapentin administration on the minimum alveolar concentration of isoflurane in cats. *Anesthesia and Analgesia* **111**, 633–637.

Steagall, P. V., Aucoin, M., Monteiro, B. P., *et al.* (2015) Clinical effects of a constant rate infusion of remifentanil, alone or in combination with ketamine, in cats anesthetized with isoflurane. *Journal of the American Veterinary Medical Association* **246**, 976–981.

Steffey, E. P., Gillespie, J. R., Berry, J. D., *et al.* (1974) Anesthetic potency (MAC) of nitrous oxide in the dog, cat, and stump-tail monkey. *Journal of Applied Physiology* **36**, 530–532.

Steffey, E. P., Mama, K. R., and Brosnan, R. J. (2015) Inhalation Anesthetics. In *Veterinary Anesthesia and Analgesia* (eds K. A. Grimm, L. A. Lamont, W. J. Tranquilli, *et al.*). Wiley Blackwell, Ames, IA, pp. 297–331.

Walsh, C. M., and Taylor, P. M. (2004) A clinical evaluation of the "mini parallel Lack" breathing system in cats and comparison with a modified Ayre's T-piece. *Veterinary Anaesthesia and Analgesia* **31**, 207–212.

Yackey, M., Ilkiw, J. E., Pascoe, P. J., *et al.* (2004) Effect of transdermally administered fentanyl on the minimum alveolar concentration of isoflurane in cats. *Veterinary Anaesthesia and Analgesia* **31**, 183–189.

7

Monitoring

Daniel Pang

Université de Montréal, Saint-Hyacinthe, Canada

Key Points

- Assessment of anesthetic depth allows the volatile anesthetic concentration to be adjusted according to the cat's needs. Avoiding unnecessarily high concentrations of volatile anesthetics reduces the risk of hypotension and hypoventilation
- The most frequently encountered adverse effects during general anesthesia can be assessed and monitored with a small number of monitors
- Capnography is the only readily available noninvasive technique for assessment of ventilation
- The pulse oximeter is the best instrument to draw immediate attention to hypoxemia but has limited value as a monitor of ventilation during general anesthesia with 100% oxygen
- When intubation is not performed or cats are breathing room air during general anesthesia, pulse oximetry provides an alternative albeit less sensitive and nonspecific monitor of ventilation
- Monitoring should be continued into the recovery period, a time when most feline anesthetic and sedation-associated mortalities occur

Introduction

Monitoring enables detection of physiological abnormalities during anesthesia and it prompts intervention before any harm is caused. Most drugs used for sedation and anesthesia produce changes in normal physiological function either directly or by blunting responses to deviations from normality. For example, surgical depth of anesthesia using volatile anesthetics may cause dose-dependent reduction in myocardial contractility and depression of the response to decreases in arterial blood pressure, resulting in hypotension. Additionally, volatile anesthetics and many sedative-analgesic combinations can cause hypoventilation and respiratory acidosis through depression of the ventilatory response to carbon dioxide (CO_2) accumulation.

This chapter describes the key monitoring equipment and techniques available to feline practitioners, focusing on body systems that are most commonly affected by sedatives, analgesics, and anesthetics.

Feline Anesthesia and Pain Management, First Edition. Edited by Paulo Steagall, Sheilah Robertson and Polly Taylor.

Clinical Monitoring using Physical Senses ("Hands On")

The senses of sight, sound, and touch are invaluable in monitoring. They often provide the first indication of physiological changes or equipment malfunction. For example, Doppler ultrasound provides audible objective information about arterial blood pressure but also continuous indication of changes in frequency or volume of the signal, indicating changes in heart rate and blood flow that should be further investigated. Similarly, if a monitor (e.g. a pulse oximeter) gives an unexpected reading (e.g. peripheral capillary oxygen saturation; $SpO_2 < 90\%$), "hands-on" assessment of the patient will often help rule out equipment malfunction (e.g. assess mucous membrane color, respiratory pattern, and oxygen supply). A proficient anesthetist integrates the information provided by physiological monitors, clinical monitoring, and a knowledge of physiology, pharmacology and physics to provide safe, efficient perioperative care.

Table 7.1 describes predicted changes in cardiopulmonary variables and neurological reflexes at different depths of general anesthesia.

Mucous membrane color and capillary refill time, typically assessed at the buccal mucosa, provide subjective information on peripheral perfusion, red blood cell concentration, oxygenation, and hydration status. However, this information should be evaluated in combination with other evidence due to its subjective nature.

Table 7.1 Anesthetic depth and cardiorespiratory variables.

Clinical sign	Depth of anesthesia		
	Light	*Appropriate*[a]	*Deep*
Palpebral reflex	Present	Absent	Absent
Eye position	Central	Ventromedial rotation	Central
Pupil diameter	Variable (drug dependent)	Variable (drug dependent)	Dilated
Jaw tone	Present	Absent	Absent
Withdrawal response to toe pinch	Present	Absent	Absent
Heart rate[b]	Possibly increased (depending on drugs given)	Steady	Possibly decreased (depending on drugs given)
Respiratory rate[b]	Possibly increased (depending on drugs given)	Steady	Possibly decreased (depending on drugs given)
Cardiopulmonary response to noxious stimulation	Yes	Variable[c]	No

Notes:
a) An appropriate depth of anesthesia will vary depending on the nature of stimulation. For example, the anesthetic depth required for diagnostic imaging will be less than for surgery.
b) Heart and respiratory rates are often affected by drugs (e.g. bradycardia and decreased respiratory rate associated with dexmedetomidine). Single observations are unreliable. It is more informative to evaluate changes in heart and respiratory rates following stimulation or over time.
c) There should be no more than a minimal response (< 10–15% of prestimulation values) when the anesthetic depth is appropriate for the degree of noxious stimulation. The depth of anesthesia should be increased or analgesics should be administered if a marked response to surgery occurs.

Healthy cats are expected to have pink, moist mucous membranes with a capillary refill time of less than 2 seconds. Pale mucous membranes may indicate anemia or vaso-constriction. Identifying the cause of deviations requires measurement of hematocrit, assessment of volume status and arterial blood pressure. Agonists of α_2-adrenergic receptors such as dexmedetomidine cause vasoconstriction, commonly resulting in pale mucous membranes, which may also appear bluish (cyanotic) due to reduced local tissue perfusion. This effect lasts approximately 20–30 minutes and is more marked after IV administration. Though apparent cyanosis is an expected side effect of administration of agonists of α_2-adrenergic receptors, cardiorespiratory function should be evaluated (heart and respiratory rates, arterial blood pressure) to confirm normal function.

Palpating peripheral pulses allows calculation of the pulse rate, assessment of pulse pressure and rhythm, and confirms that blood is being delivered to the periphery (Chapter 1). The relationship between systolic and diastolic pressures (pulse pressure) affects how a pulse feels. For example, it is usually pronounced and easily palpable with vasodilation (where diastolic pressure is decreased, widening the difference between systolic and diastolic pressures). In contrast, increased diastolic pressure following vasoconstriction (e.g. after dexmedetomidine administration) usually make peripheral pulses more difficult to palpate. This can lead to the incorrect assumption that a cat is hypotensive when it is actually a reflection of the reduced difference between systolic and diastolic pressures; the mean arterial blood pressure (MAP) may be within or above the normal range. Common sites for peripheral pulse palpation include the femoral, metacarpal, and metatarsal arteries.

The most widely used method of monitoring ventilation during anesthesia is from direct observation of the reservoir bag or movement of the body wall, or both. Observation of chest and abdominal excursions and the associated changes in reservoir bag volume is also valuable for confirming ventilatory efforts and patient connection to the breathing system. The respiratory rate (breaths per minute) can be counted and a subjective evaluation of tidal volume may be made. However, this may be difficult in cats due to their low tidal volume.

Respiratory rates for cats during general anesthesia range from 12–30 breaths per minute and are influenced by many factors including respiratory disease, pain, acid-base status, drugs, and body position. Clinical monitoring of respiratory rate provides less information than capnography, which provides a comprehensive picture. Indeed, limit-ing observations to respiratory rate alone is misleading because minute ventilation is the product of respiratory rate and tidal volume (Chapter 2). For example, hypoventilation and hypercapnia may be observed even in the presence of a reasonable respiratory rate (e.g. 15 breaths per minute) due to low tidal volume.

Providing a breath manually by squeezing the reservoir bag with the pressure-relief ("pop-off") valve temporarily closed gives an indication of lung and chest wall compli-ance. For example, noticeable changes occur during bronchoconstriction and increased resistance to air flow (e.g. anaphylaxis, feline asthma) and with reduction in thoracic volume (fluid or air in the pleural space). Auscultation of the lungs during intermittent positive pressure respiration can help identify inadvertent endobronchial intubation as well as detecting abnormal breath sounds.

Cardiovascular System

Hypotension is a common side effect of general anesthesia; it was reported to occur in 33% of clinical cases in one study. Young, healthy animals can withstand a degree of hypotension but it is impossible to state with any certainty the duration and severity that can be tolerated without resulting in complications. Mean systemic AP should be maintained between 60–120 mmHg (Chapter 2). Below 60 mmHg, there is a risk of inadequate tissue perfusion because organs are unable to regulate local blood flow to match metabolic requirements. Potential clinical consequences of hypotension include acute renal failure, diarrhea or ileus (secondary to reduced gastrointestinal tract perfusion), and blindness.

Indirect blood pressure measurement using the Doppler or oscillometric method is most common in feline clinical practice. Indirect techniques have greater variability in their accuracy over different ranges of blood pressure and are unable to provide information as rapidly or continuously compared with direct (invasive blood pressure) monitoring. In contrast, indirect techniques have the advantages of being noninvasive and simple to perform, and are associated with minimal risk of tissue damage (e.g. hematoma, infection). The advantages and disadvantages of each of these techniques are described below.

Doppler Ultrasound Probe, Pressure Cuff, and Sphygmomanometer

A Doppler ultrasound unit converts ultrasound waves, reflected by moving (pulsatile) blood, to an audible sound. It is strongly recommended that the unit remains switched

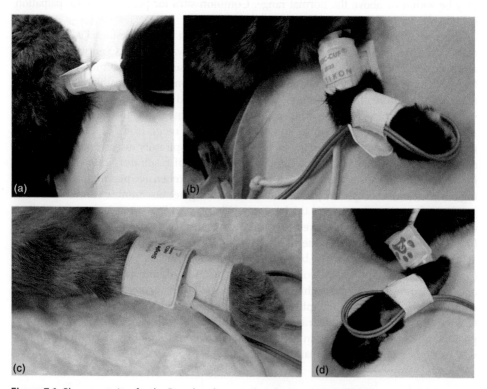

Figure 7.1 Placement sites for the Doppler ultrasound probe in cats include the ventral tail (a), ventral metacarpal area (b), ventral metatarsal area (c), and dorsomedial metatarsal area (d). Note that the blood pressure cuff is always placed proximal to the ultrasound probe to allow blood pressure measurement using a sphygmomanometer.

on throughout the anesthetic procedure so that pulsatile blood flow can be heard continuously and not only during blood-pressure monitoring.

The addition of a pressure cuff and sphygmomanometer allow measurement of arterial blood pressure. The width of the pressure cuff should be approximately 40% of the circumference of the limb or tail where it is placed. After inflating the cuff to a pressure exceeding systolic arterial blood pressure (SAP), indicated by loss of the audible signal (typically >120 mmHg during anesthesia), air is gradually released from the cuff until an audible signal returns. The pressure at which this occurs has been shown in cats to be closest to MAP. This approximation is clinically acceptable, tending to be within 10 mmHg of the true mean arterial blood pressure (*Box* 7.1; *Figure* 7.1).

Box 7.1: Advantages and disadvantages of arterial blood pressure monitoring with a Doppler ultrasound probe

Advantages

- Continuous, audible monitor of blood flow
- Minimal risk of injury to animal
- Noninvasive
- With practice, rapid to place
- Sudden changes in pitch, rhythm or volume of sound can indicate changes in cardiovascular function and should be investigated immediately

Disadvantages

- A pressure cuff that is too large will underestimate arterial blood pressure
- A pressure cuff that is too small will overestimate arterial blood pressure
- Electrical interference may occur when used with other electrical equipment, making it difficult to hear the Doppler signal
- Only provides the mean arterial blood pressure in cats
- Pressure readings must be performed manually

Oscillometric Devices

An oscillometric device measures arterial blood pressure by detecting pulsatile flow through a pressure cuff.

- An appropriately sized pressure cuff (as described for the Doppler technique) is selected
- The device is triggered manually or by setting a reading frequency (usually every 5 minutes) for automated readings; it inflates the pressure cuff to a value likely to exceed SAP (often as high as 180 mmHg)
- The pressure is then gradually released and the device detects the return of pulsatile flow. The detected return of arterial pulsations is registered as systolic pressure. Diastolic pressure is registered when pulsatile flow disappears. MAP is recorded at the point of maximum amplitude of detected pulsations
- In general, MAP is the most accurately recorded. The variation in device reliability and accuracy is likely to stem from sensitivity to detection of pulsatile blood flow and control of cuff pressure

Many oscillometric devices are available. When considering purchasing an oscillometric device practitioners should enquire whether comparison has been made with direct or Doppler methods, and, ideally, whether the device conforms to the American College of Veterinary Internal Medicine Consensus Statement on validation of blood pressure measurement devices. Clinical experience suggests that oscillometric devices vary considerably in their reliability and accuracy, where reliability indicates the ability to provide a blood pressure reading within a reasonable period of time and accuracy indicates the ability to measure blood pressure values within 10 mmHg of simultaneously recorded direct arterial blood pressure. The following devices have been assessed in cats: Cardell, Dinamap, and Datascope Passport (*Boxes* 7.2 and 7.3).

Box 7.2: Advantages and disadvantages of oscillometric devices for arterial blood pressure monitoring

Advantages

- Minimal training required for use
- Pressure-cuff size guidelines are the same as for the Doppler technique
- Provides three values of blood pressure (systolic, mean, and diastolic)
- Automatic readings
- Minimal background noise

Disadvantages

- These devices sense pulsatile flow, so they are sensitive to movement and dysrhythmias, which may result in inaccurate readings or failure to read
- Very low or high heart rate, or severe vasoconstriction may lead to failure to read
- In contrast to the Doppler, oscillometry does not provide a continuous audible indication of pulsatile flow

---

Box 7.3: Accuracy of oscillometric devices

- Cardell: mean and diastolic arterial blood pressures were within 5 mmHg of the direct (invasive) blood pressure measurement during hypotension, normotension, and hypertension. The systolic arterial blood pressure tended to underestimate direct blood pressure, although values were within 5 mmHg during hypotension, and within 12 and 17 mmHg during normotension and hypertension, respectively. This device was highly reliable
- Dinamap: overall, there was an underestimation of values compared with direct arterial blood pressure measurement of between 10–20 mmHg in 30% of measurements. Accuracy was improved during hypotension but there was a high rate of failure to provide a reading during hypotension (approximately 50% of attempts)
- Datascope Passport: this device was able to perform a measurement and provide a reading in over 97% of attempts. Its accuracy decreased when arterial blood pressure increased with underestimations ranging from 20–30 mmHg during hypertension (defined as mean arterial blood pressure of 120–140 mmHg). Its accuracy was slightly better during hypotension and normotension with underestimations ranging from 10–20 mmHg. No difference was identified whether fur was circumferentially clipped from the cuff placement site or left unclipped

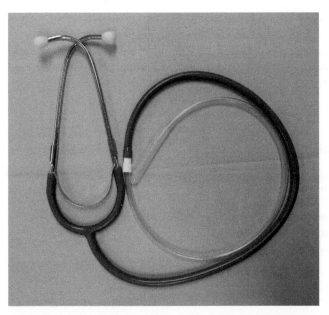

Figure 7.2 Esophageal stethoscope. The tip of the stethoscope is advanced into the esophagus until heart and lung sounds (transmitted through the air bladder) can be heard. This stethoscope allows continuous monitoring of heart rate and rhythm and respiratory rate.

Esophageal Stethoscope

Esophageal stethoscopes are often overlooked where electronic displays are the norm, yet they are simple and reliable. They are minimally invasive and can provide continuous monitoring of heart and respiratory rates (*Box 7.4; Figure 7.2*).

Box 7.4: Advantages and disadvantages of an esophageal stethoscope

Advantages

- Inexpensive
- Continuous monitoring (if worn by anesthetist or connected to an electronic transducer and speaker)
- Simple and quick to place
- Does not depend on power supply

Disadvantages

- Information is limited to heart rate and rhythm
- Provides no information on blood pressure or tissue perfusion

---

Electrocardiograph (ECG)

An ECG is the only way to diagnose a cardiac dysrhythmia definitively. While it may be tempting to purchase an ECG monitor, it should be kept in mind that dysrhythmias are much less common than hypotension and hypoventilation. Furthermore, an ECG is a measure of electrical activity; it does not provide information on contractility, blood pressure, vascular tone or tissue perfusion (Chapter 2). An acceptable trace can be obtained with an esophageal lead or adhesive ECG electrodes placed on footpads. "Crocodile" clips should be used with caution as high clamp force and serrated teeth can cause tissue damage, and when alcohol is used for electrical contact it may need to be replaced during a procedure.

Respiratory System

Box 7.5 describes the definition and methods for calculation of minute ventilation

---

Box 7.5: Minute ventilation

Minute ventilation (liters per minute) = respiratory rate (breaths per minute) × tidal volume (milliliters per breath)
There are two methods available for accurate calculation of minute ventilation:

- Measurement of volume with a flowmeter
- Indirect measurement of ventilation with capnography

Flowmeters

Several types of flowmeter are available for measurement of tidal volume. Additionally, a spirometer measures volume with rate of flow, and expiratory time. These are very useful for accurate, detailed measurements of ventilation. However, this is normally used only in the research setting and rarely in clinical anesthetic practice.

Capnography

A capnograph is the display of the partial pressure of carbon dioxide (CO_2) sampled from the anesthetic breathing circuit throughout the respiratory cycle, typically at the connection between the endotracheal tube and breathing circuit tubing (*Box* 7.6).

Box 7.6: Definitions of capnometry, capnography, hypercapnia, and hypocapnia.

- Partial pressure of exhaled CO_2 at the end of expiration ($PETCO_2$) is measured by a *capnometer*. Display of the measured level of CO_2 may be limited to a value or, more commonly, shown as a graphical waveform (*capnogram* or *capnograph*). *Capnometry* is the measurement of CO_2 and the display of the resulting measurement is *capnography*
- When a *capnogram* is displayed, it is usually accompanied by a numerical value representing the $PETCO_2$ (corresponding to highest point on the capnogram trace) Often, a value for the baseline of the trace is also displayed (corresponding to the lowest point on the trace) and may potentially indicate rebreathing of CO_2. Display of the capnogram provides useful information from waveform interpretation (*Figure* 7.3 and 7.4)
- Hypercapnia (or hypercarbia) is a greater than normal $PETCO_2$. Hypocapnia (or hypocarbia) is lower than normal $PETCO_2$

The relationship between expired carbon dioxide and ventilation is described by:

$$PETCO_2 \propto 1/V_{alv}$$

where PETCO$_2$ is the partial pressure of exhaled CO$_2$ at the end of expiration ("end tidal") and Valv is alveolar ventilation. As alveolar ventilation increases, measured expired CO$_2$ decreases proportionately, and vice versa. Accurate measurement of CO$_2$ therefore reflects ventilation.

PETCO$_2$ is closely related to PaCO$_2$ (partial pressure of arterial CO$_2$, normal range 35–45 mmHg; see Chapter 2). In principle, PETCO$_2$ should closely approximate PaCO$_2$ (difference less than 2 mmHg) as CO$_2$ is highly soluble and rapidly crosses the alveolar membrane. This is particularly true in healthy cats with normal cardiac output. However two common factors disrupt the relationship between PETCO$_2$ and PaCO$_2$: the type of anesthetic breathing system and alveolar dead space.

Breathing System

Nonrebreathing systems are commonly used in cats. They include the Bain (modified Mapleson D), T-piece (Mapleson E/F) and Lack (Mapleson A) systems and require relatively high fresh gas flow (FGF) rates (compared with a circle system) (Chapter 6). This higher FGF rate is necessary to flush away CO$_2$ in expired gas from the patient to prevent rebreathing. This may lead to dilution of CO$_2$ in exhaled gas. This effect is further exacerbated by the small tidal volume of cats leading to artificially low values for PETCO$_2$ (*Figure 7.3*).

Alveolar Dead Space

Alveolar dead space is a component of ventilation:perfusion mismatch and represents alveoli that are ventilated but poorly perfused. As a result, gas exchange between the pulmonary blood and alveolar gas is reduced so that gas leaving the alveoli contains little or no CO$_2$. The net effect of dead space is to dilute CO$_2$ from areas of lung participating in gas exchange. The diluted sample has a lower PETCO$_2$ reported by the capnometer, underestimating the PaCO$_2$.

Anesthetic equipment and techniques frequently used in cats tend to underestimate PaCO$_2$ as measured by PETCO$_2$. However, capnography is still useful to follow trends in ventilation. For example, an increase or decrease in PETCO$_2$ indicates hypoventilation or hyperventilation, respectively. Another advantage of capnography is that it allows titration of fresh gas flow rates to match individual respiratory patterns. Recommended fresh gas flow rates for breathing systems are based on typical respiratory patterns (Chapter 6). In practice, the fresh gas flow rate can be safely decreased until rebreathing of CO$_2$ is observed, indicated by an elevated baseline of the capnograph (> 2–3 mmHg).

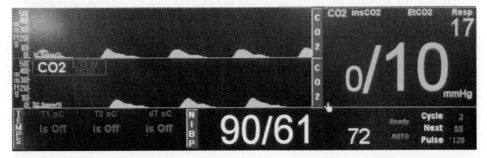

Figure 7.3 A typical capnogram observed during feline anesthesia when multiple factors (small tidal volume, mechanical dead space from the sampling chamber, high sampling rate (sidestream)) combine to cause an underestimation of PaCO$_2$ by PETCO$_2$ and an undulating waveform (loss of sharp upstroke and downstroke of Phases II and 0, respectively.) with short Phase III (see *Figure 7.4*).

Box 7.7 describes the differences between mainstream and sidestream capnometers and *Figure* 7.4 shows classic capnograms.

Box 7.7: Mainstream and sidestream capnometers

- Mainstream and sidestream capnometers use infrared technology to measure carbon dioxide. They differ in where the gas sample is analyzed: mainstream capnometers perform the measurement directly at the sampling chamber whereas sidestream capnometers draw a sample of gas from the sampling chamber and transport it to the capnometer for measurement
- Both types of capnometer are equally susceptible to loss of accuracy associated with the increased mechanical dead space caused by the presence of the sampling chamber between the endotracheal tube and the breathing circuit. This chamber provides a space in which respiratory gases mix with fresh gas flow from the anesthetic machine. This mixing, when combined with the combination of small tidal volumes and high fresh gas flows typical of feline anesthesia, results in an undulating capnogram and underestimation of PETCO$_2$ (*Figure* 7.3)
- Increased mechanical dead space also raises the likelihood of the patient rebreathing exhaled gases. This is identified on the capnogram as an elevated baseline, which does not return to zero (*Figure* 7.4c). Common causes of increased mechanical dead space are overly long ET tubes, right-angled (elbow) connectors, and capnometer sampling chambers
- Use of a pediatric sampling chamber in cats improves shape and accuracy of the capnogram trace for both systems. Larger (adult) chambers reduce accuracy as the sample is diluted by fresh gas. This is a common problem when using nonrebreathing systems and high fresh gas flow rates
- In small animals such as cats there is an additional decrease in accuracy associated with sidestream capnometers. Small tidal volumes, especially when combined with high respiratory rates and a high sampling rate lead to low values for PETCO$_2$. This can be overcome by periodically ventilating the cat manually with a slow, deep breath (approximate airway pressure of 15 cm H$_2$O). This creates a more defined sample of carbon dioxide in the sampling line and minimizes mixing of the sample
- Some capnometers allow selection of a lower sampling rate ($\leq$ 50 mL/minute, versus $\geq$ 150 mL/minute). This limits the degree of inaccuracy by reducing the proportion of fresh gas in the sample. Additionally, with sidestream capnometry, the time to transport sampled gas from the sampling chamber at the endotracheal tube to the capnometer results in a slight delay between sampling and displaying the capnograph
- Mainstream capnometers are not affected by sampling rate. The delay in displaying the measured CO$_2$ is minimal as the measurement is carried out without any transport of gas. However, sidestream capnometers have the advantage of a lightweight connector, which creates little drag on the endotracheal tube. As a consequence, in contrast to a mainstream capnograph, there is a reduced risk of tracheal damage. This is of particular relevance during any procedure where a cat's head is likely to be moved frequently, such as dentistry or orofacial surgery
- As sidestream capnometers remove a sample of gas from the breathing system, the sample should be appropriately scavenged to reduce workplace pollution. An exhaust port is typically located on the back of the capnometer and connected to the waste gas scavenging system

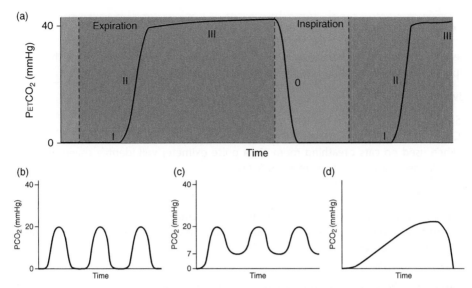

Figure 7.4 (a) Classic capnograms[1]; (b) undulating capnogram typically observed during feline anesthesia due to the combination of nonrebreathing system and sidestream capnometer with high sampling rate; (c) capnogram with an elevated baseline, which indicates rebreathing of CO_2 most commonly as a result of high respiratory rates and inadequate fresh gas flow; (d) Capnogram showing a decrease in the slope of Phase II and short alveolar plateau (Phase III) associated with bronchoconstriction (e.g. asthma).

[1]Early expired (exhaled, Phase 1) gas comes from anatomical dead space and does not contain CO_2. As expiration progresses (Phase II), CO_2 concentration increases, reflecting a mixture of anatomical and alveolar dead space gas. Phase III (alveolar plateau) reflects CO_2-rich gas from the alveoli, with the highest point representing end-tidal gas, with a CO_2 concentration approximating arterial blood. This is followed by inspiration (inhalation, Phase 0) where CO_2-free gas is inspired. *Source:* Courtesy of Vivian Leung.

Use and Interpretation of the Capnogram

- The normal range for $PaCO_2$ is 35–45 mmHg (Chapter 2). An increase in $PaCO_2$ is called hypercapnia (hypercarbia) and indicates hypoventilation. A decrease in $PaCO_2$ is called hypocapnia (hypocarbia) and indicates hyperventilation
- Hypoventilation and hypercapnia may result from neurological or respiratory disease, and drug-induced respiratory depression (e.g. anesthetics, opioids). Hyperventilation and hypocapnia may result from inadequate depth of anesthesia or a response to noxious stimulation (pain), or both. Less commonly, this may reflect low pulmonary perfusion (see below)
- Sudden loss of the capnogram wave can be caused by apnea, a disconnection between the capnometer sampling chamber and endotracheal tube, or occlusion of the endotracheal tube
- Sudden decrease in PETCO$_2$ without changes in ventilation may indicate decreased pulmonary blood flow secondary to reduced cardiac output or pulmonary thromboembolism. The former is often an early indicator of impending cardiac arrest
- The use of capnography is now recommended during cardiopulmonary resuscitation (CPR, Chapter 10). PETCO$_2$ is low (10–15 mmHg) during effective CPR and an increase in PETCO$_2$ (> 20 mmHg) may be an early indicator of return of spontaneous circulation

---

Box 7.8: Advantages and disadvantages, and the use of pulse oximetry

---

The most common type of pulse oximeter probe is the clip style, with each half of the clip apposed across a tissue bed – transmission (transmittance) pulse oximetry.

Advantages

- Specific indicator of hemoglobin saturation
- Continuous audible and visual indication of pulse rate
- When used on cats breathing room air, a pulse oximeter will identify severe hypoventilation or apnea as a decrease in SpO_2

Disadvantages

- Mistakenly assumed to be a sensitive monitor of ventilation
- Insensitive to changes in PaO_2 above 100 mmHg (as occurs when a high concentration of oxygen is delivered)
- High rate of false alarms (see below)

Locations for clip-style pulse oximeter probe placement:

- Tongue – most common site for measurements. Large probes designed for larger animals or human fingers will compress tissue over time, leading to erroneous readings, particularly in cats
- Ear
- Across toe pad (hind paw is often a useful site during dental and other oral procedures). The hind paw has been shown to be the most reliable

Other probe types

- Reflection (reflectance) pulse oximetry: probes have the light source and sensor located in-line and rely on detection of light reflected from tissue and bone. Reflection probes are commonly placed rectally although they can also be placed in the esophagus
- During states of poor peripheral perfusion (e.g. hypothermia, vasoconstriction), reflection probes may provide a more accurate reading of SpO_2

Factors interfering with pulse oximetry

- Probe too large – if the two halves of the probe clip are not parallel false low readings can occur. Additionally, tissue compression from a large probe tends to decrease local perfusion leading to inaccurate readings or failure to read
- Pigmented skin – minimal decrease in accuracy, unless pigmentation is particularly deep
- Carbon monoxide poisoning (carboxyhemaglominemia) – associated with house fires, leads to the dangerous scenario of falsely elevated SpO_2 readings. Co-oximetry is required to provide an accurate value for oxygen saturation
- Movement artifact, e.g. shivering, interferes with the pulse oximeter as sensing of pulsations is used to identify hemoglobin saturation from an arterial source
- Vasoconstriction (e.g. following administration of vasopressors or agonists of α_2-adrenergic receptors)
- Bright light, particularly from a pulsating source such as fluorescent lights can artificially elevate SpO_2 readings

<hr />

Box 7.8: (*Continued*)

Steps to take when a low SpO$_2$ is observed:

1) Assess the patient for changes in respiratory rate and quality, heart rate, and mucous membrane color
2) Reposition the pulse oximeter probe
3) Differential list for hypoxemia: low cardiac output, inadequate concentration of inspired oxygen, severe hypoventilation or apnea, impaired gas exchange (atelectasis, fluid-filled alveoli)

<hr />

Pulse Oximetry

Pulse oximeters are valuable monitors because they provide a continuous visual and audible indication of pulse rate and identify SpO$_2$ which correlates to PaO$_2$ (*Box* 7.8). However, there is widespread misunderstanding that they are sensitive monitors of ventilation.

Pulse oximetry uses the measurement of hemoglobin saturation with oxygen (SpO$_2$) as a reflection of the partial pressure of arterial oxygen (PaO$_2$). The relationship between these variables is described by the oxyhemoglobin dissociation curve (*Figure* 7.5).

During anesthesia, if high inspired concentrations (close to 100%) of oxygen are provided, the SpO$_2$ should usually be greater than 95%. A SpO$_2$ reading of less than 90% indicates hypoxemia, a physiological state that cannot be sustained for long before brainstem hypoxia and cardiovascular collapse occur. Pulse oximetry is a relatively insensitive monitor for changes in PaO$_2$ because the high concentration of inspired oxygen (close to 100%) often administered during general anesthesia results in a high

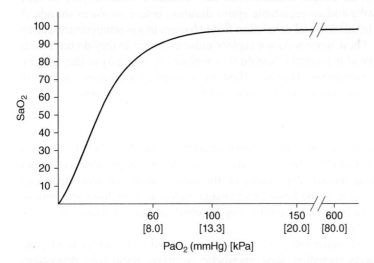

Figure 7.5 The oxyhemoglobin dissociation curve. The expected PaO$_2$ and SaO$_2$ (arterial saturation of hemoglobin with oxygen) at sea level, breathing 21% oxygen ("room air") are approximately 100 mmHg and > 95%, respectively. When breathing 100% oxygen, PaO$_2$ will be close to 600 mmHg in healthy cats with a SaO$_2$ > 95%. This illustrates the relative insensitivity of the SaO$_2$, as measured by a pulse oximeter, to large changes in PaO$_2$.

PaO$_2$ (approximately 600 mmHg) (*Figure* 7.5). At this PaO$_2$ the oxyhemoglobin disso-ciation curve is relatively flat, so that the SpO$_2$ will change little until the PaO$_2$ has decreased to a value closer to 100 mmHg. In contrast, when breathing room air (inspired oxygen of 21%), PaO$_2$ will be approximately 100 mmHg with decreases in PaO$_2$ more rapidly reflected by a decrease in SpO$_2$. Regardless of inspired oxygen concentration, a pulse oximeter should be considered a "fail safe" monitor as it is specific to the serious problem of hypoxaemia. The use of pulse co-oximeters allows identification of other types of hemoglobin (carboxyhemoglobin and methemoglobin) in addition to the oxygenated and deoxygenated hemoglobin identified by pulse oximeters (*Box* 7.9).

Box 7.9: The use of co-oximeters

Co-oximeters allow identification of other species of hemoglobin (carboxyhemoglobin and methemoglobin) in addition to the oxygenated and deoxygenated hemoglobin identified by pulse oximeters. This is achieved through the use of more light wave-lengths. This would be particularly useful in carbon monoxide intoxication (e.g. house fires) in which SaO$_2$ overestimation occurs with a pulse oximeter since carboxyhemo-globin is measured as oxygenated-hemoglobin.

Methemoglobinemia in cats is usually acquired following drug or chemical exposure, including acetaminophen, ibuprofen, skunk musk and some local anesthetics (Chapter 5). The light absorption spectrum of methemoglobin causes the pulse oximeter reading to tend towards 85%, independent of the actual PaO$_2$.

Apnea Alarm

Apnea alarms provide an audible indication of each breath, a visual display of time elapsed between breaths and an adjustable apnea duration before an alarm sounds. A thermistor identifies inhalation and exhalation from changes in gas temperature during the respiratory cycle. These devices do not replace pulse oximetry as they do not reflect SpO$_2$ and the presence of hypoxemia. Nor do they replace capnography as they give no indication of minute ventilation. However they are a simple, inexpensive method to confirm that the cat is breathing and is connected to the breathing system.

Temperature

Reference intervals for rectal temperature in healthy adult cats are 36.7–38.9 °C (Chapter 2). The majority of cats (>95%) become hypothermic under general anesthesia (Chapter 10). General anesthesia causes depression of thermoregulatory control, decreased metabolic heat production, vasodilation, and redistribution of heat from the core to periphery. Decreases in body temperature may be observed after sedation and even before general anesthesia.

Small decreases in body temperature (1–2 °C) are associated with a plethora of post-operative adverse effects including slow anesthetic recovery, respiratory depression, increased discomfort, reduced drug metabolism, increased bleeding and incidence of wound infection, and decreased renal function. Supporting evidence for these side effects in human medicine is strong, though limited research has been carried out in veterinary medicine. Intraoperative hypothermia will reduce drug metabolism and elimination, potentially leading to prolonged drug effect. Large decreases in body temperature ($\geq 5\,°C$) will produce bradycardia, dysrhythmias, and result in reduced CO_2 production and cardiac output (Chapter 10). Once body temperature has fallen it is much more difficult to correct as the physiological changes associated with anesthesia impede efforts at patient warming.

Temperature monitoring can be performed using rectal and esophageal thermometers. Temperature probes on a cable leading to a digital readout are widely available and have considerable advantages over thermometers that need to be inserted into the rectum and removed for each reading. Although alternative sites such as axillary and tympanic membrane are less stressful and better tolerated than rectal measurements in conscious cats, they are, unfortunately, inaccurate and variable.

- Studies of axillary temperature recordings have shown mixed results when compared with rectal temperature recordings and are not recommended as an alternative
- Axillary temperatures tend to underestimate rectal temperature recordings, though this difference is highly variable (approximately $-1\,°C$ to $2.6\,°C$). Body condition scores $> 5/9$ reduce accuracy further though coat length has a minimal effect on axillary temperature
- Axillary temperatures have low sensitivity (33%) to detect hyperthermia and moderate sensitivity to detect hypothermia (80%) when compared with rectal temperature recordings
- Similarly, the temperature gradient between tympanic membrane and rectal temperature recordings is highly variable (approximately $-1.6\,°C$ to $3.0\,°C$) making it unsuitable as a replacement for rectal temperature recording

Gas Analyzers

Anesthetic gas monitoring is offered as an optional module when a multiparameter monitor is purchased. Anesthetic gases are most commonly measured using infrared absorption spectroscopy, which identifies different gas molecules through their characteristic absorption of infrared light. A sample of gas is removed from the breathing system for analysis and this is usually combined with sidestream capnography. The display of expired anesthetic agent concentration confirms vaporizer function and accuracy. It also gives a subjective indication of depth of anesthesia when the minimum alveolar concentration of the anesthetic agent is taken into consideration (Chapter 6). However, this can be highly variable and the numerous factors affecting the MAC should be taken into consideration.

Monitoring of oxygen concentrations by paramagnetic or electrochemical analysis confirms the presence of an acceptable concentration of oxygen in the breathing system (usually close to 100%) ensuring integrity of the oxygen supply. More importantly, oxygen sensing is a sensitive and rapid indicator of a hypoxic inspired gas mixture. It provides an earlier warning of "impending"/"potential" hypoxemia than pulse oximetry. There is no manufacturing standard in veterinary medicine to "measure system oxygen levels or associate low" levels with an audible alarm.

Fluid Monitoring

Cats have an increased risk of fluid overload due to their relative small size, less body water and increased susceptibility to pulmonary edema when compared with dogs

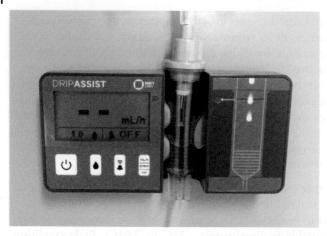

Figure 7.6 A drip counter facilitates monitoring of fluid rate and the total volume administered. Drips of fluid enter the chamber and break a photobeam. This allows the device to count the drip rate and calculate flow rate (mL/hour).

(Chapter 8). Simple measures can be taken to minimize this risk including the use of fluid pumps, syringe drivers, buretrols, and drip counters (*Figure* 7.6, *Figure* 8.1).

Accurate delivery of fluids is most easily achieved with fluid pumps or syringe drivers. However, buretrols and drip counters provide a cheap, practical alternative. A buretrol allows a limited reservoir of fluid, which limits the risk of volume overload (Chapter 8). The buretrol is connected between the fluid bag and the IV drip set. Drip counters provide a continuous monitor of delivered fluid by counting the drip (flow) rate that enters the chamber of a drip set. Importantly, drip counters do not control the flow rate, which must still be set by the user.

Fluid balance (total "ins and outs") can be monitored, taking in to account insensible losses, fluid administration and losses through any drainage tubes. Urine output can be measured by collection from litter trays (using nonabsorbent litter substrate) or more accurately by placing a urinary catheter. If urine output is measured (e.g. cats with ureteral obstruction), it should be approximately 2 mL/kg/hour in a healthy cat. *These values should be interpreted in the context of intravenous fluid administration, disease or concurrent drug administration.* For example, urine production of 2 mL/kg/hour in a cat receiving 10 mL/kg/hour of intravenous fluids could be considered low; administration of furosemide should increase urine output to greater than 2 mL/kg/hour in a normovolemic cat; or urine output may be less than 2 mL/kg/hour in a dehydrated or hypovolemic cat until hydration status is corrected.

Urine specific gravity (USG), body weight, hematocrit, and serum albumin, mucous membranes, and skin tenting are other noninvasive methods of monitoring fluid therapy and changes in volume. Urine specific gravity can aid in the assessment of hydration status. While a high USG indicates dehydration, a low value can be more difficult to interpret; it may reflect a return to normal hydration but can also be influenced by other factors. For example, dehydrated cats with diabetes mellitus and those with renal insufficiency may produce dilute urine. Furosemide can result in a low USG due to diuresis even in the presence of dehydration.

Further Reading

Binns, S. H., Sisson, D. D., Buoscio, D. A., *et al.* (1995) Doppler ultrasonographic, oscillometric sphygmomanometric, and photoplethysmographic techniques for noninvasive blood pressure measurement in anesthetized cats. *Journal of Veterinary Internal Medicine* **9**, 405–414.

Branson, K. R., Wagner-Mann, C. C., and Mann, F. A. (1997) Evaluation of an oscillometric blood pressure monitor on anesthetized cats and the effect of cuff placement and fur on accuracy. *Veterinary Surgery* **26**, 347–353.

Brodbelt, D. C., Pfeiffer, D. U., Young, L. E., *et al.* (2007) Risk factors for anaesthetic-related death in cats: Results from the confidential enquiry into perioperative small animal fatalities (CEPSAF). *British Journal of Anaesthesia* **99**, 617–623.

Brown, S., Atkins, C., Bagley, R., *et al.* (2007) Guidelines for the identification, evaluation, and management of systemic hypertension in dogs and cats. *Journal of Veterinary Internal Medicine* **21**, 542–558.

Caulkett, N. A., Cantwell, S. L., and Houston, D. M. (1998) A comparison of indirect blood pressure monitoring techniques in the anesthetized cat. *Veterinary Surgery* **27**, 370–377.

Comroe, J. H. Jr, and Botelho, S. (1947) The unreliability of cyanosis in the recognition of arterial anoxemia. *The American Journal of the Medical Sciences* **214**, 1–6.

Gaynor, J. S., Dunlop, C. I., Wagner, A., *et al.* (1999) Complications and mortality associated with anesthesia in dogs and cats. *Journal of the American Animal Hospital Association* **35**, 13–17.

Grandy, J. L., Dunlop, C. I., Hodgson, D., *et al.* (1992) Evaluation of the Doppler ultrasonic method of measuring systolic arterial pressure in cats. *American Journal of Veterinary Research* **53**, 1166–1169.

Hagerty, J. J., Kleinman, M. E., Zurakowski, D., *et al.* (2002) Accuracy of a new low-flow sidestream capnography technology in newborns: A pilot study. *Journal of Perinatology* **22**, 219–225.

Lerche, P., Muir, W. W. 3rd and Bednarski, R. M. (2000) Nonrebreathing anesthetic systems in small animal practice. *Journal of the American Veterinary Medical Association* **217**, 493–497.

Levy, J. K., Nutt, K. R., and Tucker, S. J. (2015) Reference interval for rectal temperature in healthy confined adult cats. *Journal of Feline Medicine and Surgery* **17**, 950–952.

Machon, R. G., Raffe, M. R., and Robinson, E. P. (1999) Warming with a forced air warming blanket minimizes anesthetic-induced hypothermia in cats. *Veterinary Surgery* **28**, 301–310.

Malloy, R., Marshall, M. K., Rozycki, H. J., *et al.* (1998) Mainstream end-tidal carbon dioxide monitoring in the neonatal intensive care unit. *Pediatrics* **101**, 648–653.

Pascucci, R. C., Schena, J. A., and Thompson, J. E. (1989) Comparison of a sidestream and mainstream capnometer in infants. *Critical Care Medicine* **17**, 560–562.

Pedersen, K. M., Butler, M. A., Ersbøll, A. K., *et al.* (2002) Evaluation of an oscillometric blood pressure monitor for use in anesthetized cats. *Journal of the American Veterinary Medical Association* **221**, 646–650.

Redondo, J. I., Suesta, P., Gil, L., *et al.* (2012) Retrospective study of the prevalence of postanaesthetic hypothermia in cats. *Veterinary Record* **170**, 206.

Sessler, D. I. (2001) Complications and treatment of mild hypothermia. *Anesthesiology* **95**, 531–543.

Simini, B. (1998) Cherry-red discolouration in carbon monoxide poisoning. *The Lancet* **352**, 1154.

Thomson, S. M., Burton, C. A., and Armitage-Chan, E. A. (2014) Intra-operative hyperthermia in a cat with a fatal outcome. *Veterinary Anaesthesia and Analgesia* **41**, 290–296.

Wood, A. M., Moss, C., Keenan, R., *et al.* (2014) Infection control hazards associated with the use of forced-air warming in operating theatres. *Journal of Hospital Infection* **88**, 132–140.

www.capnography.com (accessed June 24, 2017); an excellent comprehensive resource on all things related to capnography

www.frca.co.uk (accessed June 24, 2017); a free resource covering a wide range of topics, including accessible reviews of physiology relevant to anesthetic monitoring.

8

Fluid Therapy

Peter Pascoe

University of California, Davis, CA, United States

Key Points

- Cats may be more prone to fluid overload than dogs if their blood volume and latent heart disease are not accounted for
- Many types of fluids can be used but the standards are balanced electrolyte solutions, colloids, and blood or blood components
- Hydration or volume status should be normalized as much as possible before anesthesia
- Intraoperative fluids are used to replace metabolic and procedural losses
- Therapy should continue into the postoperative period until the cat can regulate its own fluid intake and output

Introduction

Fluid therapy in cats has become controversial since a large anesthesia morbidity and mortality study reported that cats receiving fluids intraoperatively had nearly a fourfold increase in the risk of death. Although there are reasons why cats may be more prone to fluid overload than similar-sized dogs, this "association" is more likely to be a result of the cats receiving intraoperative fluids being more compromised than those that did not. Every patient needs to be assessed with regard to its fluid status before anesthesia, and treated judiciously in order to achieve the best outcome.

Feline Physiology and Pathology with regard to Fluid Therapy

Cats are often described as being more likely to suffer from fluid overload than a comparable-sized dog. One of the contributing factors to this is that the blood volume of the cat is less than that of the dog (*Box* 8.1). In most instances fluid dose rates have been based on mL/kg so it is expected that if the same dose of fluid was administered to a cat and a dog that there would be a greater relative increase in blood volume in the cat than in the dog. For example, if 20 mL/kg of a crystalloid solution was administered, which

Feline Anesthesia and Pain Management, First Edition. Edited by Paulo Steagall, Sheilah Robertson and Polly Taylor.

redistributed rapidly to leave about 30% of that volume in the circulation, the relative increase in blood volume would be 7% in the dog and 11% in the cat. Such an increase would probably not cause a problem in a normal animal, but continuing to administer fluids on the same basis will overload a cat sooner than a dog. To complicate this further, these data were generated in normal healthy animals whereas many veterinary patients do not have normal body condition scores, with the prevalence of obesity estimated at about 30% of the population. Obese patients have an increased total blood volume compared with that at their normal body weight but it is decreased when expressed as a percentage of their actual body weight. In humans, blood volume decreased from 70 mL/kg to 42 mL/kg when body weight increased from normal to 200% of normal. This may make such patients even more prone to fluid overload.

Box 8.1: Cat versus dog blood volumes

Values of blood volume for the cat range from 4.1% to 6% of body weight (41–60 mL/kg), depending on the method used for measurement, whereas in dogs the reported blood volumes are in the range of 8–9% of body weight (80–90 mL/kg).

A second issue is the presence of latent cardiac disease in cats.

- In one study that examined 103 apparently healthy cats the prevalence of cardiomyopathy was 16% and only a third of these had audible murmurs
- In another study, where murmurs were ausculted in 57 apparently healthy cats, 44 of the animals had left ventricular hypertrophy, six had congenital abnormalities, and seven of the cats with a murmur had no detectable cardiac disease
- Taken together these results suggest that occult cardiac disease is prevalent in this species and that physical examination may not be an adequate screening test. A new screening test using the N-terminal prohormone of brain natriuretic peptide (NT-proBNP) shows great promise for differentiating cats with and without cardiomyopathy. That occult cardiac disease may be a contributor to pulmonary edema was demonstrated in a study examining the use of an oxygen carrying colloid in cats
- Out of 44 treated animals, eight developed respiratory changes, and of these, five were subsequently diagnosed as having hypertrophic cardiomyopathy (the other three animals were not tested for this)
- In these eight cats the mean volumes of administered crystalloid and colloid were less than in the animals that did not suffer from respiratory complications, suggesting that cardiomyopathy played a role in their pulmonary changes.

The glycocalyx is a thin layer (~1 μm) composed of endothelial bound glycoproteins such as syndecan and glycipan with side chains like heparan, chondroitin, and dermatan sulfates, which is present on the luminal side of the vasculature. Albumin is trapped in this layer at low concentrations and acts to increase the oncotic pressures favoring reabsorption of fluid. This barrier also protects or delays the effects of decreasing plasma protein concentrations that might occur during fluid resuscitation. However, damage to the glycocalyx occurs during sepsis, reperfusion injury, and the release of natriuretic peptides. The latter can occur during volume loading, suggesting that hypervolemia in and of itself may be detrimental to fluid exchange and could lead to greater loss of fluid into the interstitium.

Fluids

The fluids that may be used in the perioperative period include crystalloids and colloids. Crystalloid solutions are a mixture of water and electrolytes and may be hypo-, iso-, or hypertonic.

- Hypotonic fluids, such as 0.45% sodium chloride, are not commonly used unless the patient has a deficit of water without loss of electrolytes or it is being used to provide maintenance of ongoing losses. Because these fluids have the potential to cause hemolysis they must be administered slowly
- Isotonic fluids include 5% dextrose, 0.9% sodium chloride (normal saline), and balanced electrolyte solutions such as lactated Ringer's or Hartmann's solution (*Table* 8.1). A 5% dextrose solution is isotonic but once it is administered it provides purely water as the dextrose is metabolized. The water is then free to distribute into both the extracellular and intracellular compartments, and is a good solution to treat pure water dehydration but is not a good solution to use if the deficit also involves electrolytes
- Normal saline has a similar sodium content to cat plasma but an excess of chloride. The latter has to be excreted in exchange for bicarbonate, and so this is an acidifying solution. The balanced electrolyte solutions (Lactated Ringer's/Hartmann's, acetated solutions such as Normosol and Plasmalyte) are designed to have an electrolyte content similar to plasma and contain an anion that can be metabolized to remove acid from the circulation. However, these solutions are hypotonic when administered to cats and the sodium content is particularly low in comparison with normal values for this species. Despite this relative hypotonicity the routine use of these fluids in cats does not appear to have caused major clinical problems
- Hypertonic fluids, such as 7.5% sodium chloride, have been used to increase the circulating volume rapidly using a small volume of infusate. These fluids should ideally be used when it is possible to monitor the changes in sodium concentration and provide more dilute solutions to replace the fluid that the hypertonic solution draws from other body compartments. The benefits of hypertonic solutions appear to extend beyond the volume effect with improved microcirculatory flow, reduced intracranial pressure and modulation of the immune response
- Colloids are solutions that contain molecules large enough not to cross a semi-permeable membrane, and so the solution will stay in the vascular space rather than redistribute immediately to the interstitial volume (*Table* 8.2; *Table* 8.3). The synthetic colloids, dextrans, hydroxyethyl starches (HESs), and polygelatins have the advantage over blood products that they do not need to be kept refrigerated and have a long shelf life. The major disadvantages are that they may decrease platelet activity, clotting factors, and, in humans, the HESs have been associated with acute kidney injury. All of these molecules are, to some extent, excreted through the kidneys so there is potential for osmotic nephrosis
- Blood and its component parts are colloids and it is important that the patient receives the appropriate type of blood (*Box* 8.2)
- Hemoglobin-based oxygen carrying solutions (HBOCS) have been used in cats. The commercial solution that has been used (Oxyglobin) is an ultrapurified polymerized bovine hemoglobin containing 13 g/dL of hemoglobin with a colloid osmotic pressure

Table 8.1 Physicochemical properties of the crystalloids. Mw is the molecular weight average of all the molecule sizes present and it relates to viscosity. Mn is the average molecular weight of all the colloid particles in the solution and relates to colloid oncotic pressure.

Solution	Dextrose g/L	pH	Na (mmol/L)	Cl (mmol/L)	Ionized Ca (mmol/L)	K (mmol/L)	Mg (mmol/L)	Buffer mmol/L	Osmolality (mOsm/L)
Normal cat	0.63–1.18		151–158	117–126	1.27	3.6–4.9		NA	317–323
Dextrose 5%	50	4.0	0	0	0	0		0	252
Sodium chloride 0.9%	0	5.0	154	154	0	0		0	308
Ringer's	0	5.5	147.5	156	2.25	4			312
Lactated Ringer's/Hartmann's	0	6.5	130–131	109–112	1.5	4–5		28 lactate	272
Normosol-R (acetated solution)	0	6.5–7.6	140	98	0	5	1.5	27 acetate, 23 gluconate	294
Plasmalyte 148 (acetated solution)	0	6.5–8.0	140	98	0	5	1.5	27 acetate, 23 gluconate	295
Sodium chloride 7.5%	0	5.0	1283	1283	0	0	0	0	2566

Table 8.2 Physicochemical properties of the artificial colloids.

Colloid	Mw (kDa)	Mn (kDa)	Colloid (g/L)	pH	Relative viscosity	Na (mmol/L)	Cl (mmol/L)	Ca (mmol/L)	K (mmol/L)	Osmolality (mOsm/L)	Colloid oncotic pressure (mm Hg)
Dextran 40, NaCl	40	26	100	3.5–7	5.1–5.4	154	154	0	0	310	NM
Dextran 40, dextrose	40	26	100	3–7		0	0	0	0	255	NM
Dextran 70, NaCl	70	41	60	5.1–5.7	3.4–4	154	154	0	0	310	59
Oxypolygelatin (Vetaplasma, Gelifundol)	30	23.3	55			145	100	2	0	200	45–47
Succinylated gelatin (Gelofusine)	35	22.6	40	7.4		154	125	0.4	0.4	279	34
Urea-linked gelatin (Haemaccel)	35	24.5	35	7.2–7.3	1.7–1.8	145	145	6.26	5.1	310	25.5–28.5

Note: NM – not measurable because of diffusion of smaller molecules.

Table 8.3 Physicochemical properties of hydroxyethyl starch solutions. See table 8.2 for definitions.

Colloid	Mw (kDa)	Mn (kDa)	Molar substitution	C2:C6 ratio	Colloid (g/L)	pH	Na (mmol/L)	Cl (mmol/L)	Ca (mmol/L)	K (mmol/L)	Lactate (mmol/L)	Osmolality (mOsm/L)	Colloid oncotic pressure (mm Hg)
Hetastarch 670 (Hextend)	670		0.75	4–5:1	60	5.9	143	124	5	3	28[a]	307	31.3 ± 0.6
Hetastarch 450	450	69	0.7	4.6:1	60	5.5	154	154	0	0	0	310	29–32
Hetastarch 264 (Pentaspan)	264	63	0.45		100	5	154	154	0	0	0	326	
Hetastarch 264 (Pentalyte)	264	63	0.45		60		143	124	5	3	28[a]		32.2 ± 1
Hetastarch 200 (Expahes)	200		0.5	5:1	100	4–7	154	154	0	0	0	300	65
Hetastarch 200 (haes-steril)	240		0.4–0.55	5:1	60 or	3.5–6	154	154	0	0	0	308	
Hetastarch 200 (Elohäst)	200		0.6–0.66	5:1	100	4–7	154	154	0	0	0	308	25
Hetastarch 130 (Voluven), Vetstarch	130	70–80	0.4	9:1	60	4–5.5	154	154	0	0	0	308	
Hetastarch 70 (Expafusion)	70		0.5	4:1	60	6	138	125	1.5	4	20	290	

Note:
a) Hextend and Pentalyte also contain 0.45 mmol/L of magnesium and 99 mg/dL of dextrose.

of 42 mmHg. This particular product has had a troubled history and other similar solutions or solutions based on synthetic oxygen-carrying molecules may become available in the future. The main advantage of the HBOCS is that they are stable at room temperature and can be stored on the shelf for years rather than the 4–5 weeks' maximum storage for whole blood or PRBCs.

Box 8.2: Blood types and products in cats

Cats have three blood types: A, B, and AB, and the prevalence of these types appears to have some geographic distribution. Another antibody present in A type cats, the *Mik* antibody has recently been described as the source of a hemolytic reaction in a cat. Since blood typing is now possible in most laboratories it is feasible to ensure that the recipient and the donor have the same blood type. However, when using red cells in either whole blood or packed red blood cells (PRBCs), a cross match is still important as the resulting improvement in hematocrit is greater when cross match compatible transfusions are administered and this might prevent reactions associated with the *Mik* antibody. Fresh and fresh-frozen plasma have all the normal clotting factors so they can be used to supplement protein and help with coagulation. Plasma removed from blood after the first 24 hours and stored fresh or frozen is only useful as a source of plasma proteins as the clotting factors degrade rapidly.

Preoperative Preparation

It is beyond the scope of this chapter to describe all the pathophysiological changes that may lead to disturbances in fluid volumes, content, or distribution but it is important for the clinician to consider these changes and to correct them before proceeding to anesthetize the cat. Some common issues are discussed further.

Dehydration versus Hypovolemia

Hypovolemia refers to the circulating volume whereas dehydration refers to the total body water content of the animal. If a cat is dehydrated it is likely to be hypovolemic but a hypovolemic patient may not be dehydrated. A good example of the latter is the cat that is bleeding, where the circulating volume is reduced but there has not been enough time to pull fluids from other compartments. From a therapeutic point of view, it may be simple to restore euvolemia by rapidly administering a fluid into the circulation to replace the volume lost. The dehydrated patient needs to be rehydrated but this cannot be done rapidly because the fluids have to distribute throughout the body to restore fluid deficits in each area (*Box 8.3*).

Anemia

The reference range for hematocrit is lower in cats (30–50%) than dogs (40–55%), and it is common to see cats with hematocrits < 25% without clinical signs of disease. During anesthesia it is expected that hematocrit will decrease due to the action of drugs and changes in distribution of fluids in the body. In practice it is common to see a decrease of at least 5% and this can be exacerbated by falsely elevated values obtained from stressed

---

Box 8.3: Fluid requirements for rehydration

If a 5 kg cat was 10% dehydrated, it would need 500 mL of fluid to reverse that deficit. If such a volume was given as a bolus it could overwhelm the ability of the heart to pump this forward and result in pulmonary edema. If it is essential to anesthetize a dehydrated patient then enough fluid should be administered to restore the circulatory component of the deficit with a plan to give the rest over the next 12–24 hours. In this example, if the animal was 10% dehydrated it would have lost 10% of its circulating volume or 5–6 mL/kg. As indicated above, since only about 30% of the balanced electrolyte solution remains in the circulation a bolus of 15–18 mL/kg would have to be administered to this animal to restore circulating volume and then correction of the dehydration would be allowed to proceed more slowly.

---

cats (splenic contraction) in the preoperative period. In a laboratory study, using drugs that would not be expected to cause splenic sequestration (ketamine/diazepam without volatile anesthetics), the hematocrit of healthy cats decreased from 43% (awake) to 32% (~15 minutes after induction). A transfusion should therefore be considered in any cat presenting with a hematocrit < 25%. In the healthy dog, oxygen delivery to the tissues may not be compromised until the hemoglobin concentration is <4 g/dL (hematocrit ~12%) but this is with no decrease in cardiac output. Cats often have a significant decrease in cardiac output associated with volatile anesthetics so it is likely that hemoglobin concentrations need to be relatively higher in this species. The clinician must also consider any condition that would further limit cardiac output during anesthesia (e.g. cardiomyopathy) and adjust the target hemoglobin concentration upwards to ensure adequate oxygen delivery. In humans there is now considerable concern over the negative effects of blood transfusions on the immune system and so there is a delicate balancing act between providing adequate oxygen to the tissues without compromising the immune function of the cat. Volume overload is always a concern in cats (see above), and so it is best to use PRBCs in normovolemic cats with anemia and start the infusion slowly (< 5 mL/kg/hour). Transfusion reactions (hyperthermia, angioedema, vomiting, salivation) have been reported in about 8% of cats receiving typed (but not cross matched) transfusions. Cats that are hypovolemic and anemic should receive their transfusion rapidly in order to restore adequate oxygen delivery. Based on a retrospective study examining the expected increase in packed cell volume with whole blood transfusion the most accurate formulae are shown in *Box 8.4.*

Box 8.4: How to calculate volume of blood to transfuse

Whole blood volume to transfuse (mL) = required change in PCV% × 2 × weight (kg)

However, if PRBCs are used a more appropriate formula would be:

volume to transfuse (mL) =
(required change in PCV% × 100 × BW (kg)/(donor blood PCV%)

Hemoglobin-based oxygen carrying solutions have been used to manage cats with anemia and in two separate studies involving a total of 120 cats the overall survival to discharge was 71%. Some of these cats also received whole blood with or without PRBCs. The most serious complications occurred in cats with cardiac disease where rapid infusion rates or large volumes of PRBCs promoted pulmonary edema.

Cardiac Disease

Cats that have hypertrophic cardiomyopathy due to hyperthyroidism should be treated for their primary disease before being anesthetized if that is possible (Chapter 9). Cats with idiopathic or congenital hypertrophic cardiomyopathy and heart failure are often treated with diuretics and enalapril so these animals may be hypotensive and dehydrated. This makes fluid therapy rather difficult to plan for these patients. In such cases a central venous pressure line could be placed so that the response to fluid administration can be measured. A low cardiac output may be due to dehydration or to cardiomyopathy. If a fluid bolus (e.g. 5 mL/kg) is administered the central venous pressure will change minimally in the dehydrated patient but may increase rapidly if the heart is unable to pump the fluid forwards. Unfortunately, clinical assessment of fluid overload, such as presence of peripheral edema or pulmonary crackles due to pulmonary edema, are very late signs but need to be addressed immediately if present. Distension of the jugular veins, without holding them off, could be another indicator of increased central venous pressure but one would actively need to look for this as the jugular veins in cats are hidden by their fur.

Urethral or Ureteral Obstruction

It is important to assess the hydration status of these patients on presentation. If they are presented early in the course of the disease they may have minimal changes in fluid balance but as the duration of obstruction increases the cat may become dehydrated and hyperkalemic (Chapter 9). It is also expected that there will be a diuresis following relief of obstruction and this will need to be managed until the cat is able to drink and regulate its own fluid balance. In the face of dehydration and hyperkalemia some have argued that 0.9% saline would be the best solution as it does not contain any potassium. However, administration of lactated or acetated Ringer's has been shown to improve the acid-base status of the animal faster and still decrease potassium concentration. It is especially important to decrease potassium concentrations before anesthetizing the animal because of the increased risk of dysrhythmias. The volatile anesthetics affect L-type calcium channels in the cardiac myocytes, which may result in a lowering of the depolarization threshold towards the raised resting membrane potential caused by hyperkalemia. For the management of hyperkalemia see Chapter 9.

Head Trauma

Cats presenting with head trauma are most likely to be victims of high-rise syndrome, motor vehicle accidents, or attack by a larger animal. The high-rise cases usually present with maxillofacial trauma and may have minimal derangements or be quite dehydrated if discovery of the injury has been delayed and they have been unable to eat or drink. The motor vehicle and bite cases may present with a variety of injuries that include skull fractures with brain injury and lacerations with blood loss. Fluids that are relatively hypotonic (e.g. lactated Ringer's) should probably not be used for these animals as there is a potential for the free water in these fluids to enhance brain edema (although there is no concrete clinical evidence to support this statement). Initial resuscitation should therefore be with normal or hypertonic saline. The latter may be especially beneficial as it can not only increase cardiac output but also draws fluid from the edematous brain and enhances cerebral oxygen delivery. As indicated above a bolus of hypertonic saline should be followed by infusion of an isotonic crystalloid to prevent hypernatremia. Mannitol may also be used as an osmotic diuretic to decrease brain swelling (Chapter 9). Blood or packed red cells should be administered if the cat is anemic before or after resuscitation with crystalloids.

Intraoperative Fluids

Maintenance

Fluid administration is not always necessary especially if the cat is healthy and surgical times are short. However, an intravenous catheter allows for rapid drug administration if needed. Because of the concerns expressed above about fluid overload, it is also good practice to use an approach that will minimize the risk of inadvertent excesses. Two common methods are to use a buretrol (burette) that is only filled to a volume representing the maximum bolus allowable, or to use a fluid pump or syringe driver that is set at the desired rate, thus ensuring accurate delivery of a specified amount of fluid per unit time (*Figure* 8.1). Historically a balanced electrolyte solution at a rate of about 10 mL/kg/hour has been used routinely for anesthetized cats. This rate was based on data from people and was regarded as being enough fluid to account for normal ongoing losses, evaporative loss from the surgical site, and some hemorrhage associated with surgery. More recently the use of such high fluid rates has been questioned based again on data from humans. With liberal fluid administration rates, human patients gained weight, had delayed recovery of gastrointestinal function, altered wound healing, pulmonary complications, increased pain, and decreased muscular oxygen tension. This has led to the idea of using restrictive fluid infusions (e.g. half the above rate) but there is no strict definition of what this means, and so it is very hard to compare studies

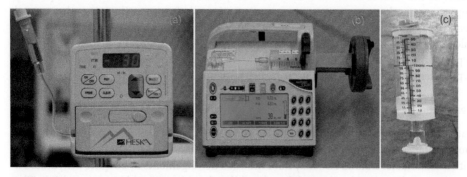

Figure 8.1 Equipment used to limit the risk of fluid overload. (a) fluid pump that can be used on a regular fluid line, (b) syringe driver, and (c) buretrol (burette).

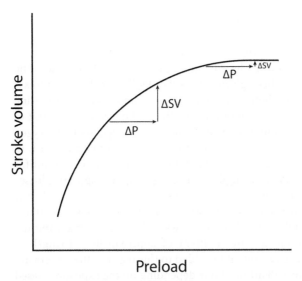

Figure 8.2 Frank–Starling curve showing the response of stroke volume to increases in preload. In the middle of the curve there is a significant ↑ increase in stroke volume (ΔSV) with an increase in preload (ΔP). At the top of the curve there is almost no increase in stroke volume with the same increase in preload.

examining "restrictive" and "liberal" fluid administration. However, complication rates have generally been lower with restrictive fluid rates. A further refinement of this is to use goal directed therapy where a measurable variable is kept within specified limits by administration of small boluses of crystalloids or colloids. A "response" to the bolus indicates that the heart is on the slope, rather than the plateau, of the Frank–Starling curve (preload versus stroke volume), and further boluses may be applied until the plateau is reached (*Figure 8.2, Box 8.5*).

Box 8.5: Developments in monitoring the effect of fluid administration

Plethysmographic variability index (PVI) is based on the pulse volume variation measured with a pulse oximeter during positive pressure ventilation. In a goal directed approach, if PVI is ≥ x% a fluid bolus is administered and the PVI checked again. If the PVI has decreased it is an indication of fluid responsiveness, if it has decreased but not to less than x% then the fluid bolus is repeated. The sensitivity of the method varies with the study conditions and the value chosen for x, with values varying from 9.5–16%. Relatively few cats are mechanically ventilated under anesthesia and there has been no validation in this species, so the value of this approach has yet to be established.

Urine production has also been used as a measure of adequate fluid therapy but this appears to be significantly affected by the drugs administered during anesthesia. Recent data suggest that the opioids and isoflurane decrease urine production to < 0.5 mL/kg/hour. Conversely agonists of α_2-adrenergic receptors increase urine production eightfold to tenfold with urine production increasing to 3–6 mL/kg/hour.

In cats it is unlikely that these technologies can be applied on a routine basis so it would be most appropriate to work out a fluid rate derived from basic principles. In the past it has been found that an animal requires roughly 1 mL of liquid per kcal of energy consumed, although this value is somewhat dependent on the source of the calories. The basal energy consumption of a dog has been given as $97 \times BW(kg)^{0.655}$ kcal/day but this is probably an overestimate for the anesthetized patient. Another approach to estimating this would be to use oxygen consumption, multiplied by the kcal consumed per unit of oxygen consumption. Data from a number of experiments in cats suggests that oxygen consumption is around 3 mL/kg/minute during anesthesia and, assuming that 1 L of oxygen produces around 5 kcal of energy, the average fluid requirement, to account for normal losses, would be approximately 1 mL/kg/hour. During surgery evaporative losses increase with exposure of tissue and the use of dry gases in breathing circuits. If it is assumed that the incoming gas is dry and that the cat has to humidify the gas to 100%, this would amount to approximately 0.25 mL/kg/hour water loss (assuming a minute ventilation of 100 mL/kg/minute and a water content of approximately 46 mg/L at 38 °C). During surgery evaporative losses might be added to this if any of the viscera are exposed, and this could range from 1–3 mL/kg/hour depending on the exposure. Based on the above calculations the minimum fluid rate should be 1–2 mL/kg/hour with additional volumes added during extensive tissue exposure. Hence the rate proposed in the recent American Animal Hospital Association (AAHA) guidelines of 3 mL/kg/hour seems reasonable. However, 11 mL/kg/minute has been administered for 60 minutes to cats without apparent harm, and even 90 mL/kg/hour produced no measurable changes except for a decrease in hematocrit, total protein, and colloid oncotic pressure. However, as many cats have latent heart disease the results may be different in each patient.

Relative Hypovolemia

Cats frequently become hypotensive during anesthesia due to the negative inotropic and vasodilatory effects of volatile anesthetics. These cats could be said to have a relative hypovolemia because of the "loss" of volume into the systemic vasculature. If a reduction of volatile agent concentration does not increase blood pressure the next step, assuming that the cat is not bradycardic, is usually to administer a bolus of fluids with the expectation that increasing preload will increase cardiac output (Chapters 9 and 10). In humans under anesthesia, it has been established that the volumes of distribution of fluids are not the same as in the awake state. However, a reasonable estimate to increase the blood volume by 10% in a cat with a blood volume of 50 mL/kg would be to administer 15 mL/kg, assuming that the crystalloid will redistribute to the interstitium in a 2:1 ratio. The rate of redistribution in cats is not known, but in humans the half-life of crystalloids in normal individuals under anesthesia is around 20 minutes, so the ongoing infusion rate would need to be of the order of 10–15 mL/kg/hour to maintain this degree of expansion. In the studies carried out in humans it has been noted that the rates of redistribution decrease if the patient is dehydrated before surgery, or hypotensive, to the extent that if the animal is severely hypotensive (e.g. a mean arterial pressure of ≤ 50 mmHg) then very little of the crystalloid will leave the vasculature.

Hypertonic saline may be used to treat hypovolemia with a dose of up to 4 mL/kg of 7.5% solution over 10–15 minutes. This dose was able to restore blood pressure and cardiac output in cats that had lost more than 50% of their blood volume but the benefits lasted less than one hour, so the infusion should be followed by other methods to maintain circulating volume (e.g. standard crystalloids). The serum sodium concentration can be expected to increase dramatically within the first 10 minutes after infusion but it will soon start to decrease due to redistribution and the addition of fluid to the circulation from the periphery.

Artificial colloids may also be used in hypovolemia. They will increase circulating volume with an efficiency that usually exceeds the volume administered because most of these solutions have osmolalities that are similar to, or exceed, plasma osmolality, and many are also hyperoncotic (*Box* 8.6).

Box 8.6: Developments in hydroxyethyl starches (HES)

There are now many HES available worldwide, and the original high molecular weight HES (450/0.7) has been succeeded by molecules with lower molecular weights and different substitution ratios that change the rate at which they are metabolized (e.g. HES 130/0.4). Some of these new molecules as well as the polygelatins have less effect on coagulation. It has been recommended for dogs that the dose of HES 450/0.7 should not exceed 20 mL/kg in 24 hours whereas with HES 130/0.4 the dose can be as high as 40 mL/kg in 24 hours with minimal effect on coagulation. These doses probably need to be reduced in cats to around 15 and 30 mL/24 hours, respectively, because of the smaller blood volume, but there are no specific studies available in this species.

Absolute Hypovolemia

The cat that is hypovolemic because of blood loss may also be treated with a rapid bolus of crystalloid at a ratio of three times the volume of blood lost. The limitation to the use of crystalloid will be the dilution of hemoglobin, and, as discussed above, the transfusion trigger point should be modified in the light of the pathophysiology of the condition and the rate of hemorrhage. Packed red blood cells may be the most efficient way to increase oxygen carrying capacity but fresh whole blood can be used, with the added advantage of containing clotting factors and proteins to maintain plasma oncotic pressure. Most blood that is collected for transfusion is prevented from clotting by the addition of citrate, which ties up calcium. The amount of citrate present usually exceeds that needed in the collected blood so it has the potential to cause hypocalcemia in the recipient. If blood is administered slowly, and only 1 or 2 units are given, the animal will compensate for this by shifting calcium from the vast stores in the body. However, if blood is given rapidly and, especially if several units are administered, the cat will become hypocalcemic. To counteract this the cat can be given 2.5–5 mg/kg of calcium chloride or 10–15 mg/kg of calcium gluconate (NB. these are not precisely equivalent doses). The use of citrate for anticoagulation is also the reason why blood should not be administered through the same line as a calcium containing solution such as lactated Ringer's – the addition of calcium could counteract the citrate and coagulate the blood. Some cats give the clinical impression that massive hypotension caused by the release of vasoactive compounds from the gut or the liver responds poorly to crystalloid administration, and appears to resolve only with the administration of blood. These animals often have a hematocrit that would normally be acceptable but crystalloids, and even artificial colloids, do not seem to improve their blood pressure.

Hemoglobin-based oxygen carrying solutions have also been used to treat hypovolemia especially where there are concerns about oxygen carrying capacity. This can be a very useful method to restore circulating volume and increase oxygen delivery. Pigmentation of the serum is an expected effect associated with the administration of these solutions.

Chronic Kidney Disease (CKD)

Many older cats have CKD, and their fluid management is complex (Chapter 9). The main aim is for the cat to emerge from anesthesia with no further damage to the kidneys. Many cats with CKD are treated with angiotensin-converting enzyme inhibitors such as benazepril or captopril and newer drugs including angiotensin II receptor antagonists (blockers) such as telmisartan. These drugs are thought to decrease proteinuria and slow the progression of the disease. In human medicine administration of these drugs on the morning before anesthesia is associated with a higher incidence of hypotension during anesthesia. This has also been seen in cats, and the drug may be withheld on the morning of anesthesia to try to avoid the increased fluid volume that might be needed to treat subsequent intraoperative hypotension. Some of these patients may also be dehydrated prior to the procedure, and so it is necessary to assess hydration status carefully before anesthesia and to monitor the effect of fluids intraoperatively using central venous pressure (see above). In the past both dopamine and mannitol have been used intraoperatively for "renal protection", but the current evidence from human anesthesia is that these therapies do not improve outcome. Dopamine is unlikely to benefit feline patients because the dopamine-1 receptors in their kidneys seem to lack a vasodilating effect. However, dopamine is very effective at increasing cardiac output, and thereby renal perfusion, in the hypotensive patient.

Postoperative Care

The postoperative period should be a time for transitioning the patient back to the awake state where the animal can function again on its own, regulating its own food and water intake. Typically in the average healthy patient, fluids will be discontinued at the start of recovery and the cat will be able to drink and eat within 2–3 hours. Sick or critically ill patients may need fluid therapy continued in order to resolve pre-existing dehydration, hypovolemia or chronic deficits or if their disease prevents them from eating or drinking. For these patients it may be appropriate to use replacement fluids such as lactated Ringer's or Hartmann's solution initially, but within a few hours the cat should be changed to a true maintenance solution that has much less sodium (40 mmol/L) and more potassium (13–16 mmol/L) (*Table* 8.1) (e.g. acetated solutions such as Normosol-M or Plasmalyte M or 56). Higher potassium concentrations may be needed if the cat is hypokalemic initially or is losing more potassium through the kidneys. Blood, plasma or colloids may also be needed to repair pre-existing deficits and further losses. Infusion solutions containing blood or plasma should be discarded after 4 hours at room temperature to decrease the risk of bacterial contamination. The volume required for 4 hours may be calculated and placed in a syringe for use, and the remainder refrigerated until needed.

Further Reading

Bahlmann, H., Hahn, R. G., and Nilsson, L. (2016) Agreement between Pleth Variability Index and oesophageal Doppler to predict fluid responsiveness. *Acta Anaesthesiologica Scandinavica* **60**, 183–192.

Bjorling, D. E., and Rawlings, C. A. (1983) Relationship of intravenous administration of Ringer's lactate solution to pulmonary edema in halothane-anesthetized cats. *American Journal of Veterinary Research* **44**, 1000–1006.

Brand, A. (2002) Immunological aspects of blood transfusions. *Transplant Immunology* **10**, 183–190.

Brandstrup, B., Tonnesen, H., Beier-Holgersen, R., et al. (2003) Effects of intravenous fluid restriction on postoperative complications: Comparison of two perioperative fluid regimens: A randomized assessor-blinded multicenter trial. *Annals of Surgery* **238**, 641–648.

Chappell, D., and Jacob, M. (2014) Role of the glycocalyx in fluid management: Small things matter. *Best Practice and Research* **28**, 227–234.

Chohan, A. S., and Davidow, E. B. (2015) Clinical pharmacology and administration of fluid, electrolyte, and blood component solutions. In *Veterinary Anesthesia and Analgesia The Fifth Edition of Lumb and Jones* (eds. K. A. Grimm, L. A. Lamont, W. J. Tranquilli, et al.) Wiley Blackwell, Ames, Iowa. pp. 386–416.

Cunha, M. G., Freitas, G. C., Carregaro, A. B., et al. (2010) Renal and cardiorespiratory effects of treatment with lactated Ringer's solution or physiologic saline (0.9% NaCl) solution in cats with experimentally induced urethral obstruction. *American Journal of Veterinary Research* **71**, 840–846.

Davis, H., Jensen, T., Johnson, A., et al. (2013) 2013 AAHA/AAFP fluid therapy guidelines for dogs and cats. *Journal of the American Animal Hospital Association* **49**, 149–159.

Dhumeaux, M. P., Snead, E. C., Epp, T. Y., et al. (2012) Effects of a standardized anesthetic protocol on hematologic variables in healthy cats. *Journal of Feline Medicine and Surgery* **14**, 701–705.

Dirven, M. J., Cornelissen, J. M., Barendse, M. A., et al. (2010) Cause of heart murmurs in 57 apparently healthy cats. *Tijdschrift voor diergeneeskunde* **135**, 840–847.

Doherty, M., and Buggy, D. J. (2012) Intraoperative fluids: How much is too much? *British Journal of Anaesthesia* **109**, 69–79.

Feldschuh, J., and Enson, Y. (1977) Prediction of the normal blood volume. Relation of blood volume to body habitus. *Circulation* **56**, 605–612.

Harris, A. N., Beatty, S. S., Estrada, A. H., et al. (2017) Investigation of an N-terminal prohormone of brain natriuretic peptide point-of-care Elisa in clinically normal cats and cats with cardiac disease. *Journal of Veterinary Internal Medicine* **31**, 994–999.

Hodgson, D. S., Dunlop, C. I., Chapman, P. L., et al. (1998) Cardiopulmonary effects of anesthesia induced and maintained with isoflurane in cats. *American Journal of Veterinary Research* **59**, 182–185.

Ingwersen, W., Allen, D. G., Dyson, D. H., et al. (1988) Cardiopulmonary effects of a halothane/oxygen combination in healthy cats. *Canadian Journal of Veterinary Research* **52**, 386–391.

Kisielewicz, C., and Self, I. A. (2014) Canine and feline blood transfusions: Controversies and recent advances in administration practices. *Veterinary Anaesthesia and Analgesia* **41**, 233–242.

Muir, W. W., 3rd and Sally, J. (1989) Small-volume resuscitation with hypertonic saline solution in hypovolemic cats. *American Journal of Veterinary Research* **50**, 1883–1888.

Murahata, Y., and Hikasa, Y. (2012) Comparison of the diuretic effects of medetomidine hydrochloride and xylazine hydrochloride in healthy cats. *American Journal of Veterinary Research* **73**, 1871–1880.

Paige, C. F., Abbott, J. A., Elvinger, F., *et al.* (2009) Prevalence of cardiomyopathy in apparently healthy cats. *Journal of the American Veterinary Medical Association* **234**, 1398–1403.

Pascoe, P. J. (2012) Perioperative management of fluid therapy. In *Fluid, Electrolyte and Acid-Base Disorders in Small Animal Practice* (ed. S. P. DiBartola). Elsevier, St. Louis, MO, pp. 405–435.

Reed, N., Espadas, I., Lalor, S. M., *et al.* (2014) Assessment of five formulae to predict post-transfusion packed cell volume in cats. *Journal of Feline Medicine and Surgery* **16**, 651–656.

Roux, F. A., Deschamps, J. Y., Blais, M. C., *et al.* (2008) Multiple red cell transfusions in 27 cats (2003–2006): Indications, complications and outcomes. *Journal of Feline Medicine and Surgery* **10**, 213–218.

Sparkes, A. H., Caney, S., and Chalhoub, S. (2016) ISFM consensus guidelines on the diagnosis and management of feline chronic kidney disease. *Journal of Feline Medicine and Surgery* **18**, 219–239.

Wehausen, C. E., Kirby, R., and Rudloff, E. (2011) Evaluation of the effects of bovine hemoglobin glutamer-200 on systolic arterial blood pressure in hypotensive cats: 44 cases (1997–2008). *Journal of the American Veterinary Medical Association* **238**, 909–914.

Wellman, M. L., DiBartola, S. P., and Kohn, C. W. (2012) Applied physiology of body fluids in dogs and cats. In *Fluid, Electrolyte and Acid-Base Disorders in Small Animal Practice* (ed. S. P. DiBartola), Elsevier, St. Louis, MO, pp. 2–25.

Weltman, J. G., Fletcher, D. J., and Rogers, C. (2014) Influence of cross-match on posttransfusion packed cell volume in feline packed red blood cell transfusion. *Journal of Veterinary Emergency and Critical Care* **24**, 429–436.

9

Anesthetic Management of Special Conditions

Paulo Steagall

Université de Montréal, Saint-Hyacinthe, Canada

Key Points

- Pathophysiological changes associated with common diseases
- General considerations and anesthetic management of cats with common diseases and conditions
- Specific goals of anesthetic management for each set of conditions
- Adjuvant therapies and their impact on anesthetic management
- Potential complications and preventive measures to reduce morbidity and mortality

Introduction

Cats with specific disease states may require general anesthesia for diagnostic, medical, or surgical procedures, which may or may not be related to the disease but will have a profound impact on homeostasis with detrimental physiological effects. Knowledge and appropriate management of disease-induced pathophysiological changes will prevent complications and reduce perioperative morbidity and mortality. It is particularly important to consider the impact of the cardiorespiratory depressant effects produced by most anesthetics. This chapter discusses anesthetic techniques and drug protocols used in the *most common* feline disease states. Except for emergency cases, the value of the medical or surgical procedure should be always weighed against the anesthetic risks.

Anesthesia of specific populations of cats is discussed in other chapters. For example, anesthesia of the fearful cat is discussed in Chapter 1, consideration of anemia and its anesthetic implications is presented in Chapter 2, anesthesia for spay-neuter programs including its relevance to kittens is described in Chapter 4, and pain management of cats with chronic pain syndrome after feline onychectomy is covered in Chapter 15.

Urethral Obstruction and Uroabdomen

General Considerations

Urethral obstruction is usually caused by proteinaceous matrix plugs, and primarily affects male cats who present with a history of hematuria and straining to urinate. Cats with urethral

Feline Anesthesia and Pain Management, First Edition. Edited by Paulo Steagall,
Sheilah Robertson and Polly Taylor.
© 2018 John Wiley & Sons, Inc. Published 2018 by John Wiley & Sons, Inc.

obstruction and lower urinary tract disease commonly require anesthesia for urethral catheterization, perineal urethrostomy or exploratory abdominal surgery because of bladder rupture and uroabdomen. These patients are often critically ill, and preanesthetic stabilization is usually required. A list of problems is presented in *Box* 9.1. Clinical presentation includes anorexia, lethargy, dehydration, depression, anuria or oliguria, halitosis, abdominal pain, vomiting, and diarrhea. Clinical signs will ultimately depend on the severity of dehydration, uremia, and hyperkalemia; acute renal failure may result. Venous catheterization is mandatory for fluid and electrolyte administration. Hematocrit, total protein, blood urea nitrogen (BUN), sodium, potassium and ionized calcium concentrations will guide appropriate treatment to reduce the risks associated with anesthesia. Reagents strips give sufficient information for BUN and a full chemical panel is not always essential.

Box 9.1: Urethral obstruction: challenges in patient stabilization and management of anesthesia

Reduced glomerular filtration rate, hypothermia, hyperkalemia, hypocalcemia, and acidemia are often present in these cats. Circulatory collapse with weak peripheral pulses must be treated before general anesthesia. Fluid therapy and adequate hydration will optimize cardiac output and renal blood flow while minimizing blood pressure variations during general anesthesia. Correction of electrolyte and acid-base imbalances in addition to severe dehydration are the most important goals of patient stabilization. Rapid fluid resuscitation (in the absence of cardiac disease) is required, especially if poor perfusion and severe dehydration are present. A bolus of balanced isotonic crystalloid fluid such as saline 0.9% is administered at 45–60 mL/kg/hour while the obstruction is relieved. Lactated Ringer's is acceptable even in hyperkalemia (Chapter 8) since saline 0.9% may worsen pre-existing metabolic acidosis because it has high chloride concentration. The rationale for aggressive fluid therapy is to promote diuresis and to treat cardiovascular collapse. Warming will prevent and treat hypothermia.

Hyperkalemia causes unique changes in the electrocardiogram (ECG). The ECG changes include bradycardia, increased T-wave amplitude, decreased R-wave amplitude, ST segment depression, decreased P wave amplitude, prolonged PR, QRS and QT intervals, and commonly, loss of P wave with possible ventricular dysrhythmias.

This bradycardia should not be treated with atropine or glycopyrrolate. Cats with a serum potassium concentration greater than 6 mEq/L should not be anesthetized until hyperkalemia is treated (*Box* 9.2).

Acidemia results in potassium ions moving extracellularly in exchange for hydrogen ions, which are buffered intracellularly.

- Metabolic acidosis decreases protein binding, increasing the availability of highly protein bound drugs
- In addition to hypovolemia, metabolic disturbances lead to electrical conductance abnormalities because hyperkalemia, raises the resting cell membrane potential; cardiac automaticity, conductivity and contractility are decreased

Azotemia may in part be produced by dehydration (prerenal). *Uremia may change protein binding and the blood-brain barrier permeability, resulting in profound drug effects.*

Box 9.2: Stepwise approach to treatment of hyperkalemia

- Calcium gluconate 10% (0.5–1 mL/kg IV) is injected over 10–15 minutes while the ECG is monitored. Administration of calcium increases cell membrane threshold potential, thereby increasing myocardial conduction and contractility
- Calcium restores the normal gradient between resting and threshold potentials of the cardiac cells and is indicated for life-threatening bradycardia. However, its effects are transient (15–20 minutes), and calcium therapy does not change potassium concentrations. Hypocalcemia potentiates the myocardial toxicity of hyperkalemia, and it should be treated
- A bolus of dextrose (0.25–0.5 g/kg IV) is diluted with two parts of saline 0.9% (by volume), and administered in combination with a bolus of insulin (0.1–0.25 U/kg IV). Insulin drives potassium into the intracellular compartment while dextrose induces endogenous insulin release
- Sodium bicarbonate (1 mEq/kg IV) is given slowly (10–15 minutes), and will also move potassium into the intracellular compartment. The effects of bicarbonate usually last a few hours, and it is recommended for severe metabolic acidosis (pH < 7.1). Judicious administration will avoid iatrogenic metabolic alkalosis, hypernatremia or paradoxic CNS acidosis

---

Anesthetic Management

Anesthesia is normally required for manipulation and placement of a urinary catheter. Sedation may not be required for catheterization in the very sick patient.

An overview of anesthetic management is provided below:

- Some cats may tolerate urinary catheterization under deep sedation using an IV combination of an opioid (e.g. methadone 0.3 mg/kg or buprenorphine 0.02 mg/kg), and midazolam (0.3 mg/kg), or low doses of propofol or alfaxalone (0.5–1 mg/kg IV for both drugs)
- Oxygen therapy is highly recommended during sedation
- Acepromazine and agonists of α_2-adrenergic receptors (dexmedetomidine) are contraindicated due to their undesirable cardiovascular effects
- Ketamine is actively excreted by the kidneys in the cat (Chapter 2), and is usually contraindicated for induction of anesthesia, especially if there are signs of acute renal failure. If ketamine is used, recovery from anesthesia may be prolonged. Anecdotally ketamine infusions (10–20 µg/kg/minute) are acceptable for perioperative analgesia after laparotomy. The doses are low (subanesthetic), and ketamine is valuable for multimodal analgesia due to its ability both to prevent and treat hyperalgesia and central sensitization
- Volatile anesthesia with isoflurane or sevoflurane is a good option if prolonged anesthesia (> 20 minutes) is required since intubation or use of a supraglottic airway device offers the best means of oxygenation, ventilation, and airway protection. However, volatile anesthetic cardiorespiratory depression is a concern

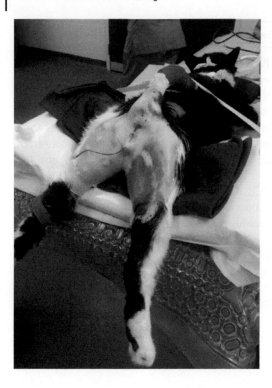

Figure 9.1 Positioning of a cat for perineal urethrostomy.

Cats undergoing perineal urethrostomy are often positioned on a tilted table (Trendelenburg) with their pelvic limbs off the table (*Figure* 9.1). This may cause respiratory impairment since abdominal viscera push on the diaphragm, limiting thoracic expansion. Respiratory depression may lead to respiratory acidosis, and worsen acidemia. Assisted ventilation may be required and a capnograph aids monitoring of ventilation (Chapter 7). Soft padding should be placed between the hind limbs and the surgical table to prevent nerve damage. Hematocrit, total protein, and lactate concentrations provide information on the effectiveness of fluid therapy and hemodilution (Chapter 8). In critically ill cats, a bolus of ephedrine (0.1 mg/kg IV) or dopamine infusions (10–20 μg/kg/minute IV) can be administered to improve cardiac contractility and promote α-adrenergic-induced peripheral vasoconstriction.

Pain management is always an important component of anesthesia:

- Analgesia is essential but NSAIDs are contraindicated due to their deleterious renal effects. NSAIDs may, however, be administered once normal hydration, perfusion, and renal function are established (Chapter 13)
- IV administration of opioids (buprenorphine, methadone or hydromorphone) is recommended since many cats present with severe abdominal pain due to a distended, tense bladder
- Opioid infusions (e.g. fentanyl or remifentanil; 5–20 μg/kg/hour) may be required during and after exploratory abdominal surgery. In contrast with dogs, opioid infusions do not substantially decrease volatile anesthetic requirements in cats

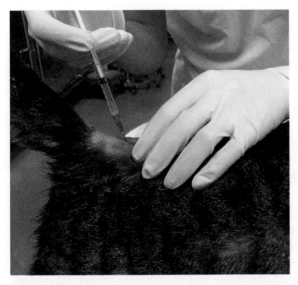

Figure 9.2 Sacrococcygeal epidural anesthesia in cats before urinary catheter placement. The technique is performed under aseptic conditions and produces anesthesia of the perineal area, penis, urethra, colon, and anus. Preservative-free lidocaine 2% (0.1–0.2 mL/kg) is injected using a 23 or 25-G 25-30mm (1.2 inch) needle. Relaxation of the tail and perineal region is usually observed.
Source: Courtesy of Dr. Edouard Martin.

- A sacrococcygeal epidural block facilitates urethral catheterization in cats with urethral obstruction (*Figure* 9.2)
- Lumbosacral epidural with local anesthetics is contraindicated in hypovolemic states due to the risk of sympathetic blockade, vasodilation, hypotension, and cardiovascular collapse

Chronic Kidney Disease (CKD)

General Considerations

Chronic kidney disease affects more than 30–40% of cats older than 10 years of age, and is a significant cause of mortality. These patients require anesthesia for a range of procedures (e.g. dental prophylaxis, imaging). The etiology of CKD has not been elucidated but it is well accepted that there is a significant inflammatory component in most cases.

The International Society of Feline Medicine has published consensus guidelines on diagnosis and management of CKD in cats (http://jfm.sagepub.com/content/18/3/219 .full.pdf+html, accessed June 25, 2017).

Common indicators of CKD vary from one patient to another and include:

- Weight loss and poor body condition
- Polyuria and polydipsia
- Azotemia (serum creatinine concentrations $\geq 140\,\mu mol/L$ or $\geq 1.6\,mg/dL$), although this may be affected by lean tissue mass and hydration

- Dehydration and hypovolemia
- Low urine specific gravity (≤ 1.030)
- Systemic hypertension (systolic blood pressure ≥ 160 mmHg)
- Long-term evidence of kidney dysfunction and decreased kidney size
- Proteinuria
- Anemia
- Hyperphosphatemia
- Hypokalemia
- Potential for "acute on chronic" CKD; metabolic and electrolyte changes will be similar to urethral obstruction leading to hyperkalemia, uremia, oliguria and anuria

Cats with CKD should be stabilized before general anesthesia with appropriate symptomatic therapy. Additional laboratory investigation and imaging may help to identify the disease severity and guide therapy. Urinary tract infection should be treated with antibiotics, ideally after bacterial culture. Fluid administration is required to correct dehydration, electrolyte, and acid-base abnormalities (*Box* 9.3) especially in cats that are uremic with anorexia, vomiting, and diarrhea. This is particularly important in order to maintain adequate blood flow during anesthesia and to eliminate uremic toxins and drugs.

Box 9.3: Patient stabilization before general anesthesia in cats with CKD: fluid therapy

- Subcutaneous fluid administration (20–30 mL/kg) is an option but hospitalization and IV treatment should be considered 24 hours before general anesthesia for IRIS stage III or IV cases
- Avoiding fluid overload is essential, and is of particular concern in geriatric cats and those with cardiomyopathy
- Cautious administration of crystalloids is also important with protein-losing nephropathy as hypoproteinemia impairs colloid oncotic pressure and may predispose patients to edema. Colloid administration is preferred for treatment of intraoperative hypotension and when large volumes are required
- Hemodilution is also an issue since many cats with CKD are anemic. This can be further aggravated by intraoperative blood loss. Severely anemic (hematocrit $\leq$ 20%) cats should be treated with erythrocyte-stimulating agents (e.g. erythropoietin) as part of patient stabilization in an attempt to increase hematocrit and meet tissue oxygen requirements. In an emergency, packed red blood cells may be indicated
- Severe metabolic acidosis (pH $\leq$ 7.1 and bicarbonate concentrations $\leq$ 15 mEq/L) may be treated with bicarbonate (0.5 mEq/kg IV over 20 minutes)

Anesthetic Management

The goal during anesthesia is to maintain renal blood flow (RBF) and minimize changes in glomerular filtration rate (GFR). Intraoperative hypotension should be avoided as it may lead to renal hypoperfusion. This is aggravated by drugs used to treat hypertension that promote vasodilation and decrease cardiac contractility such as amiodipine (calcium-channel blocker), telmisartan (angiotension receptor blocker), benazepril (angiotension-converting enzyme inhibitor) or propranolol (antagonist of β-adrenergic receptors or "β blocker"). Blood pressure should be closely monitored and hypotension treated as necessary (Chapter 10).

- Premedication of older cats with CKD includes drugs that can be reversed such as opioids and benzodiazepines
- A combination of midazolam (0.3 mg/kg) and hydromorphone (0.05–0.1 mg/kg) or methadone (0.3 mg/kg) IM will suit most of these cats unless profound sedation is required for intravenous catheterization
- Acepromazine may produce hypotension but studies in dogs have shown that it may provide renal protection by preserving RBF and GFR
- Dexmedetomidine, particularly in combination with propofol and isoflurane, decreases cardiac output leading to reduced RBF
- Local anesthesia should be always used where appropriate, especially for cats undergoing dental procedures (i.e. dental blocks; Chapter 5)
- Discussion around the use of NSAIDs in cats with CKD is beyond the scope of this chapter. However, cats with degenerative joint disease and stable CKD (controlled hypertension, lack of urinary tract infection and periodontal disease; International Renal Interest Society (IRIS) I and II) have been successfully treated with meloxicam or robenacoxib (Chapter 15). Most surgical procedures will cause inflammation, and administration of a minimum effective dose of NSAID should be considered for normovolemic cats with stable disease
- Ketamine is excreted partly unchanged by the kidneys in cats (Chapter 2) and is not an appropriate choice in most CKD cases. Based on data from humans, propofol is the drug of choice because it has minimal effects on RBF and GFR in patients with nephropathy. Alfaxalone is an alternative for induction of anesthesia
- Volatile anesthetics are widely used for maintenance of anesthesia but decrease RBF and GFR, and may produce vasodilation and hypotension. The potential for nephrotoxicity from production of inorganic fluoride ions after sevoflurane administration is not usually a clinical concern when using appropriate fresh-gas flows (Chapter 6)
- Cats have putative renal dopamine (D1) receptors and infusions have been used for inotropic support (10–20 µg/kg/minute). Low doses of dopamine (1–3 µg/kg/minute) are no longer thought to be renal protective

Hyperthyroidism

General Considerations

Hyperthyroidism is the most common endocrinopathy in geriatric cats; it is caused by adenomatous goiter or hyperplasia. Hyperthyroidism results from increased plasma concentrations of thyroid hormones (T_3 and T_4). Anesthesia is required in hyperthyroid cats either for thyroidectomy or for unrelated issues. Hyperthyroid cats are commonly cachectic because of multiple systemic disorders and a high metabolic rate which increases energy requirements and oxygen consumption. Hypothermia is likely to occur during anesthesia if not vigorously prevented.

Hyperthyroid cats may have hypertrophic cardiomyopathy (HCM) and evaluation of cardiovascular function is important, ideally with echocardiography. Cardiovascular function is over stimulated by hyperthyroidism, leading to increased myocardial contractility and cardiac output. Hypertension is common in these patients. Administration of antagonists of β-adrenergic receptors (atenolol, propranolol or esmolol) may be started 48 hours before anesthesia to minimize excessive sympathetic stimulation during surgery. Hyperthyroid cats are often treated with methimazole, which inhibits synthesis of thyroid hormones (onset of effects requires approximately one week) and this should not be stopped before anesthesia as its half-life is short. Elective procedures should be delayed until thyroid hormone concentrations have been normalized. A complete blood count (hematocrit is usually increased), serum chemistry profile (biochemical abnormalities are common), and measurement of serum thyroid hormone concentrations are recommended to guide treatment and monitor progress of the disease.

Anesthetic Management

Stimulation of thyroid function (a so-called *"thyroid storm"*) should be avoided during anesthesia as this may produce potentially life-threatening sympathetic stimulation and cardiac dysrhythmias. This is especially important in cats with HCM.

- Diagnosis of ventricular dysrhythmias before induction of anesthesia can be confirmed with judicious auscultation and an ECG recording
- Hyperthyroid cats may be difficult to handle due to increased sympathetic activity and change in behavior. Adequate sedation and a stress-free approach to handling, and induction is recommended
- Opioids alone (e.g. hydromorphone, methadone, butorphanol, buprenorphine) are commonly used for sedation. Low doses of dexmedetomidine (3–5 µg/kg IM) or alfaxalone (1–2 mg/kg IM) can be combined with opioids in the fractious cat. Acepromazine is an option in euvolemic cats where severe bleeding is not a risk during surgery (Chapter 3)
- Application of local anesthetic cream may help with venous catheterization in cats that are difficult to handle
- Preoxygenation is performed before induction. Theoretically, etomidate is the best induction agent (2 mg/kg IV) given with or without midazolam (0.25 mg/kg). These drugs do not sensitize the myocardium to the dysrythmogenic effects of catecholamines. Low doses of propofol (1–2 mg/kg IV) or alfaxalone (0.5–1 mg/kg) are more practical alternatives and suitable when given slowly to effect. Ketamine causes indirect sympathetic activity and should be avoided. Anticholinergics are not recommended
- Gold-standard monitoring of anesthesia allows early detection and treatment of potential perioperative complications. Fluid therapy must be given judiciously especially if clinical signs of HCM are present. Fluid administration should simply account for any dehydration from vomiting and diarrhea resulting from malabsorption and decreased ororectal transit time

Complications during thyroidectomy include vagal nerve stimulation (Chapter 10), hemorrhage, and excessive bandage compression of the neck and airways during recovery. Recurrent laryngeal nerve damage is also possible resulting in laryngeal paralysis and stridor and respiratory distress after extubation. Hypocalcemia is a common complication in the postoperative period if the parathyroid glands are removed accidentally. Cats are commonly hospitalized for postoperative care for 48–72 hours.

Hypertrophic Cardiomyopathy (HCM)

General Considerations

Hypertrophic cardiomyopathy is a primary idiopathic heart disease that causes structural impairment with concentric thickening of the myocardium, ventricular hypertrophy, and diastolic dysfunction (failure of relaxation). Maine Coon, Persian, and American Short Hair cats may be genetically predisposed to the disease. Hypertrophic cardio-myopathy is sometimes observed secondary to hyperthyroidism. HCM is reported to be present in around 15% of apparently normal cats, and many of these do not have a cardiac murmur. This may explain some cases of unexpected death during anesthesia (Chapter 10). The pathophysiology of HCM includes significant hemodynamic changes.

- The ventricle is thick and noncompliant. This reduces myocardial relaxation and limits end-diastolic volume, as well as affecting coronary circulation (*Figure* 9.3)
- Left-atrial enlargement, mitral regurgitation, and venous congestion are common due to high diastolic pressure. Pulmonary edema may result
- Stroke volume, and therefore cardiac output, are compromised. The systolic anterior movement of the mitral leaflets is responsible for dynamic obstruction of the left ventricular outflow tract (DOLVOT) mitral valve regurgitation and heart murmur
- If the patient is in chronic heart failure before anesthesia this should be treated. Cardiogenic edema and pleural effusion leading to dyspnea should be resolved before the anesthetic event
- Clots can form in the left atrium which may fragment, leading to arterial thrombo-embolism. Some cats are treated with clopidrogrel with or without aspirin as an attempt to decrease this risk; these drugs will result in increased bleeding during surgery

Anesthetic Management

Cats with HCM may be sedated with an opioid alone (hydromorphone 0.1 mg/kg, butorphanol 0.4 mg/kg, buprenorphine 0.02 mg/kg or methadone 0.3 mg/kg IM), or in combination with midazolam (0.25 mg/kg IM) or acepromazine (0.02 mg/kg). Cats

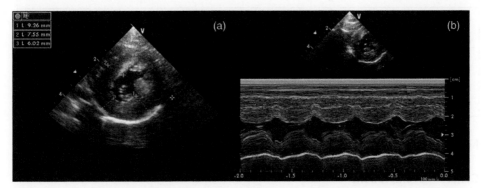

Figure 9.3 Echocardiography with signs of left sided obstructive hypertrophic cardiomyopathy. The aortic ejection fraction was turbulent and increased. (a) Right-parasternal short-axis view showing left ventricle hypertrophy with thickened interventricular septum and left ventricular wall. (b) M-mode echocardiogram at the level of the left ventricle showing the thickened myocardium and small left-ventricle cavity.

should be preoxygenated. The electrocardiogram and blood pressure (Doppler ultrasound) are best monitored before induction of anesthesia as these will reveal any dysrhythmia and hypertension.

- Ideally anesthesia can be induced with etomidate (1–2 mg/kg IV). However, propofol or alfaxalone titrated slowly and to effect are acceptable in the early stages of HCM. Combinations of intravenous fentanyl-midazolam (Chapter 4) can be used in critically ill cats to induce anesthesia or to minimize doses of propofol and alfaxalone
- Isoflurane or sevoflurane are used for maintenance of anesthesia in combination with an ultra-short opioid agonist (e.g. fentanyl or remifentanil; 5–20 μg/kg/hour). Balanced anesthesia (Chapter 6) will allow small decreases in volatile anesthetic requirements, and better cardiovascular stability (*Box* 9.4)
- Ketamine and anticholinergics are contraindicated because they increase heart rate and diastolic filling time and increase sympathetic activity. Dexmedetomidine or medetomidine may be used if necessary in cats that are difficult to handle and in cats with documented DOLVOT. Both drugs produce bradycardia and increase diastolic filling time
- Intravenous fluids should be administered judiciously (1–2 mL/kg/hour); higher rates may cause pulmonary edema
- Cats in heart failure are commonly treated with an angiotensin-converting enzyme inhibitor (e.g. enalapril) to decrease renal retention of salt and water, and diltiazem (calcium channel antagonist) to reduce heart rate and induce myocardial relaxation. It is common practice to continue their administration prior to the anesthetic procedure. If hypotension develops, vasopressors such as phenylephrine (0.25–0.5 μg/kg/minute) may be infused to effect
- Use of inotropes (e.g. dobutamine) to increase myocardial contractility is controversial as this may increase myocardial oxygen consumption and worsen DOLVET
- An inhibitor of sarcomere contractility (MYK-461) has been tested in the laboratory setting in cats with HCM and left-ventricular outflow obstruction. Reduction of contractility eliminated systolic anterior motion of the mitral valve and decreased pressure gradients in a concentration-dependent manner. This may be a therapeutic option in the future

---

Box 9.4: Anesthetic management of cats with HCM

The challenge of anesthesia in cats with HCM: *The goal is to maximize diastolic function and minimize myocardial oxygen consumption by inducing mild decreases in heart rate, and to allow adequate coronary perfusion with appropriate cardiac output.* Tachycardia must be avoided by all possible means because it reduces end-diastolic ventricular volume and does not allow time for adequate diastolic filling. A low heart rate is much preferred over tachycardia.

Neuroanesthesia

General Considerations

The blood-brain barrier is disrupted by inflammation, trauma and acute hypertension. Central nervous system (CNS) injury may lead to hypoxia, hypercapnia, hypoglycemia, hypotension, cerebral arterial spasm and transtentorial or cerebellar herniation. Blood flow and autoregulation can be severely affected and changes in flow-metabolism coupling may occur. In addition, anesthetic and sedative drugs may contribute to significant physiological changes. In normal conditions, *autoregulation* maintains constant cerebral blood flow (CBF) over a range of cerebral perfusion pressure (CPP) between 50–150 mmHg (Chapter 2). This complex integration of perfusion pressure, vascular resistance, and flow is described in *Box* 9.5. Cats with CNS injury can easily decompensate during anesthesia (*Figure* 9.4).

Box 9.5: Integration of cerebral perfusion pressure, vascular resistance and flow

Cerebral blood flow (CBF) is dependent on cerebral perfusion pressure (CPP) and cerebral vascular resistance (CVR) (CPP = CPP/CVR). CPP is dependent on mean blood pressure (MAP) and intracranial pressure (ICP) (CPP = MAP − ICC). Under clinical conditions, the anesthetist can only monitor MAP to predict changes in ICP and CPP, and ultimately CBF. CPP should be maintained around 70 mmHg in patients with a space-occupying lesion or head trauma; this correlates with a MAP of 80 mmHg. Increased ICC leads to hypertension and reflex bradycardia (Cushing's reflex), and changes in respiratory pattern (Cheyne–Stokes breathing).

Anesthetic Management

Anesthesia for patients with traumatic brain injury (TBI), space-occupying lesions, and during neurosurgery, should *optimize CBF and cerebral perfusion while minimizing increases in intracranial pressure (ICP)* (*Box* 9.6).

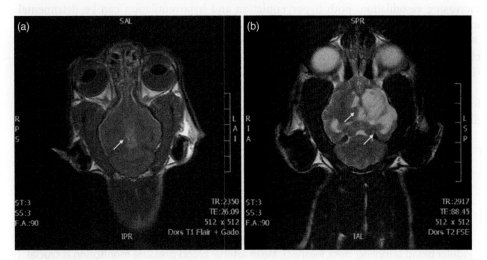

Figure 9.4 Magnetic resonance imaging in two cats. (a) A T1 flair dorsal sequence after administration of gadolinium. Necropsy revealed a meningioma of the third ventricle (area of the hippocampus, thalamus, and part of the cerebellum), and an adenocarcinoma in the frontal sinus. The image shows a 12 × 7.5 × 5 mm multilobed, well defined structure (white arrow) with areas of enhancement and meningitis after administration of gadolinium. Such patients are at risk of brain herniation during anesthesia. This may also occur after traumatic brain injury (e.g. intracranial bleeding). (b) Ischemic brain injury of the left cerebral hemisphere in a cat. There is hyperintensity (white arrow) of the rostrolateral part of the left temporal and frontal lobe, mainly in the cortical region.

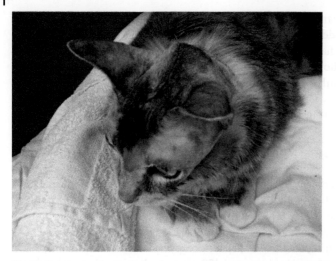

Figure 9.5 A cat recovering from surgery after removal of a meningioma.

Cerebral blood flow is altered by changes in partial pressures of carbon dioxide and oxygen in blood ($PaCO_2$ and PaO_2, respectively) (Chapter 2). Hypercapnia affects CBF via pH-dependent changes in extracellular fluid in the brain resulting in cerebral vasodilation. This vasodilation is induced by nitric oxide and prostaglandin release. Hypocapnia causes cerebral vasoconstriction and reduces CBF. Severe vasoconstriction can lead to neuronal death and deteriorating neurological function. Increases in $PaCO_2$ produce linearly increasing vasodilation. Both hyperventilation and hypoventilation can be detrimental in patients with head trauma. For this reason, $PaCO_2$ should be maintained between 30–33 mmHg using intermittent positive pressure ventilation (IPPV). The response to changes in PaO_2 is less dramatic because cerebral vasodilation occurs only with hypoxemia ($PaO_2 < 60$ mmHg). After TBI, oxygen should be administered to prevent hypoxemia.

General anesthesia may be required for decompression of the cranium after head trauma, for shunt placement in hydrocephalus, for diagnostic imaging such as MRI in intracranial disease and idiopathic epilepsy, and for surgical interventions for tumor removal (*Figure 9.5*).

Box 9.6: Goals of neuroanesthesia

The aim during neuroanesthesia is to maintain cerebral perfusion pressure and autoregulation. This dictates adequate ventilation, appropriate venous drainage, hemodynamic stability, as well as reduction of intracranial pressure (ICP) and cerebral metabolic rate while avoiding sudden increases in ICP (coughing during intubation, jugular blood sampling, neck leashes). Mean arterial blood pressure monitoring is crucial in these patients. Cerebral vasoconstriction leads to decreased oxygen demand and ICP; vasodilation has the opposite effect.

- Intravenous opioids alone are normally administered for sedation. Vomiting should be avoided to prevent any increases in ICP. Butorphanol, methadone, and buprenorphine are drugs of choice, and the precise choice depends on the invasiveness of the procedure. Maropitant (1.0 mg/kg SC or IV) will prevent vomiting and can be included in the anesthetic protocol

- Short-acting agonists of μ-opioid receptors (e.g. fentanyl) are administered to prevent increases in ICP in response to surgical stimulation. Opioid infusions can be stopped or adjusted to effect to minimize impairment of neurological function and allow assessment of function. Doses should be adjusted to avoid respiratory depression and increased $PaCO_2$
- Drugs causing cerebral vasodilation such as acepromazine and calcium channel blockers are best avoided. Volatile anesthetics cause vasodilation and should be used cautiously
- Anesthesia is best induced with alfaxalone, propofol or barbiturates, and maintained using propofol or alfaxalone and mechanical ventilation for critical cases. Anesthetic maintenance with propofol may lead to prolonged recoveries. An intravenous bolus of lidocaine (1 mg/kg) has been advocated to minimize coughing during endotracheal intubation
- Use of ketamine for neuroanesthesia is controversial (*Box* 9.7)
- Hypothermia, by decreasing metabolic rate and release of glutamate, has been employed for neuroprotection. Other therapies and maneuvers to decrease ICP include appropriate head positioning, care to avoid jugular occlusion, administration of mannitol (0.5–1 g/kg) and hypertonic saline (2–3 mL/kg), as well as adequate fluid administration to improve rheology and optimize tissue oxygen delivery

---

Box 9.7: The use of ketamine in neuroanesthesia

Ketamine has historically been contraindicated in dogs and cats with traumatic brain injury due to the likelihood of increasing ICP and seizure activity. Recent studies show that subanesthetic doses of ketamine may in fact have neuroprotective effects against ischemic and glutamate-induced brain injury because NMDA receptors are stimulated during brain injury. Other studies reported that low doses of ketamine (1 mg/kg) did not increase ICP. However, controversy remains, and anesthetic doses of ketamine are rarely given to patients with increased ICP since sympathetic activation could increase MAP, CBF, and CPP, potentially increasing ICP.

Diaphragmatic Rupture

General Considerations

Diaphragmatic rupture is caused by trauma, including high-rise syndrome or attacks by dogs (Chapter 10). This can cause significant morbidity and mortality in cats; trauma per se is associated with multiple fractures and organ rupture (i.e. spleen or bladder). Organs that are commonly displaced into the thoracic cavity include liver, stomach, and small intestines. Physical examination will detect areas of borborygmi or silence on thoracic auscultation and the abdomen may feel empty when palpated. Patient stabilization should address decompensation of the cardiorespiratory system.

A list of problems is described below, and their significance will depend on the severity of the clinical signs.

- Respiratory distress and tachypnea
- Lung collapse and pleural effusion
- Hypoxemia
- Cardiovascular collapse
- Decreased venous return, hypotension, and poor tissue delivery
- Strangulated viscera with tissue necrosis and pain
- Hypothermia
- Release of endotoxins and re-expansion pulmonary edema

A stepwise approach for patient stabilization includes administration of 100% oxygen, fluid therapy, administration of analgesics and further diagnosis with laboratory and radiographic examination.

Anesthetic Management

Stress-free handling and induction is paramount in these cases. Cats should be allowed to stay in sternal recumbency or to simply sit; in some cases, holding them in a standing position relieves respiratory distress. Radiographs should not be performed with the cat in dorsal recumbency. Reverse Trendelenburg position may help in cases of respiratory distress.

- Drugs with minimal impact on cardiorespiratory function should be used (e.g. midazolam, opioids). Preoxygenation can be provided gently without stress to the cat (*Figure* 9.6)
- Sedation and pain management are initially addressed by administration of opioids. The IV route is preferred once a catheter has been placed. The choice of opioid drug will depend on the degree of pain, and whether there has been multiple trauma (Chapter 13)
- In the perioperative period, balanced anesthesia should be employed, including administration of opioids and ketamine infusions. Intercostal blocks are used if a thoracic drain is placed and if there is thoracic trauma (e.g. fractured ribs)
- Rapid intubation and initiation of IPPV is recommended. Ventilation should be gentle, with low inflation pressure (12–15 mmHg) and inspiratory flow rate, since re-expansion pulmonary edema is a potential complication. Attempts to reinflate atelectic lung tissue should be avoided as these will re-expand postoperatively once the integrity of the thoracic cavity is restored
- Airway obstruction (Chapter 10) can occur if the endotracheal tube becomes filled with blood and debris; in this scenario, increased resistance to breathing and hypercapnia will develop and the tube should be replaced
- Mortality may be up to 20% after diaphragmatic hernia repair in cats. Postoperative care is of major importance in these cases. Mortality usually correlates with other complications and concurrent injuries
- Interpleural anesthesia with bupivacaine (2 mg/kg) can be administered via the thoracic drain for up to 96 hours after surgery. The thoracic drain is flushed with sterile saline 0.9% (same volume as bupivacaine) to deposit the local anesthetic within the thoracic cavity. Postoperatively cats are ideally placed in an oxygen cage where pulse oximetry can be used and inspired oxygen concentrations monitored

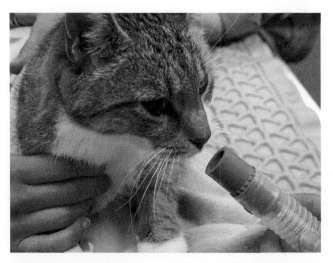

Figure 9.6 Preoxygenation in a cat before induction of anesthesia.

Gastrointestinal Emergencies

General Considerations

Emergency abdominal surgery is required to treat a range of conditions including intestinal obstruction (foreign body, intussusception, neoplasia, megacolon), gastrointestinal (GI) ulceration, uroabdomen (see urinary obstruction and uroabdomen). Complications include fluid losses (vomiting and diarrhea, and changes in fluid distribution), proliferation of intestinal bacteria and secondary intestinal inflammation, GI perforation, peritonitis, systemic inflammatory response syndrome (SIRS), sepsis, severe hypotension, hypovolemia, and shock.

Clinical findings are variable but tachycardia is observed in hypovolemic patients. Bradycardia may be observed in cats with increased vagal tone. The list of problems includes:

- Hyperthermia or hypothermia, electrolyte imbalance, and acid-base abnormalities
- Hypochloremia, hypokalemia, hypoglycemia, and hyperlactatemia are common, but fluid imbalance will vary with the condition (vomiting versus diarrhea, dehydration, hypovolemia, septic versus nonseptic)
- Cats presenting for this type of surgery are usually critically ill and should be stabilized with appropriate fluid therapy (Chapter 8) using crystalloid and colloid solutions. Electrolyte imbalance should be addressed accordingly, and antibiotics should be administered when the intestinal wall is damaged and if bacteremia and septicemia have developed
- Hypotension should ideally be treated before general anesthesia but this is not always possible. Colloid or hypertonic saline can be given IV immediately before induction to restore the circulating blood volume at least briefly

• Hypothermia is potentially harmful (Chapter 10) and every attempt should be made to rewarm the cat during stabilization

Anesthetic Management

Drugs with minimal impact on cardiorespiratory function should be used (e.g. midazolam, opioids, ketamine). Ketamine may be beneficial because of its sympathomimetic, NMDA antagonist, anti-inflammatory, and anti-endotoxic properties (Chapter 4). The combination of ketamine and midazolam is sufficient for induction of anesthesia, and will increase heart rate and blood pressure. If cats are normotensive, propofol and alfaxalone are good alternatives. Regurgitation followed by aspiration pneumonia is a common complication after induction of anesthesia (Chapter 10). The cat should remain in sternal recumbency throughout induction and intubation until the airway is secured. Suction should be available and a stomach tube can be used after intubation to empty GI contents.

Severe abdominal pain is treated with opioid and ketamine infusions because NSAIDs are generally contraindicated (Chapter 13). Intraperitoneal bupivacaine (2 mg/kg) (Chapter 5) is recommended at the end of the surgery as it provides postoperative analgesia for up to 8 hours. Epidural anesthesia (morphine ± local anesthetic) for abdominal analgesia is an option once hypovolemia and cardiovascular collapse have been treated (Chapter 5). Administration of colloids is particularly important if protein-losing enteropathy occurs and hypoproteinemia has developed. Early postoperative management addresses oxygenation, analgesic requirements, urine output, nausea, vomiting, appetite, laboratory monitoring, and nutrition. Measurement of lactate concentration may guide prognosis.

Idiopathic Hepatic Lipidosis

General Considerations

Hepatic lipidosis is a hepatobiliary disease commonly associated with inappetence and poor nutrition in cats. Successful treatment requires nutritional support, and anesthesia is typically required for feeding tube placement (i.e. percutaneous endoscopic gastrostomy (PEG) or esophagostomy tube). Cats with lipidosis may develop a range of effects (from behavioral changes to hepatic encephalopathy and coma). These cats may be obese but some will present with severe weight loss, dehydration, vomiting and diarrhea, predisposing them to hypothermia. Correction of dehydration and electrolyte disorders is highly recommended prior to general anesthesia for tube-placement surgery. Hypokalemia is common due to anorexia, and anemia, hypoproteinemia, hypoglycemia, and coagulation disorders are often a consequence of liver failure.

Anesthetic Management

The goals of anesthetic management are described in *Box* 9.8.

Box 9.8: Anesthesia for cats with hepatic lipidosis

Management of anesthesia in patients with idiopathic hepatic lipidosis should maintain hepatic blood flow while drugs requiring *hepatic metabolism* are avoided (i.e. acepromazine, agonists of α_2-adrenergic receptors, benzodiazepines, and alfaxalone). Cats with hepatopathy have altered pharmacokinetics, and general anesthetics should be given slowly to effect. Preference is given to short-acting drugs, which can be antagonized. Hypothermia is a particular concern in these cases.

Anesthetic management incorporates administration of low doses of short-acting opioids (e.g. fentanyl) for premedication. Methadone, buprenorphine, hydromorphone, and butorphanol are all acceptable, and choice depends on the proposed surgical or medical procedure. Cats generally have low glucuronidation potential, and when coupled with hepatic disease, metabolism of phenolic compounds such as propofol may be slow, increasing oxidative stress of feline red blood cells and formation of Heinz bodies. However, this is probably of concern *only* with repeated and daily injections of propofol at high doses. Propofol is a suitable anesthetic for cats with primary hepatic lipidosis undergoing feeding tube placement. Administration of NSAIDs is contraindicated since these drugs are metabolized in the liver. Anesthesia is maintained with either isoflurane or sevoflurane, which undergo little or no hepatic metabolism. Fluid therapy should be adjusted to avoid hemodilution in anemic cats.

Diabetes Mellitus

General Considerations

Cats with diabetes mellitus may require anesthesia for procedures unrelated to the disease. Type II diabetes is the most common in cats, with decreased insulin secretion and sensitivity (insulin resistance). This results in increased serum glucose levels and more than 50% of these cats require exogenous insulin administration. Geriatric male cats are commonly affected. Clinical signs include polyuria, polydipsia, polyphagia, and weight loss. Patient hydration and serum-glucose concentration should be stabilized before general anesthesia except for emergency procedures. Laboratory findings include hypercholesterolemia and hypertriglyceridemia. Urine specific gravity is reduced due to hyperglycemia-induced osmotic diuresis.

Complications of diabetes mellitus can include diabetic neuropathy (Chapters 11, 14, and 15), hypertension, infection, and diabetic ketoacidosis (DKA). *Clinical presentation of peripheral neuropathy includes pain on manipulation of the distal limbs with signs of central sensitization and allodynia that are caused by ischemic episodes and demyelination.* In most of these cases, anesthesia is uneventful, however DKA may occur in poorly controlled diabetes leading to severe dehydration, metabolic acidosis, hypokalemia, and cardiovascular collapse, and it is one of the main concerns in the postoperative period. These cats should be monitored for ketonuria.

Anesthetic Management

Anesthetic protocols will generally be based on individual requirements, health status, and the proposed procedure. Opioids and local anesthetic techniques blunt physiological stress response to surgery and anesthesia, and should prevent intraoperative hyperglycemia. Use of dexmedetomidine or other agonists of α_2-adrenergic receptors is controversial since these drugs inhibit insulin release, and themselves induce hyperglycemia and osmotic diuresis. Ketamine may have an indirect effect on serum glucose concentrations due to its sympathomimetic effects.

Fasting should be limited to 2–4 hours since it can influence insulin requirements. Water is provided *ad libitum*. The anesthetic procedure should be scheduled in the morning to facilitate convenient glucose monitoring and potential insulin therapy. The protocol for insulin administration is also controversial in cats with diabetes mellitus. The following is a suggestion:

- Half-dose of insulin is administered in the morning approximately 1–2 hours before the procedure
- The anesthetist can either administer a crystalloid solution with dextrose 2.5% if the cat is hypoglycemic (≤ 150 mg/dL), or administer another half-dose of insulin if the cat is hyperglycemic (≥ 250 mg/dL) during anesthesia
- Glucose concentrations can be monitored throughout the procedure, or at least before extubation at the end of the procedure. Blood sampling should be from a dedicated IV catheter to avoid erroneous results when dextrose solutions are being administered IV
- An infusion of KCl at 0.25–0.5 mEq/kg/hour can be included for hypokalemic patients. Serum glucose concentrations should be monitored continually until the cat will eat

Other Conditions

Cesarean section is not as common a procedure in cats as it is in dogs. General considerations and anesthetic management of these cases are largely extrapolated from the canine literature. In brief, anesthetic drugs cross the placenta and will affect fetal physiology and health of the newborn kittens. Pregnancy-induced changes in maternal physiology such as slow gastric emptying, increased cardiac output and oxygen demand are similar in cats to other species (Chapter 10). Premedication with opioids is controversial due to the potential for respiratory depression in the kittens. However, opioids can be reversed with naloxone, and are important in maternal pain management. Given preoperatively they probably reduce requirements for volatile anesthetic, which improves kitten vigor at birth. In general, preoxygenation is recommended followed by induction with propofol or alfaxalone, and maintenance with volatile anesthetics. This protocol has minimal effect on the new born kittens. Epidural anesthesia minimizes isoflurane requirements, and is an excellent choice for perioperative pain relief because it does not produce cardiorespiratory depression. A protocol for neonatal resuscitation should be in place.

Anesthesia of cats with *oral and maxillofacial disorders* and *ophthalmic disease* is performed on a routine basis. Anesthetic management depends primarily on patient health status and concomitant diseases. Administration of neuromuscular blocking agents might be required to obtain a central eye position and ventilation is mandatory if they are used. Potential hazards of vagal simulation during ophthalmic surgery and any systemic effects of topical drugs such as catecholamines are described in Chapter 10. Local anesthetic techniques are employed unless contraindicated (Chapter 5). A multimodal approach with opioids and NSAIDs is strongly recommended (Chapter 13).

Further Reading

Cooper, E. S. (2015) Controversies in the management of feline urethral obstruction. *Journal of Veterinary Emergency and Critical Care* **25**, 130–137.

Costello, M. F., Drobatz, K. J., Aronson, L. R., *et al.* (2004) Underlying cause, pathophysiologic abnormalities, and response to treatment in cats with septic peritonitis: 51 cases (1990–2001). *Journal of the American Veterinary Medical Association* **225**, 897–902.

Cunha, M. G., Freitas, G. C., Carregaro, A. B., *et al.* (2010) Renal and cardiorespiratory effects of treatment with lactated Ringer's solution or physiologic saline (0.9% NaCl) solution in cats with experimentally induced urethral obstruction. *American Journal of Veterinary Research* **71**, 840–846.

Garosi, L., and Adamantos, S. (2011) Head trauma in the cat: 2. Assessment and management of traumatic brain injury. *Journal of Feline Medicine and Surgery* **13**, 815–823.

Gowan, R. A., Baral, R. M., Lingard, A. E., *et al.* (2012) A retrospective analysis of the effects of meloxicam on the longevity of aged cats with and without overt chronic kidney disease. *Journal of Feline Medicine and Surgery* **14**, 876–881.

Lamont, L. A., Bulmer, B. J., Sisson, D. D., *et al.* (2002) Doppler echocardiographic effects of medetomidine on dynamic left ventricular outflow tract obstruction in cats. *Journal of the American Veterinary Medical Association* **221**, 1276–1281.

Marks, S. L., Straeter-Knowlen, I. M., Moore, M., *et al.* (1996) Effects of acepromazine maleate and phenoxybenzamine on urethral pressure profiles of anesthetized, healthy, sexually intact male cats. *American Journal of Veterinary Research* **57**, 1497–1500.

O'Hearn, A. K., and Wright, B. D. (2011) Coccygeal epidural with local anesthetic for catheterization and pain management in the treatment of feline urethral obstruction. *Journal of Veterinary Emergency and Critical Care* **21**, 50–52.

Pascoe, P. J., Ilkiw, J. E., and Pypendop, B. H. (2006) Effects of increasing infusion rates of dopamine, dobutamine, epinephrine, and phenylephrine in healthy anesthetized cats. *American Journal of Veterinary Research* **67**, 1491–1499.

Payne, J. R., Brodbelt, D. C., and Luis Fuentes, V. (2015) Cardiomyopathy prevalence in 780 apparently healthy cats in rehoming centres (the CatScan study). *Journal of Veterinary Cardiology* **1**, S244–S257.

Posner, L. P., Asakawa, M., and Erb, H. N. (2008) Use of propofol for anesthesia in cats with primary hepatic lipidosis: 44 cases (1995–2004). *Journal of the American Veterinary Medical Association* **232**, 1841–1843.

Reimer, S. B., Kyles, A. E., Filipowicz, D. E., *et al.* (2004) Long-term outcome of cats treated conservatively or surgically for peritoneopericardial diaphragmatic hernia: 66

cases (1987–2002). *Journal of the American Veterinary Medical Association* **224**, 728–732.

Rush, J. E., Freeman, L. M., Fenollosa, N. K., *et al.* (2002) Population and survival characteristics of cats with hypertrophic cardiomyopathy: 260 cases (1990–1999). *Journal of the American Veterinary Medical Association* **220**, 202–207.

Schmiedt, C. W., Tobias, K. M., and Stevenson, M. A. (2003) Traumatic diaphragmatic hernia in cats: 34 cases (1991–2001). *Journal of the American Veterinary Medical Association* **222**, 1237–1240.

Sparkes, A. H., Caney, S., Chalhoub, S., *et al.* (2016) ISFM consensus guidelines on the diagnosis and management of feline chronic kidney disease. *Journal of Feline Medicine and Surgery* **18**, 219–239.

Stern, J. A., Markova, S., Ueda, Y., *et al.* (2016) A small molecule inhibitor of sarcomere contractility acutely relieves left ventricular outflow tract obstruction in feline hypertrophic cardiomyopathy. *PlosOne* **11**, e0168407.

Wiese, A. J., Barter, L. S., Ilkiw, J. E., *et al.* (2012) Cardiovascular and respiratory effects of incremental doses of dopamine and phenylephrine in the management of isoflurane-induced hypotension in cats with hypertrophic cardiomyopathy. *American Journal of Veterinary Research* **73**, 908–916.

10

Anesthetic Complications

Polly Taylor[1] and Sheilah Robertson[2]

[1]Taylor Monroe, Little Downham, Ely, United Kingdom
[2]Lap of Love Veterinary Hospice, Lutz, FL, United States

Key Points

- Anesthesia always has the potential to cause death or morbidity, particularly in high-risk cases. Good preparation reduces these to a minimum
- Cats have unique characteristics, which may lead to complications: Small size; unique metabolism and temperament; potential for airway trauma, fluid overload, and hypothermia; undiagnosed HCM
- Mishaps with airway management are a common cause of anesthetic complications in cats
- Inadequate respiration has many causes; if detected early this is usually straightforward to treat
- Failure of the circulation, whatever the cause, is always a serious and life-threatening complication
- Hypothermia is common in cats; it is easier to prevent than to treat
- A protocol for cardiopulmonary resuscitation should be planned and described on a simple wall chart anywhere that sedation or anesthesia is performed

Introduction

In 1990, a survey of anesthesia in small animal practice in the United Kingdom reported that around one in 500 healthy cats and one in 30 sick cats died during or just after anesthesia. Many of these deaths occurred when the animals were not being monitored, particularly during recovery. Almost 20 years later a much larger study, the Confidential Enquiry into Perioperative Small Animal Fatalities (CEPSAF) reported an overall mortality rate associated with anesthesia and sedation of approximately one in 1000 healthy cats. This mortality rate remains similar in smaller but more recent studies (Chapter 1). Although the risk of anesthetic mortality in cats has improved, it is higher than in dogs and the complications arising from feline anesthesia are not trivial. According to the CEPSAF study, increased risk of mortality in cats was associated with:

- Poor health status
- Increasing age

Feline Anesthesia and Pain Management, First Edition. Edited by Paulo Steagall, Sheilah Robertson and Polly Taylor.
© 2018 John Wiley & Sons, Inc. Published 2018 by John Wiley & Sons, Inc.

- Extremes of body weight
- Emergency or complex surgery
- Endotracheal intubation
- Fluid therapy

Monitoring the pulse and using pulse oximetry decreased the risk. Of note, 60% of feline deaths occurred in the postanesthetic period, the majority of these in the first three hours.

Adverse events are more difficult to document because there are no universal definitions nor mandatory reporting in veterinary medicine. According to a recent report adverse events occur in approximately 35% of feline anesthetics. These include but are not limited to arousal, hypoventilation, desaturation, hypotension, hypertension, dysrhythmias, hyperthermia, hypothermia, airway complications, and excitation during recovery.

There is no doubt that prevention is better than cure; many complications can be prevented or at least made manageable if procedure-related problems are anticipated and careful preparation made before induction of anesthesia (*Box* 10.1). It is now well established that the preoperative check list prevents complications resulting from human error and a simple system adapted for each clinic should be used as described in Chapter 1. Thereafter constant observation throughout the course of anesthesia and recovery has been shown to reduce the risk of mortality.

Box 10.1: Prevention is always better than intervention

- Assign anesthetic risk
- Use check lists
- Monitor during anesthesia
- Monitor during recovery at least until the cat is sitting up and the temperature is normal

---

Allocation of anesthetic risk (ASA status, Chapter 1) is not just an academic exercise. It alerts the anesthetist to the likelihood of complications developing, and focuses the preparation for a specific procedure onto the most appropriate anesthetic and analgesic protocols, supportive equipment, and expertise required. Since the evidence shows that high risk cats are more likely to die or to develop serious complications than healthy cats, they warrant particularly careful preanesthetic preparation and perianesthetic monitoring. This includes the very thin or fat, very young or old, cats with comorbidities (e.g. hyperthyroidism or diabetes mellitus; Chapter 9), emergency or trauma cases as well as the sick cat.

The cat has unique physiological characteristics that lead to their own particular problems during anesthesia.

- Cats have a unique temperament and, as described in Chapter 1, stress, fear, and anxiety coupled with inappropriate handling may lead to stormy induction of anesthesia, and difficult maintenance and recovery
- Use of feline-friendly handling techniques (Chapter 1) contributes positively to reducing anesthetic complications

- Among the domestic species most commonly treated the cat is surprisingly small; a 5 kg dog is a small dog, but a 5 kg cat is a large cat. This feature may be inadvertently overlooked and lead to use of inappropriately large equipment, overvigorous manipulation, and to drug overdose and fluid overload
- Failure to make allowance for the feline deficiencies in metabolism of some drug groups (Chapter 2) will also contribute to perioperative complications

Complications are less likely to occur if vital functions and equipment are frequently and systematically checked (*Box* 10.2).

Box 10.2: Top priorities to prevent complications

Check:

- Airway
- Breathing
- Circulation
- Temperature
- Positioning
- Equipment

Airway Management

The cat has a small and delicate airway, and the larynx and trachea are easily damaged by overvigorous intubation. The small diameter of the trachea makes it vulnerable to blockage by low surface tension fluids and relatively small objects such as pieces of food or mucus. A small amount of swelling will have a significant effect on airway diameter. The cat also has a well developed laryngeal reflex, which may lead to laryngeal spasm if inappropriately stimulated (*Box* 10.3). Airway trauma and its consequences account for a significant proportion of anesthetic-related mortality and morbidity in cats, and feature high on the list of common claims against malpractice. The CEPSAF study identified endotracheal intubation as a factor associated with an increased risk of anesthetic death especially when procedures were short (< 30 minutes). Clearly the cat's larynx and trachea are easily damaged and should be treated gently.

Maintenance of a clear airway is essential. Complete obstruction rapidly causes death through hypoxia. Partial obstruction is more common and causes insidious respiratory insufficiency leading to hypercapnia and hypoxia. In a conscious cat this often leads to panic, increased oxygen demand, more respiratory effort, and a vicious cycle of worsening obstruction. During anesthesia, a partially obstructed airway leads to labored attempts to breathe so that it may appear as though anesthesia is too light. This may progress to shallow breathing, and even apnea, particularly during deep anesthesia. Careful frequent and regular monitoring (Chapter 7) should detect a change in respiratory effort and pattern and prompt investigation of the cause and subsequent appropriate action.

The unprotected airway may be obstructed by fluids such as saliva, blood, flushing fluids or gastrointestinal contents. Low surface-tension fluids, such as saliva and mucus may produce bubbles big enough to block the trachea of a small cat completely.

Box 10.3: Laryngospasm

- The cat has a well developed protective laryngeal reflex (Chapter 2)
- Spasm is easily provoked at intubation
- Spasm is more likely if anesthesia is too light
- Spasm is more likely if the larynx is already inflamed (pre-existing disease or injury)
- May be triggered when the tube is removed (especially if the tube is not removed before swallowing and coughing occur)
- Good practice to remove the tube while the cat is still well anesthetized:
  - Tube is more easily replaced if a problem occurs
  - Less likely to trigger spasm
  - The cat should be carefully observed until fully conscious

Treatment of laryngeal spasm

Immediate remedial action is essential for laryngeal spasm that does not relax within 10 to 20 seconds.

- The larynx must not be stimulated further - no further attempts to intubate should be made (Some serious medical accidents at intubation have been associated with failure to *stop* trying to intubate as this has made the situation worse)
- Oxygen should be given by mask or "flow-by" (the patient end of the breathing circuit is placed close to the cat's nose) so that any gas able to enter the trachea is oxygen-enriched
- More local anesthetic may exacerbate the problem. It should be used if none has already been tried
- If the obstruction is incomplete, spasm may be resolved if:
  - anesthesia is deepened
  - extra time is allowed
- If obstruction is complete or it does not resolve spontaneously:
  - IV muscle relaxant (e.g. atracurium 0.2 mg/kg) if immediately available
  - NB: IPPV then required until spontaneous respiration is restored
  - No guarantee that spasm will not reoccur when anesthesia lightens, and the tube is removed

If all else fails, a temporary airway can be provided with a large (14-G) needle or catheter placed percutaneously between two tracheal rings (a tracheotomy can be performed but these are extremely difficult to manage in cats, and are best avoided if possible)

Anticholinergics, although no longer routinely used in premedication may help to prevent an excessive volume of saliva in the mouth, but may be detrimental by making it more viscous. Anticholinergic premedication may be beneficial in some cases and should be chosen on a case-by-case basis (Chapter 3). If a cat is not intubated or a supraglottic airway device (SGAD) is not used, it is important to keep the cat's head and neck extended to prevent airway obstruction. Brachycephalic cats should always have a protected airway.

Vomiting and inhalation of stomach contents may occur both at induction and intubation, as well as when the tube is removed at the end of the procedure. It is probably more likely to occur if intubation and tube removal are attempted during very light anesthesia. Pieces of food can cause complete obstruction and rapid death unless the obstruction is removed very quickly. If there is any likelihood that the cat has a full stomach extreme care is required to ensure that *vomitus* is not aspirated; all equipment to deal with this event should be set up ready for use. Regurgitation and gastroesophageal reflux are common complications in cats undergoing abdominal laparotomy for foreign body removal or intestinal obstruction. They should be quickly intubated after anesthetic induction. In addition, vomiting at induction or extubation may occur in queens presenting for cesarean section, even if they have been fasted, as stomach emptying is delayed close to parturition. This problem can also occur in greedy cats who had food withheld for surgery but escaped and gorged on anything they could find (without the owner's knowledge) before presentation at the clinic.

- If vomiting does occur it is more easily managed if anesthesia is maintained, or even deepened. This reduces the likelihood of more vomiting, and allows any obstruction to be removed without causing gagging or struggling
- It is helpful to hold the cat's head lower than the body (i.e. off the edge of the table) to let gravity empty the mouth and make aspiration less likely
- Mechanical suction or a large syringe can be attached to a urinary catheter, esophageal feeding tube or "whistle-tip" suction catheter to clear the airway. Q-tips and small crocodile forceps that fit into the oropharynx and trachea are all valuable aids to rapid clearance of the obstruction
- If agonists of α_2-adrenergic receptors are used as part of the anesthetic protocol, ondansetron has been shown to decrease vomiting associated with dexmedetomidine, but they must be given together; the effect is not seen if ondansetron is given first
- In high-risk cases, maropitant can be given 45–60 minutes before induction

Acute effects of vomiting at induction relate primarily to airway obstruction, but inhalation of stomach contents and bile into the lungs causes serious aspiration pneumonitis due to direct chemical damage. Subsequent bacterial growth and inflammatory response result in aspiration pneumonia. Aspiration may also occur as a result of gastroesophageal reflux occurring during anaesthesia without active vomiting. In a review of cats with aspiration pneumonia admitted to a referral center 11 of 28 had a history of recent anesthesia. Gastroesophageal reflux can result in esophagitis and esophageal stricture. Suctioning (*Figure* 10.1) and flushing of the esophagus with saline after a regurgitation or vomiting event may be performed but the benefits are uncertain.

Complications from Intubation

Although a tracheal tube should always be placed if there is any doubt about maintenance of the airway, endotracheal intubation is associated with an increased risk of mortality in cats (*Box* 10.4). Hence it may be better to use discretion and choose not to intubate for short, non-head-and-neck procedures in otherwise healthy animals undergoing injectable anesthesia. The cat has no excess pharyngeal tissue and generally maintains a good airway without an endotracheal tube; a mask can be used to administer

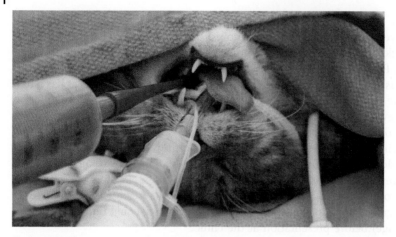

Figure 10.1 If regurgitation occurs the esophagus can be suctioned using a soft catheter (in this image a red rubber urethral catheter is being used) attached to a catheter tipped syringe. The esophagus can also be flushed with saline and suctioned with the same equipment. The endotracheal tube should be tested to verify an adequate seal prior to this procedure (Chapter 1).

oxygen and any inhaled anesthetic. Masks should be of appropriate size to prevent rebreathing and should be close fitting and well secured to prevent leakage of waste anesthetic gases (*Figure* 10.2).

Endotracheal intubation is the best way to ensure a clear airway as it less likely than an unprotected airway to be blocked with unwanted fluid or other debris. However, intubation does not guarantee a clear airway, as problems with the tube itself may occur (*Box* 10.4).

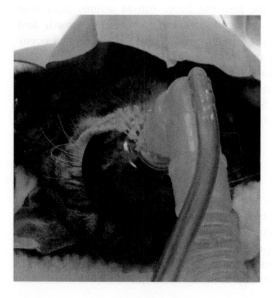

Figure 10.2 Face masks should be an appropriate size to prevent rebreathing and leakage of waste anesthetic gases.

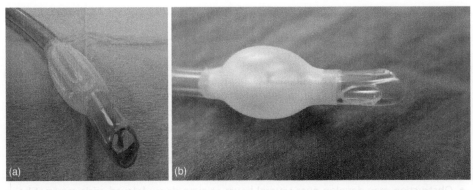

Figure 10.3 (a) The tip of an endotracheal tube can become partially or fully occluded by mucus and blood. (b) All endotracheal tubes should have a Murphy eye to allow an alternative route for passage of gases if the tip becomes occluded.

Box 10.4: Complications from endotracheal tubes

Blocked endotracheal tube

- Kinked tube
- Obstructed by malfunctioning cuffs
- Blocked with fluid (mucus, saliva, blood, lubricant gel)
  - The tube itself may be blocked by sticky secretions from airway infection (*Figure* 10.3a), which enter the tube during intubation and accumulate during anesthesia
  - Endotracheal tubes should always have a Murphy eye (*Figure* 10.3b) to provide an alternative gas route should the tip become blocked
- Inadvertent esophageal intubation
  - Oxygen and inhaled anesthetics are not directed into the lungs
  - Leads to hypoxemia because the cat is breathing air
  - Hypoxemia exacerbated by the gas-inflated stomach, pressing on the diaphragm and reducing lung volume
  - No uptake of inhaled anesthetics; the cat will not remain anesthetized
- Proper intubation should be verified immediately after intubation (Chapter 4). Capnography is very useful and considered the "gold standard" (Chapter 7)

Endotracheal tube lost in the trachea

- Endotracheal tube bitten off and the tip lost into the trachea
  - Occurs if anesthesia becomes too light or the tube is left in too long during recovery
  - No cat should be left unattended during recovery with an ETT in place
- Connector detached and the whole tube is lost in the trachea
  - Tight connector fit should be part of the preanesthetic equipment check
- The cat must be kept anesthetized or reanesthetized with an intravenous agent while the tube is retrieved. This may be possible with a laryngoscope and crocodile forceps, but if lost deep into the trachea will require a cat-sized endoscope and appropriate forceps

Box 10.4: (*Continued*)

Damage to pharynx, larynx, and trachea

- Caused by over vigorous intubation technique
- May lead to serious, often ultimately fatal complications
- Pharyngeal damage may be unnoticed at intubation, and manifest several days later as a necrotic retro-pharyngeal abscess. These are notoriously difficult to resolve, and are best prevented by using gentle intubation techniques (Chapter 1)
- Trauma-induced hemorrhage and disruption of normal anatomy may obstruct the airway
- Obstruction may develop over several hours or even days; delayed crisis may not be recognized as associated with anesthesia and intubation
- The "crackle cat" presents a few days (or even longer) after anesthesia
  - Usually associated with difficult intubation
  - Damage to the airway in the pharyngeal region or cervical trachea leads to escape of gas into the subcutaneous tissues. The gas accumulates subcutaneously and spreads progressively over most of the body so the cat "crackles" when it is handled
  - If the lesion resolves or is located and repaired, the gas will slowly be absorbed and the cat will return to normal
  - If the damage is associated with a pharyngeal abscess or a large tracheal tear the prognosis is guarded
  - Intrathoracic tracheal tears leading to a pneumothorax carry a worse prognosis and are more difficult to treat
- The trachea may be torn by over inflating the cuff
  - Large volume low pressure cuffs are less likely to tear the trachea than the low volume high pressure type
  - The cat is small, the volume within a so-called large-volume low- pressure cuff is still relatively small, and it is surprisingly easy to produce a high pressure. In this case the ensuing tear will be bigger (tears occur along the length of the cuff), and the prognosis more guarded
- Measuring the cuff pressure (Chapter 1) is the only reliable preventive measure

Tube too long (Chapter 1, *Figure* 1.4a, b, c)

- Tracheal tears
- Endobronchial intubation
  - Effectively removes the remaining lung tissue from gas exchange. Low SpO_2 detected immediately after intubation in a cat breathing oxygen enriched gas should always prompt a check on the ETT placement (using a laryngoscope). Breath sounds are heard equally on both sides of the thorax if the ETT is correctly placed.
- Increases airway dead space (excessive length of tube between teeth and breathing circuit)

Respiratory Insufficiency

Inadequate respiration, whatever the cause, leads to hypoxemia and hypercapnia (Chapter 7) (*Box* 10.5). Although a limited degree of either may be tolerated, both may lead to postoperative complications or death if prolonged or more severe. Inadequate ventilation should be detected by monitoring, and respiration supported as necessary.

Box 10.5: Causes of inadequate ventilation

- Anesthetic-induced respiratory depression
- Increased abdominal pressure restricting diaphragmatic movement:
  - Obesity, late pregnancy, ascites, abdominal mass; worse in dorsal recumbency
- Reduced lung volume:
  - Ruptured diaphragm (Chapter 9). Cats may present without history of trauma or signs of respiratory distress. Marked hypoxemia develops at induction when the cat's position is changed and abdominal viscera in the thorax compress the lungs and thoracic blood vessels. Labored respiration and desaturation should prompt re-evaluation of the cat's lung function, further investigation and a quick decision about the surgical plan
  - Pleural fluid or pneumothorax. Occasionally occurs in association with oesophageal or tracheal damage. Hypoxemia detected by pulse oximetry is often the first warning
  - Inadvertent pressure on the thorax from surgical assistants, instruments, heavy cloth drapes. Lightweight, transparent plastic drapes are better for cats
- Inadequate oxygen supply:
  - Air, 21% oxygen (inspired fraction of oxygen, $FiO_2 = 0.21$), is often inadequate with anesthetic-induced respiratory depression
  - Bronchial intubation
  - Inadvertent repositioning of the oxygen flow control or complete failure of the oxygen supply; rapidly fatal unless immediately detected. Increased risk of fatality if nitrous oxide is in use, as more difficult to detect immediately (still has gas to breathe, remains anesthetized, no immediate change in the respiratory pattern). Equipment without low oxygen alarms should *not* be used without other means of detecting oxygen supply failure (Chapter 6, 7)
  - Leak in the breathing system; entrains air, and delivers a lower FiO_2 than anticipated. Pulse oximetry detects hypoxemia but measurement of inspired oxygen concentration is needed to identify the cause (Chapter 6)
- Inadequate fresh gas flow rate:
  - Nonrebreathing circuits (Chapter 6) depend on sufficient flow rate to prevent rebreathing of CO_2 and consequent hypercapnia; most easily detected with capnography (Chapter 7)
- Breathing circuits inappropriate for cats (Chapter 6)

Hypoxemia

Severe hypoxemia will cause immediate death, and a hypoxic incident during anesthesia, whatever the etiology, is a well recognized cause of anesthetic death. Less marked hypoxemia may be insidious, and its effects only apparent during recovery when consciousness does not return as expected, or the cat exhibits neurological abnormalities once awake.

Hypoxemia is readily detected by pulse oximetry as described in Chapter 7; its use in conjunction with pulse monitoring reduces the risks of anesthetic-related mortality. Use of agonists of α_2-adrenergic receptors may lead to low or unobtainable pulse oximeter readings because of peripheral vasoconstriction without hypoxemia being present; however this is the only instance where low readings may not indicate a problem. Low pulse oximeter readings should always prompt immediate investigation (*Box* 10.6). It is of note that an anemic cat will not have low peripheral capillary oxygen saturation (SpO_2) if all the hemoglobin it has is fully saturated. However, oxygen delivery may still be inadequate because of low blood oxygen content. Management of these cases is described in Chapter 2 and 9.

Box 10.6: Troubleshooting a low pulse oximeter reading

When a low SpO_2 reading is noted it is vital to troubleshoot quickly. Check:

- Positioning and patency of the endotracheal tube or SGAD
- Hypoventilation, apnea
- Gas supply/breathing system disconnection
- Compression of the thorax/inappropriate thoracic expansion (e.g. external compression by surgery/surgeon)
- Fluid in the lungs? (e.g. aspiration pneumonia, inflammatory exudate)
- Pneumothorax or pleural fluid
- Device error; consider repositioning

Hypercapnia

Hypercapnia is less likely to be fatal than hypoxemia, and a limited increase in carbon dioxide (CO_2) tension from anesthetic-induced respiratory depression is very common during otherwise uneventful anesthesia. However prolonged or severe hypercapnia causes respiratory acidosis, which may lead to life-threatening sympathetic stimulation, organ malfunction, and hyperkalemia. Hypercapnia is almost impossible to detect under clinical conditions without measuring end-tidal CO_2 or blood gases (*Box* 10.7). Hypercapnia may be severe in a well oxygenated cat, making sudden deterioration because of acidosis appear unexpected. CO_2 at high concentrations (> 80 mmHg) produces narcosis and is additive to the inhalant agent, resulting in overdose. A very high inspired oxygen fraction leading to high arterial oxygen tension depresses respiration and increases hypercapnia; 100% oxygen is better replaced with oxygen-air mixtures, which are more physiological, but not yet commonly used in veterinary anesthesia.

Box 10.7: Troubleshooting high end-tidal concentrations of CO_2

When a high end-tidal CO_2 develops check:

- Positioning and patency of the endotracheal tube
- Any obstruction to expiration
- Dead space
- Depth of anesthesia
- Inspired oxygen fraction

Inadequate respiration may be caused by inappropriate use of anesthetic equipment, particularly when designed for larger animals. For instance, excessive suction on the waste gas scavenging system increases the work of breathing and prevents the cat from inhaling a sufficient tidal volume. The negative pressure in the thorax during inspiration increases as the cat tries to breathe against the suction system. Depending on the system design, air may be entrained, which might lead to inadequate inspired oxygen tension. However, the usual scenario from this system misuse is hypercapnia rather than hypoxemia.

Increased dead space leads to hypercapnia, and is present when unsuitably large circuits with large connectors are used as well as with an overlong endotracheal tube. Endotracheal tubes that are too long should not simply be advanced further as this may risk endobronchial intubation or tracheal damage. The tube should be premeasured and cut if needed (Chapter 1, *Figure* 1.4c).

In addition to dead space, rebreathing circuits designed for larger animals may have a heavy expiratory valve, which the cat's respiratory effort cannot operate. This exacerbates hypercapnia as the cat rebreathes from the expiratory side of the circuit and CO_2 is retained. Although rebreathing circuits are less commonly used in cats (Chapter 6), suitable smaller models are available (*Figure* 6.5b). The hazards of such systems recognized in other species may occur in cats, including exhausted absorbent and sticking valves, which will lead to hypercapnia. If 100% oxygen is the carrier gas, hypoxemia is unlikely to occur unless there is a leak in the system and the oxygen is diluted with air. Inhalation of absorbent crystals is another potential hazard of a rebreathing system. Although inhalation is rare, the crystals are irritants and may cause tracheal irritation or even erosion. Nonrebreathing systems are more commonly used in cats but if the oxygen flow rates are inadequate rebreathing will occur.

Circulation

Complications leading to failure of the circulation make a significant contribution to anesthetic mortality and morbidity (*Box* 10.8). Adequate delivery of oxygen to tissues depends on blood oxygen content and circulation. Circulatory failure, regardless of cause, leads to complications, which may be fatal, because the tissues do not receive sufficient oxygen and nutrients, nor are waste products removed.

Box 10.8: Diagnosing the cause of hypotension, pale mucous membranes, and decreased end-tidal carbon dioxide without hyperventilation

Check for:

- Hypovolemia
- Anesthetic overdose
- Hemorrhage
- Bradycardia
- Circulatory collapse

Hypovolemia

Low circulating volume affects tissue perfusion. Normal homeostatic compensation such as vasoconstriction is likely to be depressed by anesthetic agents, and hypotension results. Driving pressure for perfusion is lost and the microcirculation becomes inadequate to sustain normal organ function.

During anesthesia hypovolemia may develop insidiously through undetected and unmeasured hemorrhage. Slow venous and capillary ooze is deceptive and can lead to significant blood loss particularly during prolonged surgery. Crisis may occur apparently suddenly when tissue perfusion reaches a critical low point. Hemorrhage should always be monitored by counting swabs, measuring the volume collected in the suction bottle and by educated estimation of unknown volumes. Volume should be replaced as it is lost. Replacement fluids (crystalloids or colloids) may be sufficient for losses up to 10% (6 mL/kg) of the normal circulating volume (around 60 mL/kg) but blood or red blood cells should be used before 25% (15 mL/kg) has been lost (Chapter 8).

Pre-existing hypovolemia which was not detected from the history and preanesthetic examination may lead to a crisis at induction, as most anesthetics cause peripheral vasodilation; hypotension develops when compensatory vasoconstriction is suddenly lost at induction. Treatment is performed with rapid infusion of crystalloid or colloid fluids. Careful preoperative evaluation of the cat's fluid status and preoperative restoration of at least some of the circulating volume is the only way to prevent this complication of anesthesia.

Hypotension

Hypotension is very common in anesthetized cats and is usually defined in this species as a mean arterial pressure below 60 mmHg (Chapter 7). Blood pressure is relatively easy to measure by indirect methods in cats. Taking action when blood pressure is low or when it starts to decrease will prevent the deterioration in tissue perfusion that leads to perioperative complications. Noting the development of hypotension should prompt investigation of the cause, such as anesthetic overdose or hypovolemia, to guide treatment. Reduction in the inspired volatile agent concentration at this stage will often prevent a major crisis. Similarly, appropriate IV therapy is most effective if started before hypotension becomes severe; pre-existing dehydration, and hypovolemia should ideally be corrected before anesthesia.

Hypertension

Hypertension (systolic arterial pressure >160 mmHg) may be detected during anesthesia, and is most likely to be associated with renal disease, hyperthyroidism (Chapter 9) or administration of agonists of α_2-adrenergic receptors (Chapter 3). Detection of hypertension should prompt evaluation of these potential problems to allow appropriate treatment (Chapter 9).

Phenylephrine and epinephrine used topically during some ophthalmic procedures are absorbed systemically and may cause hypertension and dysrhythmias; this emphasizes the importance of communication between surgeon and anesthetist.

Cardiac Disease

Recent studies indicate that around 15–18% of cats have hypertrophic cardiomyopathy (HCM), and a significant proportion of these do not show any clinical signs and do not have a heart murmur. Hence some will go undetected at a preoperative examination and a crisis will occur when the symptom-free case is anesthetized. Echocardiography is currently the "gold standard" for diagnosis, however biomarkers such as NT-proBNP may prove to be valuable screening tools. Calm induction and immediate oxygenation is desirable for all cats, and should reduce the severity of any crisis in cats with undetected HCM. Careful and accurate administration of fluids is essential (Chapter 8, 9). Management of cats that have been diagnosed with HCM is described in Chapter 9.

Dysrhythmias

Bradydysrhythmias induced by agonists of α_2-adrenergic receptors are probably the most commonly encountered. The effect is critical when cardiac output and therefore tissue perfusion becomes inadequate. Treatment of bradycardia caused by these drugs with anticholinergics does not improve cardiac output but may be lifesaving if the rate approaches cardiac arrest (Chapter 3). Reversal with atipamezole is most appropriate for bradycardia induced by these drugs.

Bradycardia may develop for several reasons and should prompt investigation of all causes of circulatory and respiratory failure. Bradycardia often provides evidence of anesthetic overdose (or hypothermia), and should prompt reduction in inspired volatile agent concentration before circulatory failure occurs.

A vagal reflex from pressure on the eye, abdominal, especially intestinal and bladder surgery and direct vagal stimulation during neck surgery is serious and should prompt removal of the stimulus and administration of an anticholinergic agent.

Rising intrathoracic pressure induces a marked vagal response due to pulmonary stretching, and the brief period of bradycardia before cardiac arrest is a warning sign that immediate action to relieve the intrathoracic pressure is required. This is most commonly caused by complete closure of the expiratory arm of the breathing circuit, usually a closed pop-off (adjustable pressure limiting) valve. If the expiratory gas route is completely closed and the relatively high fresh gas flows required by a nonrebreathing circuit (multiples of the minute volume) are running, pressure in the breathing circuit and thorax builds up very quickly and causes cardiac arrest. Positive end expiratory pressure (PEEP) valves can be used to ensure this does not occur; when placed as shown in *Figure* 10.4 they act as anti-PEEP valves. Older T-piece circuits have only a waste gas tube attached on the expiratory port of the reservoir bag, which is easily twisted (*Figure* 10.5), particularly when the cat's position is changed or it is moved onto the operating table. Modern T-piece circuits (*Figure* 10.6) incorporate a relief valve, which, even if fully closed, opens at a pressure unlikely to cause lung damage.

Fluid Overload

The CEPSAF reported a fourfold increase in the odds of anesthetic death in cats given fluid therapy during anesthesia. This is presumably a result of fluid overload in an animal whose circulating blood volume is usually under 300 mL and appropriately low

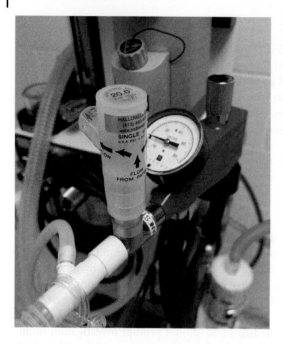

Figure 10.4 A 20 cm H_2O PEEP valve has been placed in the circuit to prevent development of excessive thoracic pressure when the expiratory port is closed or obstructed. When placed at this location it acts as an anti-PEEP valve. High intrathoracic pressures are often fatal, and may otherwise develop rapidly when flows appropriate for non rebreathing systems are in use.

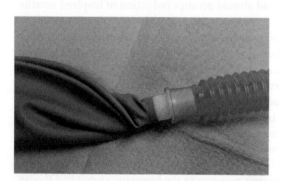

Figure 10.5 The reservoir bag can easily twist at the expiratory port in older T-piece circuits causing occlusion and a rapid increase in pressure.
Source: Courtesy of Patrick Burns.

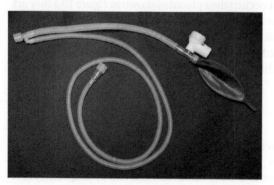

Figure 10.6 A relief valve is a built-in safety feature of newer T-piece circuits.

infusion rates are difficult to deliver accurately. The cat's circulating blood volume, even on a mL/kg basis, is considerably lower than the dog's, so the required lower infusion rates are in considerable contrast. In addition, cats with HCM (known or unknown) will not cope with excessive fluids (Chapter 9). The current American Animal Hospital Association (AAHA) fluid guidelines recommend 2–5 mL/kg/hour as maintenance rate during anesthesia. For accurate administration in the cat this requires a syringe pump or controlled infusion device (*Figure* 8.1a and *Figure* 8.1b). A buretrol (burette) where enough fluid for a predetermined time (e.g. one hour) can be used (*Figure* 8.1c).

Trauma

The anesthetized animal loses all protective reflexes and numerous forms of physical damage may occur during anesthesia. The cat is no exception, and being small may be particularly vulnerable. Burning from heating devices is probably the most frequently reported. Uncontrolled heat sources such as hot water bottles, wheat bags and electric blankets have all been reported to produce serious burns during anesthesia and should not be used (*Figure* 10.7). High-flow, low-pressure warm air heaters produce effective heating without causing skin damage, and can be used during and after anesthesia (*Figure* 10.8). It is imperative to use the correct blankets (which dissipate the heated air) recommended for these units and to ensure the nozzle of the hose and blanket are securely in place. Using just the end of the hose tucked under blankets or towels blows hot air directly on a small area of the patient and can cause severe focal burns.

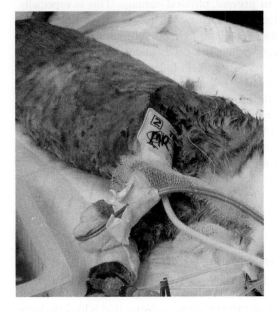

Figure 10.7 Electric blankets can cause serious burns.

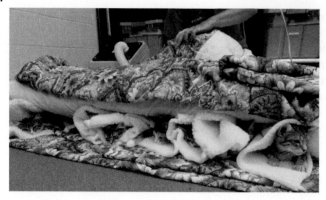

Figure 10.8 Forced warm air blankets provide a safe and effective source of heat.

The eyes are easily damaged when the palpebral reflex is absent, particularly by contact with the operating table, drapes and surgical scrub solution. Prevention of eye damage simply needs care in positioning and constant awareness of the potential hazard. Eye lubricant or corn oil (an inexpensive alternative) helps to protect the cornea from drying but does not protect against direct physical trauma. It is important not to touch the eye with the tip of lubricant tubes or bottles during application as this itself can cause damage but can also transmit infection between patients.

Rough handling as well as clumsy positioning and restraint for surgery can cause damage. Nerve damage is rare in cats as they do not have significant weight to compress dependent body parts; however, vigorous tying down of limbs may lead to neurological damage or swelling and loss of adequate blood flow distal to the tie. Common sense and gentle handling is all that is required to prevent physical damage. This is especially important in animals with degenerative joint disease who may suffer serious postoperative pain if positioned badly or placed on hard surfaces during anesthesia.

Venous access sites are easily damaged when the cat is unconscious. Inadvertent perivascular injection will occur if the catheter is dislodged during repositioning. Infusion sites should be examined regularly to ensure that infusions are genuinely being administered IV. At the very least the infusion should be stopped if administration has become perivascular, because this may cause local damage and will not give the intended benefit of IV administration. In critical cases a second IV catheter should be placed; this can be used if the first catheter fails or if blood products, which cannot be mixed with lactated Ringers solution are required.

Recovery

Airway Obstruction and Hypoxemia

All the potential hazards of anesthesia remain during recovery until the cat has regained consciousness. Airway obstruction is probably the greatest hazard; death during unobserved recovery was reported as a significant cause of mortality in the 1990 and CEPSAF reports of anesthetic death in small animals. Airway obstruction is likely to have been responsible for at least some of these. Close observation until the cat has reached a sternal position should ensure that any airway obstruction occurring during recovery will be spotted immediately and resolved appropriately. Hypoxemia may occur, particularly in the early stages when the cat is still quite deeply anesthetized but is now breathing room air. Oxygen by mask, oxygen cage, or nasal tube will resolve this. Cats that are shivering have increased oxygen requirements due to muscle activity and should receive supplemental oxygen until normothermic.

Postanesthetic Blindness

Postanesthetic blindness is an uncommon but well recognized complication, which is seen soon after the cat regains consciousness and may be temporary or permanent (Chapter 2). It is thought to be associated with a hypoxic or critical cardiovascular (ischemic) event during anesthesia and other neurological effects resulting from this may include altered mentation, head tilt, and ataxia. Post anesthetic blindness is a common sequel to successful cardiopulmonary resuscitation (CPR).

A more specific cause of post anesthetic blindness (unilateral or bilateral) is now recognized as a result of maxillary artery occlusion when a cat's mouth is open (Chapter 2) (*Figure* 10.9a). Spring loaded mouth gags and needle caps (42 mm) placed between the upper and lower canine teeth can alter blood flow in some cats (*Figure* 10.9b). Smaller (20 and 30 mm) plastic mouth gags have minimal effects; these can be made from needle caps or syringe barrels (*Figure* 10.9c). The cat's mouth should be opened only as far as needed for a procedure and only intermittently (less than 3–5 minutes at a time). Spring-loaded mouth gags should never be used.

Excitement

Emergence delirium, dysphoria, and excitement may be seen during the recovery period and it is often difficult to ascertain the reason. Sudden arousal, for example when no preanesthetic sedation was used or a reversal drug has been given can lead to explosive recoveries where cats thrash around, can injure themselves and be difficult to restrain. Dysphoria may be linked to the use of opioids, for example prolonged fentanyl infusions. Sedation with low dose dexmedetomidine, medetomidine, acepromazine, propofol (0.5 mg/kg) or alfaxalone calms the cat, reduces oxygen demand, and usually

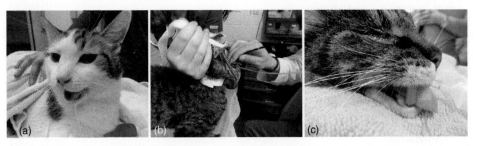

Figure 10.9 (a) Spring-loaded mouth gags can result in postanesthetic blindness and other neurological deficits. (b) Inappropriate use of a spring-loaded mouth gag. (c) Home made mouth gags (20–30 mm) can easily be substituted for spring-loaded gags.

resolves the condition. Excitement, restlessness and dysphoria may be a manifestation of pain in the recovery period, and this should be evaluated and treated as described in Chapters 12 and 13.

Prolonged Recovery

Although hypothermia is a common cause of prolonged recovery it may also be drug induced. Anesthetic overdose, heavy premedication, phenotypic failure to metabolize a drug and use of barbiturates (especially if "topped up") or propofol infusions may all prolong recovery. Reversal of dexmedetomidine and medetomidine with atipamezole reduce recovery time considerably without apparently affecting pain. If a benzodiazepine is thought to be the reason for the delayed recovery, administration of flumazenil will verify this. Where there is no means of antagonism of the anesthetic the cat must be provided with supportive care and monitored as during anesthesia until consciousness returns.

Body Temperature

Hypothermia

Small decreases in body temperature (1–2 °C) are associated with a multitude of intraoperative and postoperative adverse effects (*Box* 10.9). Supporting evidence for these side effects in human medicine is strong, although there is limited research in veterinary medicine. Large decreases in body temperature (≥ 5 °C) cause bradycardia, dysrhythmias, reduced metabolism and CO_2 production, decreased cardiac output, and eventually cardiac arrest.

Cats often seek heat and it must be assumed that being cold is unpleasant for them; in addition, as they warm up and begin to shiver after anesthesia this adds to the discomfort of surgery due to movement around the surgical site with increased muscle activity and rigidity. Shivering also increases oxygen demand, induces hypoglycemia and exacerbates hypoxemia; supplemental oxygen should be provided until cats are normothermic.

Box 10.9: Hypothermia has far reaching negative effects

- Reduced anesthetic requirements
- Reduced drug metabolism
- Delayed recovery
- Respiratory depression
- Increased bleeding
- Impaired immune function
- Increased postoperative wound infection
- Bradycardia
- Decreased cardiac output
- Dysrhythmias
- Postoperative shivering and discomfort

Once body temperature has fallen it is much more difficult to correct so the focus must be on prevention of hypothermia. When used with care, circulating warm water blankets, forced warm-air devices (*Figure* 10.8) and blankets made from semiconductive polymer fabric are all effective. Simple interventions such as keeping the preoperative and recovery areas warm, providing protection from drafts, using low fresh gas flows (only in rebreathing systems), boxes with blankets (creating a warm individual microclimate), heated cages, avoiding placing cats on cold surfaces, and keeping them dry, will all help maintain body temperature.

Hyperthermia

Opioid-induced hyperthermia has been reported in cats recovering from anesthesia. This appears to be primarily associated with hydromorphone where temperatures as high as 42.2 °C have been reported, but other opioids have been implicated (Chapter 13). This condition appears to be a North American phenomenon, and is rarely seen in the United Kingdom and other parts of Europe. This is consistent with it being primarily associated with hydromorphone, which is not available in Europe. Hyperthermia may also result from overzealous use of warming devices during anesthesia or in heavily sedated cats who cannot move from the source of heat; therefore monitoring temperature on a regular basis is important. Malfunctioning equipment, for example a heated water blanket with a faulty thermostat, can result in overheating.

Postanesthetic Renal Failure

Renal failure can be a consequence of hypotension and hypovolemia during anesthesia but may not become apparent for several days. The link between anesthesia and renal failure may not be made because of the time delay. In dogs, preoperative NSAID administration has been associated with postoperative renal failure when hypotension and hypovolemia have occurred during anesthesia. The association has not been proven in cats, but ensuring that they do not become hypotensive or hypovolemic during anesthesia is a wise precaution.

Cardiopulmonary Resuscitation (CPR)

Survival after cardiopulmonary arrest (CPA) requires rapid recognition that it has occurred, and immediate initiation of cardiopulmonary resuscitation (CPR) (*Box* 10.10). The Reassessment Campaign on Veterinary Resuscitation (RECOVER) was developed following in the footsteps of human medicine where success rates after CPA were improved with evidence-based guidelines and training. The guidelines, including user friendly algorithms and emergency drug charts were published in 2012, and are available for download (http://onlinelibrary.wiley.com/doi/10.1111/vec.2012.22.issue-s1/issuetoc, accessed June 25, 2017). Basic life-support and drug therapy is discussed here. The RECOVER guidelines provide detail for advanced life support and post-resuscitation care.

Box 10.10: Cardiopulmonary arrest

- Survival rate for patients that arrest under anesthesia is much higher than under other circumstances:
  - prompt recognition
  - most cases are receiving oxygen
- Use of pulse oximeters and monitoring the pulse (e.g. Doppler) decreases feline mortality
- Emergency drugs should be calculated before anesthesia and recorded on the patient's chart
- Chart should remain with the cat at all times
- Charts of emergency drug doses should be attached to each anesthetic machine, and walls of operating rooms and clinical areas
- Emergency "crash" carts, or portable "pick-up-and-go" boxes should be in the anesthesia and surgical areas
  - restock after use
  - inventory at least once a week

Recognition of Cardiopulmonary Arrest

Apnea may precede cardiac arrest therefore all cats that are or become apneic should be checked for the presence of a pulse or heart beat by palpation or auscultation. If a pulse oximeter or Doppler is in place, loss of the auditory signal should alert the anesthetist to check the patient immediately. End-tidal concentrations of CO_2 ($ETCO_2$) can indicate apnea or cardiac arrest; if the patient is apneic and a breath is given but $ETCO_2$ is low or zero, it is most likely that circulatory collapse has occurred. Although an ECG may be in place this is not a reliable indicator of circulation (Chapter 7). Even if CPA is not confirmed it is recommended to proceed with CPR if there is a strong suspicion.

Treatment – Basic Life Support (*Box 10.11*)

- The first CPR step is cardiac compressions, even if the cat is not intubated. Ideally this is performed with the cat in right lateral recumbency. Many cats will be in dorsal recumbency during surgery with the abdomen open therefore start chest compressions in that position;
  - The anesthetist can use one hand to stabilize the chest wall on one side, and the other to compress over the heart. An alternative method is to use the thumb on one side and the other four fingers on the other and compress from both sides over the heart (circumferential compression)
- The cat's chest is compliant so the recommended depth of compression (50% of the width of the chest) should be achievable. It is important to allow full chest recoil to maximize intrathoracic blood flow
- The surgeon may be able to close the abdomen quickly with a laparotomy sponge and towel clamps so the cat can be moved to a lateral position, or the surgeon may access the heart via the diaphragm and begin direct cardiac compressions

- If the cat is not already intubated, a cuffed endotracheal tube should be placed using a laryngoscope and without stopping cardiac compressions unless necessary
- If available a capnograph is connected between the ETT and circuit
- Ventilation at ten breaths per minute and short inspiratory time (1 second) allows for adequate cardiac filling time
- The person performing ventilation should focus on their rate and timing; it does not need to be synchronized with cardiac compressions
- The size of the reservoir bag is controlled by manipulating the adjustable pressure limiting (APL) valve ("pop-off" valve); on some machines this requires rotating the valve to close it and then turning it back to the open position repeatedly; this takes time but leaving it closed by mistake is disastrous
- An easier and safer approach is to use a pop-off occlusion valve, which only requires the operator to press down on it while administering a breath, then releasing it (*Figure* 10.10)
- If a heartbeat and pulse do not return spontaneously and quickly after starting basic life support, drug therapy is indicated

---

Box 10.11: Cardiopulmonary resuscitation

- Step 1: Note the time. Turn off the vaporizer and stop anesthetic drug infusions. Empty the circuit of inhalant agent
- Step 2: Cardiac compression; 100–120 times/minute. Compress 50% of the depth of the chest and allow full recoil
- Step 3: If not already in place, intubate with a cuffed endotracheal tube. Ventilate 10 times/minute with an inspiratory phase of 1 second ($\leq 10\,cmH_2O$)
- Step 4: Consider antagonism of sedative and analgesic drugs

---

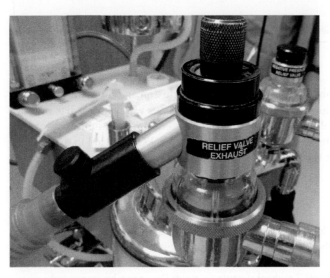

Figure 10.10 A pop-off occlusion valve allows easy and rapid ventilation without the risk of the pop-off valve being left closed.

Drug Therapy (*Box* 10.12)

The goal of drug therapy is to increase systemic vascular resistance and improve cerebral and coronary artery perfusion. Low dose epinephrine (adrenaline) (0.01 mg/kg) is given every 3–5 minutes. Epinephrine has both α and β adrenergic receptor activity, resulting in peripheral vasoconstriction, increased cardiac contractility and rate and is the most commonly used vasopressor in CPR. Vasopressin (0.8 U/kg) is a pressor that does not increase heart rate or contractility, and therefore myocardial oxygen demand, which is a side effect of epinephrine. However, there are no clear reported benefits to its use, and it is significantly more expensive. If increased vagal tone is thought to be a cause of CPA or if bradycardia preceded the arrest, atropine (0.02–0.04 mg/kg) should be administered.

Box 10.12: Drugs for cardiopulmonary resuscitation

IV:

- Epinephrine 0.01 mg/kg
- Vasopressin 0.8 U/kg
- Atropine 0.02–0.04 mg/kg

If no IV access – through endotracheal tube:

- Epinephrine 0.1 mg/kg
- Dilute all drugs in saline or normal saline (to 2 mL)
- Use a catheter or tube (e.g. urinary catheter) narrow enough to fit into the endotracheal tube, and long enough to reach the carina – this should be in the emergency kit

If no IV access – intraosseous route (IO):

- Tibia or humerus
- Needs IO needle or IO placement device (hypodermic needle sufficient for kittens)

Monitoring During CPR

Creating sufficient circulation for cerebral and cardiac perfusion and ultimately return of spontaneous circulation is the goal of CPR. $ETCO_2$ correlates well with cardiac output, and should be used if possible. A pulse oximeter will detect flow and indicate oxygenation. A Doppler will indicate flow in peripheral arteries. An ECG will aid in diagnosing the type of arrest but is not the first monitor to apply or to rely on.

Further Reading

Barton-Lamb, A. L., Martin-Flores, M., Scrivani, P. V., *et al.* (2013) Evaluation of maxillary arterial blood flow in anesthetized cats with the mouth closed and open. *Veterinary Journal* **196**, 325–331.

Bhandal, J., and Kuzma, A. (2008) Tracheal rupture in a cat: Diagnosis by computed tomography. *Canadian Veterinary Journal* **49**, 595–597.

Blunt, M. C., Young, P. J., Patil, A., *et al.* (2001) Gel lubrication of the tracheal tube cuff reduces pulmonary aspiration. *Anesthesiology* **95**, 377–381.

Brodbelt, D. (2009) Perioperative mortality in small animal anaesthesia. *Veterinary Journal* **182**, 152–161.

Brodbelt, D. C., Pfeiffer, D. U., Young, L. E., *et al.* (2007) Risk factors for anaesthetic-related death in cats: Results from the confidential enquiry into perioperative small animal fatalities (CEPSAF). *British Journal of Anaesthesia* **99**, 617–623.

Bukoski, A., Winter, M., Bandt, C., *et al.* (2010) Comparison of three intraosseous access techniques in cats. *Journal of Veterinary Emergency Critical Care* **20**, 393–397.

Clarke, K. W., and Hall, L. W. (1990) A survey of anaesthesia in small animal practice: AVA/BSAVA report. *Journal of Veterinary Anaesthesia* **17**, 4–10.

Fox, P. R., and Schober, K. A. (2015) Management of asymptomatic (occult) feline cardiomyopathy: Challenges and realities. *Journal of Veterinary Cardiology* **17**, S150–158.

Franci, P., Leece, E. A., and McConnell, J. F. (2011) Arrhythmias and transient changes in cardiac function after topical administration of one drop of phenylephrine 10% in an adult cat undergoing conjunctival graft. *Veterinary Anaesthesia and Analgesia* **38**, 208–212.

Gordon, A. M., and Wagner, A. E. (2006) Anesthesia-related hypotension in a small-animal practice. *Veterinary Medicine* **101**, 22–24.

Hardie, E. M., Spodnick, G. J., Gilson, S. D., *et al.* (1999) Tracheal rupture in cats: 16 cases (1983–1998). *Journal of the American Veterinary Medical Association* **214**, 508–512.

Hofmeister, E. H., Trim, C. M., Kley, S., *et al.* (2007) Traumatic endotracheal intubation in the cat. *Veterinary Anaesthesia and Analgesia* **34**, 213–216.

Machon, R. G., Raffe, M. R., and Robinson, E. P. (1999) Warming with a forced air warming blanket minimizes anesthetic-induced hypothermia in cats. *Veterinary Surgery* **28**, 301–310.

Martin-Flores, M., Scrivani, P. V., Loew, E., *et al.* (2014) Maximal and submaximal mouth opening with mouth gags in cats: Implications for maxillary artery blood flow. *Veterinary Journal* **200**, 60–64.

McMillan, M., and Darcy, Y. H. (2016) Adverse event surveillance in small animal anaesthesia: An intervention-based, voluntary reporting audit. *Veterinary Anaesthesia and Analgesia* **43**, 128–135.

McNeil, P. E. (1992) Acute tubulo-interstitial nephritis in a dog after halothane anaesthesia and administration of flunixin meglumine and trimethoprim-sulphadiazine. *Veterinary Record* **131**, 148–151.

Mitchell, S. L., McCarthy, R., Rudloff, E. *et al.* (2000) Tracheal rupture associated with intubation in cats: 20 cases (1996–1998). *Journal of the American Veterinary Medical Association* **216**, 1592–1595.

Prasse, S. A., Schrack, J., Wenger, S., *et al.* (2016) Clinical evaluation of the v-gel supraglottic airway device in comparison with a classical laryngeal mask and endotracheal intubation in cats during spontaneous and controlled mechanical ventilation. *Veterinary Anaesthesia and Analgesia* **43**, 55–62.

Reassessment campaign on veterinary resuscitation: Evidence and knowledge gap analysis on veterinary CPR (2012) *Journal of Veterinary Emergency and Critical Care* (special

182 Feline Anesthesia and Pain Management

issue) **22** (s1), S1–S131, http://onlinelibrary.wiley.com/doi/10.1111/vec.2012.22.issue-s1/ issuetoc (accessed June 25, 2017).

Redondo, J. I., Suesta, P., Gil, L., *et al.* (2012) Retrospective study of the prevalence of postanaesthetic hypothermia in cats. *Veterinary Record* **170**, 206–210.

Santos, L. C., Ludders, J. W., Erb, B. H. N., *et al.* (2011). A randomized, blinded, controlled trial of the antiemetic effect of ondansetron on dexmedetomidine-induced emesis in cats. *Veterinary Anaesthesia and Analgesia* **38**, 320–327.

Scrivani, P. V., Martin-Flores, M., Van Hatten, R., *et al.* (2014) Structural and functional changes relevant to maxillary arterial flow observed during computed tomography and nonselective digital subtraction angiography in cats with the mouth closed and opened. *Veterinary Radiology and Ultrasound* **55**, 263–271.

Stiles, J,. Weil, A. B., Packer, R. A., *et al.* (2012) Post-anesthetic cortical blindness in cats: Twenty cases. *Veterinary Journal* **193**, 367–373.

Van Oostrom, H., Krauass, M. W., and Sap, R. (2013) A comparison between the v-gel supraglottic airway device and the cuffed endotracheal tube for airway management in spontaneously breathing cats during isoflurane anaesthesia. *Veterinary Anaesthesia and Analgesia* **40**, 265–271.

11

Mechanisms of Pain

Craig B. Johnson

Massey University, Palmerston North, New Zealand

Key Points

- Pain is a multifactorial modality comprising perceptive and emotive components
- Pain ranges from physiological to neuropathic
- The experience of pain requires consciousness
- Nociception occurs without consciousness and causes numerous autonomic responses
- Numerous mechanisms contribute to the experience and physiological consequences of pain

Introduction

Pain is a multifactorial modality comprising perceptive and emotive components (*Figure* 11.1) (*Boxes* 11.1 and 11.2). This complexity leads to a spectrum of pain ranging from the wholly physiological, such as A-fiber or fast pain through to phenomena such as neuropathic and cancer pain that are deeply pathological. Although pain itself is considered to exist only at cognitive levels within the central nervous system, there are a multitude of peripheral mechanisms that lead to its perception.

It is the nature of clinical medicine that treatment of pain focuses on the pathological end of the pain spectrum, and that many analgesic therapies target peripheral mechanisms. For this reason, most of this chapter will deal with pain from these perspectives. The mechanisms of pain are intimately linked with those of inflammation, and it should be noted that many of the neuromodulators discussed in this chapter are also integral components of the inflammatory response to tissue damage.

Mechanisms of Modulation in Tissues

The somatic parts of the body are innervated with two distinct populations of nociceptors, known as A-fiber and C-fiber mechano-heat-sensitive nociceptors (AMHs and CMHs respectively). There are numerous nerve endings of these neurons in the superficial layers of the skin, and other structures such as synovial joints and the dura mater. They are also distributed throughout other somatic tissues although more sparsely.

Feline Anesthesia and Pain Management, First Edition. Edited by Paulo Steagall, Sheilah Robertson and Polly Taylor.

Box 11.1: Definitions of acronyms and glossary

- *Allodynia* – pain due to a stimulus that does not normally provoke pain
- *AMH* – A fiber mechano-heat-sensitive nociceptor
- *AMP, ADP, ATP* – adenosine mono-, di-, and triphosphate. Involved in cellular energy systems and also used as signaling molecules
- *Analgesia* – absence of pain in response to stimulation that would normally be painful
- *ASIC* – acid-sensing ion channel
- *CB1* – cannabinoid 1 receptor
- *CCK* – cholecystokinin
- *CMH* – C fiber mechano-heat-sensitive nociceptor
- *COX-1 COX-2* – cyclooxygenase 1 and 2
- *Eicosanoids* – a family of signaling molecules made by oxidation of 20-carbon fatty acids and usually derived from the cell membrane of damaged cells
- *GABA* – γ amino-butyric acid
- *5-HT* – 5-hydroxytryptamine (synonym for serotonin)
- *Hyperalgesia* – increased pain from a stimulus that normally provokes pain
- *Hypoalgesia* – diminished pain in response to a normally painful stimulus
- *NGF* – nerve growth factor
- *NMDA* – N-methyl-D-aspartate
- *nNOS* – neuronal nitric oxide synthase
- *Nociceptor* – a high-threshold sensory receptor of the peripheral somatosensory nervous system that is capable of transducing and encoding noxious stimuli
- *Noxious stimulus* – a stimulus that is damaging or threatens damage to normal tissues
- *NTR* – neurotensin receptor
- *PAG* – periaqueductal grey matter
- *Pain* – pain is a distressing experience associated with actual or potential tissue damage with sensory, emotional, cognitive, and social components
- *Pruriceptor* – a sensory receptor of the peripheral somatosensory nervous system that is capable of transducing and encoding pruritic stimuli
- *Pruritic stimulus* – a sensation that causes the desire or reflex to scratch
- *RVM* – rostral ventromedial medulla
- *TLR4* – toll-like receptor 4
- *TNF* – tumor necrosis factor
- *TRPV 1* – transient receptor potential vanilloid 1
- *Wind-up* – perceived increase in pain intensity over time when a given stimulus is delivered repeatedly above a critical rate or intensity

---

Box 11.2: The phenomenon of pain

Pain cannot be perceived by animals while they are unconscious, *but* the nociceptive mechanisms that lead to its perception are still active unless they are specifically blocked; noxious stimuli during anesthesia can dramatically increase the pain perceived when an animal regains consciousness.

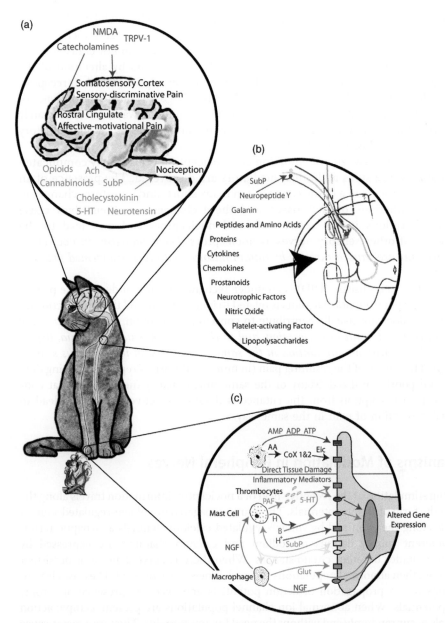

Figure 11.1 Nociceptive pathways. (a) Neuromodulators acting in the brain – red text acting on higher centers, blue text acting on periaqueductal grey matter and rostro-ventral medulla. (b) Neuromodulators acting at the spinal cord – red text acting at spinal ganglion, black text acting in dorsal horn. Pathways indicated by color – yellow: C-fiber acute pain, purple: A-fiber touch, pink: A-fiber fast pain, red: representative interneuron, green: descending modulatory fiber of reticulospinal system.

(c) Neuromodulators acting in peripheral tissues. Rectangular receptors are ionotropic – red: purinergic receptors, orange: voltage-activated sodium channels, purple: acid-sensing ion channels, blue: N-methyl-D-aspartate receptors. Ovoid receptors are metabotropic – red: serotonin, orange: bradykinin, yellow: cytokine, green: nerve growth factor.

Key to abbreviations – AMP, ADP and AMP: adenosine mono, di and tri phosphate, AA: arachidonic acid, Eic: eicosanoids, SubP: substance P, PAF: platelet-activating factor, H: histamine, H+: protons, B: bradykinin, Cyt: cytokines, Glut: glutamate, NGF: nerve growth factor, 5-HT: serotonin (5-hydroxy-tryptamine), Ach: acetyl choline, NMDA: N-methyl-D-aspartate, TRPV-1: *1* transient receptor potential vanilloid 1.

Nociception also occurs in the viscera, where it is thought to be modulated largely by mechanoreceptors operating at the high end of their sensory range rather than by primary nociceptors. For this reason visceral pain is largely due to bowel distension.

In both somatic and visceral tissues, pain modulation occurs by alteration of the threshold and sensitivity of these nerve endings as well as by expansion of their receptive fields. Modulation of nociception at the tissue level is in large part due to the presence of a vast number of molecules that affect nerve endings in different ways, and is intimately linked with inflammation. Some of the more important classes of inflammatory mediators are described in *Table* 11.1.

The interaction between inflammation and nociception is extremely complicated and becomes more so as additional mediators are discovered. The presence of an inflammatory process in a tissue can result in many short- and long-term changes in the cellular functions of that tissue and these changes can themselves cause dramatic alterations in the activity of local nociceptors and may lead to the recruitment of other sensory nerves as nociceptors. *Local increases in nociceptor sensitivity that are caused directly by inflammatory mediators are termed primary hyperalgesia.*

Degenerative joint disease (DJD) is an under-recognized cause of deep tissue pain in cats. Sensory input from normal joints is related to joint position and the forces acting on the joint, and does not usually contribute to conscious perception. *Overstimulation of these pathways can result in nociception, and in the long term cause allodynia, hyper-algesia and pain without stimulation in the same way as is seen in cutaneous sensory pathways.* The nature of the resulting pain (in humans at least) is reported as being dull, aching, and poorly localized. Many of the same inflammatory mechanisms that con-tribute to pain perception from the cutaneous tissues are active in DJD and lead to increased perception of pain in the same way.

Mechanisms of Modulation in Peripheral Nerves

Following stimulation of the receptive field of a nociceptor, information travels along the nerve in the form of action potentials. These are propagated by voltage-regulated sodium channels along the axon and by voltage-regulated calcium channels at synaptic termi-nals. Different subpopulations of sodium and calcium channels are expressed by nociceptors under different circumstances. When there is nerve damage or persistent stimulation, then abnormal populations of ion channels are expressed. These can lead to alterations in the propagation of action potentials and even the presence of ectopic action potentials. When abnormal ion channel populations are present, ectopic action potentials occur randomly and without the need for any stimulus. They are a major cause of *neuropathic pain.*

In addition to the propagation of sensory information to the central nervous system, nociceptor stimulation has a number of local effects that are thought to be due to peripheral axon reflexes. These include arteriolar vasodilatation, mast cell degranulation, and the activation of other immune cells, keratinocyte stimulation, and smooth-muscle

Table 11.1 Examples of the more important classes of inflammatory mediators.

Eicosanoid	These are metabolites of arachidonic acid, a component of the plasma membrane, which are released into the extracellular fluid following cell lysis. They include molecules such as prostaglandins, thromboxanes, and leukotrienes. Prostaglandins are produced by both constitutive and induced forms of the enzyme cyclooxygenase (COX-1 and COX-2, respectively) (Chapter 13). They reduce the threshold of nociceptors and increase their sensitivity via activation of nociceptor-specific voltage-activated sodium channels.
Bradykinins	These are present in inflammatory exudates and have an important role in the inflammatory process. They reduce the threshold and increase the sensitivity of nociceptors to natural stimuli and stimulate nociceptive activity in their own right acting at the β_1 and β_2 receptors via intracellular second messenger systems involving phospholipase C and protein kinase C.
Protons	A reduction in extracellular pH is a consequence of inflammatory processes and results in pain and hyperalgesia. A group of ASICs appear to be responsible for this effect when the reduction in pH is moderate. During severe acidosis TRPV1 is also involved. Both are sodium channels whose expression is increased by inflammation and nerve injury.
Serotonin	Degranulating mast cells release platelet-activating factor and this in turn causes serotonin (also known as 5-HT) to be released from platelets. Serotonin can activate nociceptors directly, and can also potentiate the effects of bradykinin.
Histamine	Release of substance P from nociceptor terminals causes local mast cells to secrete histamine. This has a role in the local inflammatory response, where it is responsible for vasodilatation and edema, and potentiates responses to bradykinin and heat. Injection of histamine into normal tissue causes the sensation of itch rather than pain.
Purines	Cellular degeneration causes the release of purines such as AMP, ADP and ATP into the extracellular space. The presence of these molecules stimulates nociception and application of purines is painful even when there is no additional stimulation. Purinergic receptors have been found on nociceptors in the periphery and in spinal ganglia, but the role of purines in the modulation of nociception appears to be closely linked to capsaicin receptor activity.
Cytokines	These are released by a variety of cells and are involved in regulation of the inflammatory process. They may excite nociceptors by rapid alterations in the sensitivity of ion channels, by stimulating the release of other inflammatory mediators or by intracellular effects that alter the gene expression of the nociceptor.
Excitatory amino acids	The most studied excitatory amino acid is glutamate. Glutamate receptors can activate ligand-gated ion channels (NMDA receptors) or act via G-protein coupled metabotropic receptors, both of which have been identified on CMH neurons in the skin. Glutamate is released by macrophages, endothelial cells and Schwann cells among others and can also be released from the nerve terminals of the nociceptors themselves.
Nerve growth factor	Pro-inflammatory cytokines induce the release of nerve growth factor (NGF) from many cells including fibroblasts and keratinocytes. In turn, NGF stimulates the release of histamine and serotonin from mast cells, and can also induce hyperalgesia to heat by a direct effect on nociceptive nerve terminals.

contraction. Stimulation of one branch of a nociceptor causes antidromic propagation of action potentials into adjacent branches, and this in turn contributes to these local inflammatory effects.

There is increasing evidence that neuronal cell bodies in the spinal ganglia have an important role to play in the modulation of nociception. The spinal ganglia are not themselves innervated with nerve endings, but functional peptide receptors have been found on the cell body membrane for neurotransmitters such as substance P, neuropeptide Y, and galanin. These have all been shown to modulate excitability in the somatic membrane, and so are implicated in the development of hyperalgesia and neuropathic pain. Neuropeptides can only cross the blood-brain barrier to a very limited extent, and so it is possible that the spinal ganglion is their main site of action. Upregulation of these receptors in states of neuropathic pain has recently been demonstrated.

Mechanisms of Modulation in The Spinal Cord

The dorsal horn of the spinal cord is a major site of modulation of nociception. The neuronal circuits of the dorsal horn are very complex and not fully understood, but in general there are several kinds of neurons that are involved in the perception and modulation of pain.

Primary afferent neurons convey sensory information from the periphery and project into the dorsal layers of the spinal cord (laminae I–V). They include myelinated low-threshold mechanoreceptors conveying sensory information that can become nociceptive when stimulation is intense, myelinated nociceptive fibers responsible for pin-prick pain and unmyelinated nociceptive fibers, which are sensitive to a wide range of stimuli such as mechanical, thermal and chemical modalities.

Spinal interneurons comprise the vast majority of the cell population of the dorsal horn and account for the complexity of the spinal neuronal circuits both in terms of their anatomical complexity and the large number of molecules for which they can express receptors (e.g. neuropeptides, nNOS etc.). Most of the connections made by interneurons are to other neurons in the same dermatome, but a smaller number of connections, particularly in laminae I–III, interact with neurons at a distance of one or two segments. Interneurons can be either inhibitory (GABA-minergic or glycinergic) or excitatory (glutaminergic).

Projection neurons project cranially to target regions of the brain including the thalamus, midbrain periaqueductal grey matter, pons, and medulla oblongata. Individual projection neurons often have multiple axons, and project to more than one of the above regions.

Descending neurons – descending pathways project from many areas of the brain including the medulla and locus coeruleus. They can be either facilitatory or inhibitory. This descending inhibitory system involves modulation in the brain and is discussed in more detail below.

Non-neuronal cells – glial cells such as astrocytes and microglia can profoundly influence nociceptive pathways. Their role is discussed in a later section of this chapter.

Table 11.2 Examples of the more important mediators that act in the dorsal horn to induce or inhibit hyperalgesia and allodynia.

Peptides and amino acids	Examples include: substance P, neurokinins A and B, calcitonin gene-related peptide, dynorphin, endorphin, galanin, nociception/orphanin, bradykinin, adrenomedullin, glutamate, endogenous opioids, purines, and serotonin.
Proteins	Examples include: glycoprotein GP120, thrombin; fibronectin and secretory protein Bv8.
Cytokines	Examples include: TNF-α, interleukin-1β, interleukin-6, and interseron-γ.
Chemokines	Examples include: fractalkine, and monocyte chemoattractant protein-1.
Prostanoids	Examples include: prostaglandins E_1, E_2, D_2 $F_2\alpha$
Neurotrophic factors	Examples include: brain-derived neurotrophic factor and nerve growth factor
Miscellaneous molecules	Examples include: nitric oxide, lipopolysaccharides, and platelet-activating factor.

The complexity of the architecture of the dorsal horn makes it difficult to provide a brief description that is informative in terms of the nociceptive function of this region of the central nervous system. It is more useful to consider the effects of neurotransmitters and other mediators in terms of their ability to induce plasticity by mechanisms in the dorsal horn, and so induce or inhibit hyperalgesia and allodynia. Examples of the more important mediators are given in *Table* 11.2.

Some of these substances are capable of inducing hyperalgesia when applied to the spinal cord as single agents, others do not cause hyperalgesia alone, but facilitate the actions of other agents. In the whole animal the balance of these mediators is constantly changing and the relative concentrations of different mediators is distinct for different types of pain. Some of these mediators have even been shown to promote hyperalgesia or hypoalgesia depending on the experimental context in which they are studied. Plasticity in the dorsal horn of the spinal cord can be induced in a number of ways that are modulated by altered concentrations of these neuromodulators. Sustained activation of C-fiber inputs seen in chronic painful conditions can induce hyperalgesia and allodynia, but the absence or long-term reduction of these inputs as seen following damage to peripheral nerves may also cause this. Neuronal mechanisms of long-lasting plasticity include processes such as long-term potentiation and long-term depression of particular pathways as well as remodeling of networks by synaptic growth and trimming or even apoptosis of particular neurons. All of these mechanisms are initiated and maintained by the balance of neuronal modulators in the dorsal horn.

Mechanisms of Modulation in the Brain

The experience of pain is complex and involves the participation of many regions of the brain. Functional imaging (e.g. functional magnetic resonance imaging (fMRI)) studies in humans give an overall picture of pain perception that involves an extensive cortical and subcortical network including sensory, limbic, associative, and motor areas of the forebrain. Different aspects of pain perception are dealt with by different areas of the forebrain; the somatosensory cortex processes sensory-discriminative components and the rostral cingulate cortex processes affective-motivational components. The insula cortex appears to have an important role in both aspects of pain perception.

The relationship between a stimulus and its perception depends on the interaction of these different centers and is both complex and context-specific. Experimental stimulation of brain regions such as the PAG and the RVM produce subjective analgesia and it has been demonstrated that these sites are primary CNS targets of opioid analgesics (*Box* 11.3). In addition to their ability to reduce the cognitive perception of pain, the PAG and RVM stimulate descending pathways that inhibit the response of nociceptive systems in the dorsal horn. Agonists of the α_{-2} adrenergic receptor are active in this area (*Box* 11.3). These cyclical mechanisms play a large role in context-specific hypoalgesia as well as in the hyperalgesia and allodynia seen in persistent pain states.

Box 11.3: Sites and mechanisms of action of analgesic agents

Site of action	Agent
Peripheral tissue	NSAIDs, cannabinoids, opioids
Peripheral nerves	
Tissue nerve endings	Local anesthetics, SSRIs, piprants
Axons	Local anesthetics, carbamazepine, capsaicin
Spinal ganglion	
Presynaptic modulation	Opioids, nitrous oxide, gabapentinoids
Spinal cord	Opioids, nitrous oxide, local anesthetics, agonists of the α_{-2} adrenergic receptor, gabapentinoids, ziconotide, cannabinoids, dopamine antagonists, tramadol
Brain	Opioids, nitrous oxide, SSRIs, NSAIDs, local anesthetics, ketamine (additional sites of action and mechanisms probable), gabapentinoids, cannabinoids, dopamine antagonists, tramadol, amantadine, amitriptyline, piprants
Non-neuronal mechanisms	Bisphosphonates, astrocyte inhibitors, immune modulators

---

Similar to the dorsal horn of the spinal cord, many neuromodulators act in the higher centers to provide analgesia. Important examples are given in *Table* 11.3.

The link between anxiety and hyperalgesia may be mediated by cholecystokinin. It is important to reduce fear and anxiety for many reasons in a clinical setting (Chapter 1), not least for their negative impact on pain.

There are many other neurotransmitters and neuromodulators that interact with the nociceptive system elsewhere within the higher centers of the central nervous system. These include the catecholamines (especially dopamine and norepinephrine (noradrenaline)), NMDA and vanilloids (via the TRPV1 receptor).

Table 11.3 Examples of the more important mediators that act in the brain to induce or inhibit hyperalgesia and allodynia

Opioids	The PAG/RVM system has a high density of opioid receptors and endogenous opioids are potent analgesics at this site. It is interesting to note that the other major site of these receptors, the dorsal horn, is the other main component of the cyclical nociceptive system that is largely responsible for the amplification and reduction of pain sensations seen in hyperalgesia and allodynia. The clinical application of opioids is discussed in Chapter 13.
Cannabinoids	The distribution of CB1 receptors in the PAG/RVM and the dorsal horn of the spinal cord is similar to that of the opioid receptors. Endo-cannabinoids are involved in the central modulation of nociception in a separate, but parallel manner to endogenous opioids.
Acetylcholine	The RVM contains nicotinic acetylcholine receptors that contribute to antinociception in conjunction with serotonergic neurons.
Cholecystokinin	This peptide has both anti-opioid and pronociceptive actions at many levels of the central nervous system via the CCK2 receptor. Its cellular actions appear to be the converse of those of the opioids, and it has been demonstrated that CCK2 antagonists can potentiate the analgesic actions of opioids. CCK contributes to anxiety and its effects on the perception of noxious stimuli may form the link between anxiety and hyperalgesia.
Neurotensin	Similarly to CCK, neurotensin co-locates with opioid receptors. Low doses of neurotensin activate pain-facilitating neurons, but higher doses also activate pain-inhibiting neurons leading to an overall biphasic effect. This may be mediated by differential receptor affinities of the NTR 1 and 2 receptors. Neurotensin appears to be a necessary mediator of hyperalgesia caused by inflammation since this effect can be blocked by microinjection of an NTR1 antagonist into the RVM.
Substance P	Substance P receptors are found in the RVM where its direct application produces hypoalgesia, but other studies have demonstrated pro-nociceptive activity. The details of the role of substance P at this level in the nociceptive pathways are not yet clear, but it is likely that it has a complex modulating role similar to that of neurotensin.

The Role of Glial Cells (Glia, Neuroglia) and the Immune System

In addition to the neuronal components of nociceptive pathways, the role of glia has been increasingly identified as an important modulator of pain perception.

- Astrocytes constitute approximately half of all glial cells and are intimately associated with the neurons that they support
- Astrocytes play vital roles in the regulation of the extracellular environment of the neurons and modulate availability of extracellular ions, neurotransmitter release, release of inflammatory mediators, synapse formation, and ultimately neuronal survival
- Microglia originate from macrophage precursors and are found throughout the central nervous system. Under normal circumstances they are inactive and

unobtrusive cells, but on activation they perform very similar roles in the inflammatory process to those played by the macrophage outside the central nervous system, and are part of the reticuloendothelial system

• Noxious stimulation of C-fibers is sufficient to stimulate some microglial activation and all models of neuropathic pain currently envisage a degree of microglial response (*Box* 11.4)

Box 11.4: The contribution to pain from microglial activity

It is uncertain whether microglial activation contributes directly to the perception of pain, but there is evidence that microglial responses amplify the output of neural networks in the spinal cord that are active in pain perception. It is likely that reducing microglial activation will have some analgesic effect. This critical role of microglia in pain perception further illustrates the intimate associations between pain and inflammation apparent at every level of the nociceptive system.

Activation of an innate immune receptor expressed by microglia and astrocytes, TLR4, can dramatically amplify pain, and it is associated with the development and maintenance of neuropathic pain. Antagonists of TLR4 could be stand-alone treatments for various pathological pain states, and enhance the magnitude and duration of opioid analgesia while minimizing their adverse effects. However, these experimental drugs have not been tested in cats and it is not yet clear what the clinical applications may be. The persistent hyperalgesia and pain-related behavior seen following tissue and particularly nerve injury is associated with activation of both microglia and astrocytes. These actions have been demonstrated in the dorsal horn of the spinal cord and also more recently in higher centers of the central nervous system.

Mechanisms of Cancer Pain

Cats are affected by a wide variety of cancers, which can be painful for a number of reasons. Pain may also be associated with secretion of eicosanoids either directly by the tumor or via an immune response to its presence, direct effects on central nociceptive pathways and invasion of or pressure from the tumor into muscle, bone or neurological tissues (*Figure* 11.2 and *Figure* 11.3). Therapeutic protocols for cancer such as chemotherapy and radiotherapy may themselves cause pain. Moreover, many of the mechanisms causing cancer pain lead to allodynia, which exacerbates the existing pain from concurrent diseases.

Pain caused by Cancers in Bone

Although tumors in bone are less common in cats than dogs, when they occur, pain may be particularly severe as a result of the unique mechanism of pain in this tissue. The pain of both primary neoplasms of bone and metastatic tumors within bone appears to be due to an increase in bone resorption without corresponding formation of new bone. This

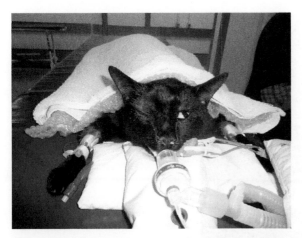

Figure 11.2 A common mechanism of cancer pain is the increasing size of the mass stretching surrounding normal tissues. Distention of the globe as caused by this intraocular neoplasm is often associated with severe pain.
Source: Courtesy of Professor Jane Dobson.

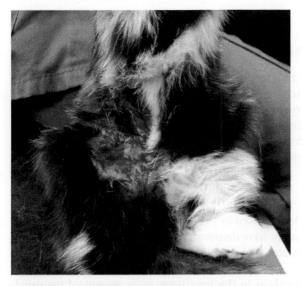

Figure 11.3 Inflammatory processes in the adjacent tissues to superficial tumors such as this mammary carcinoma can result in chronic pain and discomfort.
Source: Courtesy of Dr. Malcolm Brearley.

relative excess of osteoclast activity results in reduced bone density and can lead to the formation of microfractures and eventually macrofractures.

Sarcomas and mammary tumors are common in cats and cause pain through expansion, stretching, invasion, ulceration, and inflammation. Although it ultimately removes the source of the pain, surgical excision adds acute pain to the ongoing cancer pain (*Figure* 11.4).

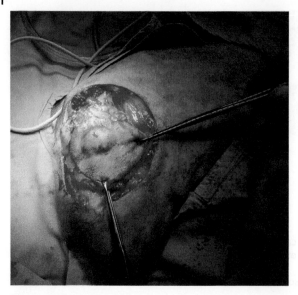

Figure 11.4 Acute surgical pain is usually easier to manage than pain of neoplastic origin and surgical removal of painful neoplasms should be considered as a component of analgesic therapy.
Source: Courtesy of Dr. Bryden Stanley.

Secretion of Eicosanoids and Inflammatory Responses

Tumors and their associated inflammatory responses secrete a large number of neuro-chemical mediators many of which are associated with allodynia. Examples include endothelin-1, bradykinin, nerve growth factor, cytokines such as tumor necrosis factor and protons. These factors sensitize nociceptors in the tissues local to the tumor and can also contribute to central mechanisms of wind up.

Endothelin-1 is a vasoactive peptide acting via receptors found on spinal ganglion neurons and Schwann calls and possibly directly on nociceptive fibers via TRPV1 receptors. Endothelin-1 has been associated with oral squamous cell carcinomas and renal, ovarian, and mammary carcinomas.

Bradykinin is a vasoactive peptide produced by melanomas with receptors on primary afferent neurons. Experimental studies have demonstrated that administration of both endothelin and bradykinin receptor antagonists reduce pain-related behaviors in animal models of cancer.

Nerve growth factor (NGF) is involved in the long-term management of neuronal function, acting by regulation of synaptic plasticity and apoptosis of neurons and the proliferation of their processes. Chronic exposure of sensory neurons to NGF results in allodynia and the formation of neuroma-like structures that are seen in some tumors.

Cytokines are released directly by tumor cells as well as by the inflammatory cells that generate local tissue responses to them. This increase in cytokine concentrations in the local tissue causes allodynia by the mechanisms described earlier. The local inflammation leads to a relatively acidic environment in the tumor, and surrounding tissues and this itself contributes to allodynia acting via ASICs and TRPV1 receptors.

Central Nociceptive Mechanisms

The mechanisms of central wind-up have been described earlier in this chapter. Cancers associated with allodynia through peripheral mechanisms result in a prolonged barrage of increased nociceptive input to the spinal cord and higher centers of the brain. This can cause very profound changes in the central nociceptive pathways and result in widespread sensitization with many effects including upregulation of receptors in the spinal cord, an increase in the size of sensory fields of nociceptors, and facilitation of both ascending nociceptive pathways and descending excitatory pathways. In severe cases, these mechanisms can lead to spontaneous activity in the nociceptive pathways resulting in "spontaneous pain" that is no longer temporally limited to response to noxious stimulation.

Many neoplasms have been associated with hypertrophy of astrocytes in the ipsilateral spinal cord that is rarely seen with other painful lesions. There is evidence that this hypertrophy results in activation of the astrocytes and contributes to central sensitization.

Pain from Cancer Treatment

Chemotherapeutic agents such as vincristine, paclitaxel, and cisplatin can induce peripheral neuropathies that cause changes in sensation, may be painful, and can be dose limiting in humans. It can be assumed that the same happens to cats, however this has not been well documented. The mechanisms of these neuropathies are not well understood, but they are distinct from each other and so it is likely that each drug is acting by a unique mechanism. Radiotherapy can also have painful consequences due to such side effects as tissue burns, bone necrosis, and nerve damage.

Diabetic Neuropathy

Pain due to neuropathy may be present in cats with diabetes. (*Figure* 11.5) (Chapter 9, Chapter 14). The mechanisms of this pain are poorly understood and a detailed

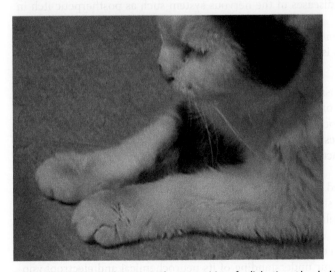

Figure 11.5 Neuropathic pain in the extremities of a diabetic cat has led to intense licking and staining of the paws

discussion is beyond the scope of this chapter. Schreiber *et al.* reviewed the possible mechanisms in 2015.

Pruritus (Itch)

Pruritus is distinct from pain, but the two sensations have mechanisms that are remarkably similar to each other. A noxious stimulus elicits a very strong withdrawal reflex with the obvious aim of removing the stimulated area from a potentially damaging situation. An itch stimulus elicits a similarly strong scratch reflex and it has been postulated that this has the function of removing a noxious agent such as a thorn that has already attached to the skin.

The sensation of itch is mediated via a particular population of C-fibers (pruriceptors) that are poorly sensitive to mechanical stimulation, but very sensitive to pruritic chemicals such as histamine. The mechanisms of pruriception parallel the nociceptive pathways in the central nervous system and there is very close correlation between the central sensitization pathways of chronic pain and chronic pruritus. The role of the anterior cingulate gyrus in changing the perception of a pruriceptive stimulus from pleasant to unpleasant seems to parallel its role in the attribution of pain during stimulation of nociceptive pathways.

Pruritus has been classified into four categories based on the underlying mechanism:

Pruriceptive itch – pruriceptive mediators such as histamine activate peripheral pruriceptors. Examples in cats include ectopic parasites and allergic dermatitis, and some skin infections.

Neurogenic itch – generated by central stimulation of nondiseased pruritic pathways. The itch mediated by opioids is an example of this. Opioid-induced pruritus has been described after epidural administration of morphine in the cat; however this is not common.

Neuropathic itch – due to diseases of the nervous system such as postherpetic itch in humans.

Psychogenic itch – in humans this is related to illusional conditions such as parasitophobia. Whether this is related to the rare cases of intractable pruiritis in cats is unknown.

Feline ulcerative dermatosis is associated with self-trauma resulting in nonhealing deep ulcers most often seen on the neck and between the scapulae. The underlying cause is currently unknown. Glucocorticoids and surgical resection may be successful in some cases but protective bandages are often required to prevent self-mutilation. Topiramate, a drug used to treat refractory epilepsy, was successful in one cat after all other treatments failed.

Sensations of pruritus and pain can interact with each other in the central nervous system. Applying an itch stimulus such as scratching or rubbing can reduce the perception of pain and similarly the application of a painful stimulus can reduce the perception of itch.

Progress has been made in elucidating the mechanisms of pruritus in recent years, but there are still large gaps in our understanding of its neurochemical and electrophysiological aspects as well as its association with nociception.

Further Reading

AAHA/AAFP Pain Management Guidelines, http://www.catvets.com/guidelines/practice-guidelines/pain-management-guidelines (accessed June 25, 2017).

Davis, K. M., Hardie, E. M., Lascelles, B. D., *et al.* (2007) Feline fibrosarcoma: Perioperative management. *Compendium of Continuing Veterinary Education* **29**, 712–714, 716–720, 722–729.

Dawes, J. M., Andersson, D. A., Bennett, D. L. H., *et al.* (2013) Inflammatory mediators and modulators of pain. In *Wall and Melzack's Textbook of Pain*, 6th edn. (eds. S. B. McMahon, M. Koltzenburg, I. Tracey, and D. C. Turk). Elsevier, Philadelphia, PA, pp. 48–67.

Fan, T. M. (2015) Cancer patients. In *Veterinary Anesthesia and Analgesia the Fifth Edition of Lumb and Jones* (eds. K. A. Grimm, L. A. Lamont, W. J. Tranquilli, *et al.*) Wiley Blackwell, Ames, IA, pp. 993–1003.

Grant, D. and Rusbridge, C. (2014) Topiramate in the treatment of feline idiopathic ulcerative dermatitis in a two-year old cat. *Veterinary Dermatology* **25**, 222–e60.

Heinricher, M. M. and Fields, H. L. (2013) Central nervous system mechanisms of pain modulation. In *Wall and Melzack's Textbook of Pain, 6th edn.* (eds. S. B. McMahon, M. Koltzenburg, I. Tracey, and D. C. Turk). Elsevier, Philadelphia, PA, pp. 129–142.

Morris, J. (2013) Mammary tumours in the cat: Size matters, so early intervention saves lives. *Journal of Feline Medicine and Surgery* **15**, 391–400.

Pacharinsak, C., and Beitz, A. J. (2014) Mechanisms of cancer pain. In *Pain Management in Veterinary Practice* (eds. C. M. Egger, L. Love, and T. Doherty). Wiley Blackwell, Ames, IA, pp. 29–37.

Sandkühler, J. (2013) Spinal cord plasticity and pain. In *Wall and Melzack's Textbook of Pain*, 6th edn. (eds. S. B. McMahon, M. Koltzenburg, I. Tracey, and D. C. Turk). Elsevier, Philadelphia, PA, pp. 94–110.

Schmelz, M. and Handwerker, H. O. (2013) Itch. In *Wall and Melzack's Textbook of Pain, 6th edn.* (eds. S. B. McMahon, M. Koltzenburg, I. Tracey, and D. C. Turk). Elsevier, Philadelphia, PA, pp. 211–220.

Schreiber, A. K., Nones, C. F. M., Reis, R. C., *et al.* (2015) Diabetic neuropathic pain: Physiopathology and treatment. *World Journal of Diabetes* **6**, 432–444.

Williams, A. C., and Craig, K. D. (2016) Updating the definition of pain. *Pain* **157**, 2420–2423.

Woolf, C. J. (2010) What is this thing called pain? *The Journal of Clinical Investigation* **120**, 3742–3744.

12

Assessment and Recognition of Acute Pain

Sheilah Robertson

Lap of Love Veterinary Hospice, Lutz, FL, United States

Key Points

- Pain is an emotion and always unpleasant
- Behavioral indicators of acute pain in cats
- Pain scoring tools for use in clinical practice
- Differentiating pain, fear, and stress

Introduction

One of the first challenges in treating pain in cats is recognizing and quantifying it. The International Association for the Study of Pain (IASP) has proposed the following definition of pain: *Pain is a distressing experience associated with actual or potential tissue damage with sensory, emotional, cognitive, and social components.* The sensory component includes the type of pain, its source, location, and intensity. The affective or emotional components can be thought of as "how it makes the patient feel."

Because cats cannot directly tell us how they feel, proxy decisions are made for them and their pain is what the assessor says it is. The veterinary care team must understand behaviors resulting from pain because failure to treat has a negative effect on a cat's welfare.

Pain-assessment Tools

> *"If you cannot measure it, you cannot improve it"* – Lord Kelvin

There is currently no gold standard for assessing acute pain in cats. Several scoring methods that include physiological and behavioral variables have been and continue to be developed and validated.

Feline Anesthesia and Pain Management, First Edition. Edited by Paulo Steagall, Sheilah Robertson and Polly Taylor.

Physiological Indicators of Pain

No single physiological measurement is a sensitive or reliable correlate of pain in a clinical setting. There is a weak correlation between pain scores and systolic blood pressure, heart rate or respiratory rate in cats after ovariohysterectomy. Physiological variables can be affected by many factors other than pain. The stress of a journey to a veterinary hospital will alter heart rate, blood pressure, and respiratory rate in most cats (Chapter 1). Stress, anxiety, and fear are well documented in clinical settings and these are accompanied by cardiovascular changes.

Mechanical Threshold Testing

Following surgery or acute injury, changes occur locally, resulting in peripheral or primary sensitization. Changes in the central nervous system may also occur (*central* or *secondary sensitization*), leading to a decrease in the mechanical threshold required to elicit a response in areas remote from the primary injury (Chapter 11). Sensitivity of a wound can be measured by quantifying the stimulus required to produce a response in the patient (e.g. turning to look at the site, turning to bite, or vocalizing). Application of mechanical pressure is termed *algometry*. Mechanical threshold testing with devices such as algometers, von Frey filaments and palpometers are used to measure both primary (wound), and secondary (remote areas) hyperalgesia. Using a finger-mounted pressure device, researchers could demonstrate a reduction in scrotal hyperalgesia following castration when cats were treated with meperidine (pethidine) compared with no analgesics. Mechanical devices that accurately measure applied force can be valuable research tools (*Figure* 12.1). In clinical practice, physical palpation often provides important information (*Figures* 12.2a and 12.2b).

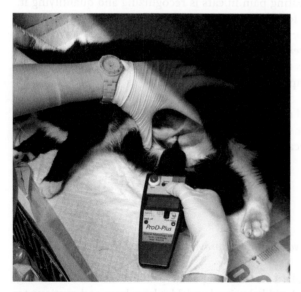

Figure 12.1 Various devices can be used to measure mechanical thresholds; in this example an algometer is being used on the ventral abdomen to measure the force on a 2 mm probe required to elicit a response.
Source: Courtesy of Dr. David Yates.

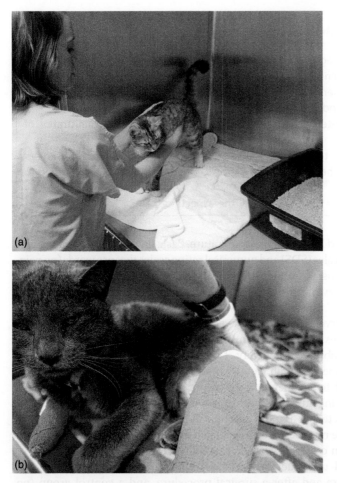

Figure 12.2 In a clinical setting the cat's response to palpation can provide valuable information: (a) abdominal palpation; (b) palpation around a wound following surgery.

Attributes of Pain-Assessment Tools

A scoring system, often termed a tool, scale, or instrument, should have the following attributes:

- Be based on a recognizable response to pain by the cat
- Have a human goal in mind; for example, if specific behaviors are seen, these prompt treatment
- Data collected are as objective and specific as possible
- Any tool used must be tested for validity, reliability, repeatability, and sensitivity (*Box 12.1*). Without strictly defined criteria of what to look for, and observations by trained observers, scoring systems are highly variable, with observers disagreeing about what they see

> **Box 12.1: Essential attributes of a pain-assessment tool**
>
> **Reliability** – is there close agreement between different observers?
> **Repeatability** – also described as "test retest" variability. This is the variation in measurement by an observer of the same item under the same conditions between different time periods and it should be small
> **Sensitivity** – can the tool detect changes, for example over time or after administration of an analgesic?
> **Utility** – easy to use, quick to perform, and suitable for a range of different observers
> **Construct validity** – does the test measure the concept or construct it was intended to measure?
> **Content validity** – does the tool measure all the aspects of pain?

Several scales are described in the veterinary literature. Basic unidimensional pain scales include simple descriptive scales (SDS) and numerical rating scales that use words (no pain, mild pain, severe pain) or assign numbers to levels of pain, for example, "no pain"=0. Visual analog scales (VAS) have been widely used in cats. This tool consists of a continuous line, anchored with "no pain" at one end and "worst imaginable for this condition" at the opposite end, with the observer placing a mark vertically through the horizontal line at a point they consider correlates to pain in the animal under observation. All these scales are associated with significant observer variability. These scales are unidimensional, and do not account for the many aspects of pain. Purely observational studies without interaction with the animal may lead to erroneous assessments: inactivity may be a protective mechanism or because moving hurts therefore unless there is interaction with the patient their pain may go undetected. It is now accepted that quantitative measurement of behavior is the most reliable method for assessing pain in animals. The key questions are "what does pain look like in cats, and what do cats do when they are in pain?"

Scales can be developed using detailed behavior ethograms. With this technique, animals are observed before and after a surgical procedure, and a control group (no surgery) can also be included. Good knowledge of normal cat behavior and that of the individual are important for assessment. Three simple things to consider when assessing a cat after surgery are: is the cat showing normal behaviors, have normal behaviors been lost or have new behaviors developed (*Box* 12.2)?

> **Box 12.2: Three key points when assessing pain in cats**
>
> • Is the cat demonstrating normal behaviors?
> • Are any of the cat's normal behaviors lost after surgery or injury?
> • Does the cat develop new behaviors after surgery or injury?

Some pain tools have been developed based on cats undergoing ovariohysterectomy; however, different types and sources of pain, such as abdominal versus musculoskeletal or oral pain, may result in different behaviors and must be considered when using these tools. For clinical use, the tool must have utility, meaning that it should be easy to use, quick to perform, and suitable for a range of different observers (veterinarians, nurses, technicians) (*Box* 12.1).

Based on current knowledge, the major domains that should be assessed are shown in *Box* 12.3

Box 12.3: The major behavior-based domains for assessing acute pain in cats

- Posture and comfort
- Activity
- Attitude and demeanor
- Interaction with people
- Response to touch, pressure, and palpation
- Attention to the wound
- Vocalization
- Facial expression

Data should be recorded preoperatively (baseline) for later comparison whenever possible. However, there are specific behaviors that occur almost exclusively in painful cats. The UNESP-Botucatu Multidimensional Composite Pain Scale (UNESP-Botucatu MCPS) is available along with examples (videos) and explanations of behaviors via a dedicated website (www.animalpain.com.br/en-us/, accessed June 25, 2017). The scale was developed in Brazilian Portuguese, and it has been validated in English, French, Spanish, and Italian. The UNESP-Botucatu MCPS is a valid, reliable, and responsive instrument that involves different domains such as "pain expression" and "psychomotor change." On the other hand, this scale has only been validated for evaluating cats after ovariohysterectomy and is time consuming. It is not known whether this tool is suitable or would have the same "performance" in cats undergoing other types of surgical procedure, trauma, or with medical or neuropathic pain. Currently, a short-form of the scale is under investigation and may circumvent some of the above issues.

The Glasgow Composite Measures Pain Scale-Feline (CMPS-Feline) includes many of the same assessment domains but was developed independently using cats with surgical, traumatic, and medical conditions to test validity. Since it was first published in 2014, it has been revised (rCMPS-F), and now contains assessment of facial expressions (see later) and guidance for use (*Figure* 12.3). This tool is available for download in English and Spanish at: www.newmetrica.com/acute-pain-measurement/ (accessed June 25, 2017).

Construct validity (i.e. *does the test measure the concept or construct it was intended to measure, in this case pain?*), and content validity (i.e. *does the tool measure all the aspects of pain?*) were reported (*Box* 12.1). The instrument is practical and easy to use in the clinical setting.

A clinical trial involving cats undergoing ovariohysterectomy found that the Glasgow rCMPS and UNESP-Botucatu MCPS had a strong association when used by the same observer. However, in that study, the use of rescue analgesia would have been significantly different depending on the scale used. Therefore, the results of a study, or treatment of a patient might change depending on the instrument used even when using validated tools. This emphasizes that these pain scales should be used to guide treatment decisions and that clinical judgement remains important.

Other pain scales are available for use such as the Colorado State University Feline Acute Pain Scale but these have not been validated.

Glasgow Composite Measure Pain Scale: CMPS - Feline

Guidance for use

The Glasgow Feline Composite Measure Pain Scale (CMPS-Feline), which can be applied quickly and reliably in a clinical setting, has been designed as a clinical decision making tool for use in cats in acute pain. It includes 28 descriptor options within 7 behavioral categories. Within each category, the descriptors are ranked numerically according to their associated pain severity and the person carrying out the assessment chooses the descriptor within each category which best fits the cat's behavior/condition. It is important to carry out the assessment procedure as described on the questionnaire, following the protocol closely. The pain score is the sum of the rank scores. The maximum score for the 7 categories is 20. The total CMPS-Feline score has been shown to be a useful indicator of analgesic requirement and the recommended analgesic intervention level is 5/20.

Glasgow Feline Composite Measure Pain Scale: CMPS - Feline

Choose the most appropriate expression from each section and total the scores to calculate the pain score for the cat. If more than one expression applies choose the higher score

LOOK AT THE CAT IN ITS CAGE:

Is it?
Question 1

Silent / purring / meowing	0
Crying/growling / groaning	1

Question 2

Relaxed	0
Licking lips	1
Restless/cowering at back of cage	2
Tense/crouched	3
Rigid/hunched	4

Question 3

Ignoring any wound or painful area	0
Attention to wound	1

Question 4

(a)   Look at the following caricatures. Circle the drawing which best depicts the cat's ear position?

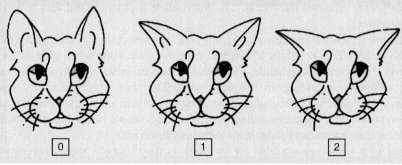

| 0 | 1 | 2 |

(b) Look at the shape of the muzzle in the following caricatures. Circle the drawing which appears most like that of the cat?

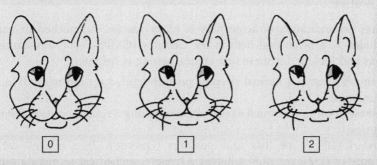

APPROACH THE CAGE, CALL THE CAT BY NAME & STROKE ALONG ITS BACK FROM HEAD TO TAIL

<u>Question 5</u>
Does it?
    Respond to stroking   0

Is it?
    Unresponsive   1
    Aggressive   2

IF IT HAS A WOUND OR PAINFUL AREA, APPLY GENTLE PRESSURE 5 CM AROUND THE SITE. IN THE ABSENCE OF ANY PAINFUL AREA APPLY SIMILAR PRESSURE AROUND THE HIND LEG ABOVE THE KNEE

<u>Question 6</u>
Does it?
    Do nothing   0
    Swish tail/flatten ears   1
    Cry/hiss   2
    Growl   3
    Bite/lash out   4

<u>Question 7</u>
General impression
Is the cat?
    Happy and content   0
    Disinterested/quiet   1
    Anxious/fearful   2
    Dull   3
    Depressed/grumpy   4

Pain Score … /20

Figure 12.3 The refined Glasgow Composite Measures Pain Scale (rCMPS) –Feline, and guidance for use. *Source:* University of Glasgow & Edinburgh Napier. Reproduced with permission of NewMetrica Ltd.

Behavior-based Indicators of Pain (*Box* 12.3)

Posture and Comfort

Specific postures are indicators of acute pain in many species. A hunched or tense posture is included as a behavioral item in the Glasgow rCMPS-Feline. Recognizing normal postures and looking for these in a clinical setting is helpful.

- *Figure* 12.4 shows a cat in a normal sleeping posture (curled up and relaxed) in its home surroundings
- *Figure* 12.5 shows a cat in a hospital environment adopting a similar position despite multiple injuries
- The Glasgow rCMPS-Feline lists four postures (Question 2); a relaxed cat is assigned a score of 0 (*Figure* 12.5) whereas a tense/crouched cat receives a score of 3 (*Figure* 12.6)

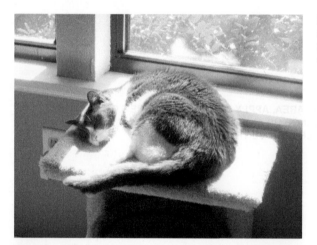

Figure 12.4 A normal resting or sleeping posture in the home environment; the cat is relaxed and curled up.

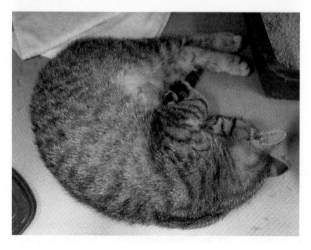

Figure 12.5 The cat in this image has adopted a normal relaxed posture following surgery; this is a positive sign during the initial observational stage of pain assessment.

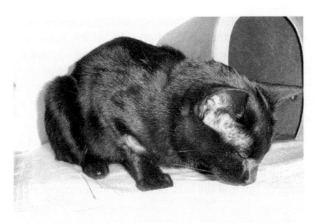

Figure 12.6 Using the Glasgow rCMPS-Feline scale this cat would score 3 (tense/crouched) for question 2.

Activity

Activity or movement should be assessed. The cat is observed to see if it moves normally, especially when it gets up or lies down.

- When cats first wake up, they perform a deep stretch (head down, front limbs extended, and hind end held in the air) (*Figure* 12.7); if they are in pain, this behavior is often absent or restricted
- Cats often stretch in this way when stroked from head to tail. It is usually necessary to open the cage door and allow the cat to leave the cage to assess mobility fully. If there is a step down from the cage to the floor, the cat is watched to see if it jumps down freely, hesitates or uses a strategy that decreases pain

Attitude and Demeanor

Attitude and demeanor encompass psychological elements of pain. Veterinarians and nurses often use words such as *depressed, uninterested, indifferent, content,* and *happy* in

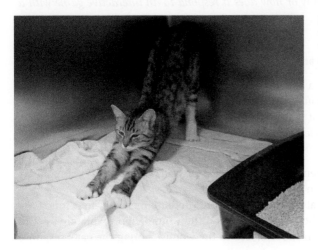

Figure 12.7 When cats wake up they usually perform a deep stretch; when in pain this behavior is often absent or altered.

reference to animals and how they might feel. The words *satisfied, uninterested, indifferent, anxious,* and *aggressive* are used in the UNESP-Botucatu MCPS. However, as everyone who works with cats knows each one has a unique personality which makes scoring demeanor difficult. A recent study showed that a cat's demeanor had a significant effect on the overall score of the Glasgow rCMPS-F and the psychomotor but not pain expression section of the UNESP-Botucatu MCPS. Behavior including demeanor is altered by hospitalization (see below).

- Position in the cage may not be a useful detail to note if considered in isolation or at a single time point. Fearful cats, whether in pain or not, may stay at the back of the cage
- However, if a cat is noted to be at the front of the cage, inquisitive, and engaged with activity outside the cage before surgery, but is at the back of the cage after surgery, this is significant

Unfamiliar surroundings such as a veterinary clinic can cause negative emotional states including anxiety and fear, resulting in freezing, hiding, and hypervigilance. These behaviors may also be noted in a cat that is in pain, so should be evaluated even though they are not specific indicators of pain. However, when taken in context (the cat has had surgery), these behaviors are valuable indicators of the cat's overall psychological state. Differentiating between fear, anxiety, stress, and pain is not straightforward, and is discussed again later.

Interaction with People

In cats that are not feral, willingness to interact with a caregiver should be assessed. Again, this is more meaningful if the responses before and after a painful event are known. Asking the owner about the cat's normal interactions with people can be helpful, and changes from what is normal for that cat can be documented. The Glasgow rCMPS-Feline includes response to being stroked along the back from head to tail. Positive responses to this maneuver include arching of the back, raising the tail, and standing on tiptoes, whereas a negative response is no response or aggression. The response to toys can also be included in the evaluation; *what does the cat do when offered a toy or how does it respond to an interactive game with a person?*

Response to Touch, Pressure, and Palpation

Testing wound sensitivity is a validated and objective assessment method. With appropriate analgesic use, it should be possible to palpate wounds and the surrounding area gently. This is an important component of assessment because many animals may be very reluctant to move because of pain; without interaction, it could easily be assumed that they are comfortable.

- This part of the pain assessment should take place after all observational components and after assessing interaction with the assessor
- If the cat has undergone an abdominal procedure (midline incision), first touch the flank using two fingers and then the area around the wound, approximately 5 cm (2 inches) from the incision, then move closer to the wound, noting the cat's response

- If there is no response, repeat this procedure, but this time apply gentle pressure. Palpation of the abdomen, the wound, and the area around the wound will elicit a range of responses
- The Glasgow rCMPS-Feline tool uses the following responses and scores:
  - Do nothing = 0
  - Swish tail/flatten ears = 1
  - Cry/hiss = 2
  - Growl = 3
  - Bite/lash out = 4

There are clearly times when palpation cannot be included in an assessment, such as when working with unsocialized or extremely fearful cats. In this case, the rest of the assessment is performed and the maximum possible score altered to compensate.

Attention to the Wound or Painful Site

The attention an animal pays to a wound can provide information about spontaneous pain and should be noted carefully. Both licking excessively and biting at a wound are "red flags" and should be investigated. These may be a response to sutures that are pulling on the skin or a wound that is itchy. Testing wound sensitivity (see above) will provide further information. Cats are fastidious groomers; it is therefore important to observe them carefully to differentiate between normal "whole body" grooming behavior and paying too much attention to one area.

Vocalization

Cats have a large and varied vocal repertoire. They may be silent, or they may purr, meow, cry, howl, groan, hiss, or spit. Purring occurs when a female cat nurses her kittens and during social contact (petting, stroking, or feeding) with humans. Purring is often associated with what we assume are pleasurable events and may be a means of communication between adult cats and kittens. However, purring also occurs during more stressful events, such as a physical examination or after an injury. Changes in vocalization such as distress meowing, growling, hissing, and spitting may suggest that the cat is anxious or fearful. Silence does not necessarily mean the cat is not anxious or that it is not in pain. Despite the ambiguity of feline vocalization, it is still widely accepted as a meaningful component of pain assessment. Spontaneous vocalizations (*is the cat meowing when observed?*) and evoked vocalizations (*does the cat cry or groan when palpated?*) are useful in an overall assessment.

Facial Expression

As early as 1872, Darwin wrote about the expression of emotions in humans and animals, noting that pain was recognizable through facial expression. Since then, significant effort has been made to validate facial indicators of pain in many species including humans.

Cats subjected to a brief noxious stimulus often narrow their palpebral fissure, alter their ear position and bunch and flatten their whiskers against their face. The UNESP-Botucatu MCPS includes "partially closed/half closed eyes" or "squinty eyes" as indicators of pain (*Figure* 12.8, 12.9a). The updated Glasgow rCMPS-Feline includes cartoons of ear and

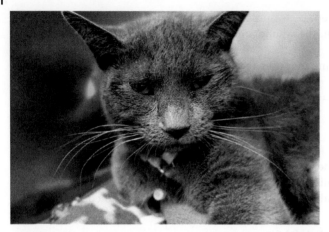

Figure 12.8 The UNESP-Botucatu Multidimensional Composite Pain Scale (UNESP-Botucatu MCPS) includes "partially closed/half-closed eyes" or "squinty eyes" as indicators of pain. This cat also has its ears in an abnormal position and a slightly tense muzzle; scoring of facial expressions are included in the Glasgow rCMPS-Feline scale; see *Figure* 12.3 for details.

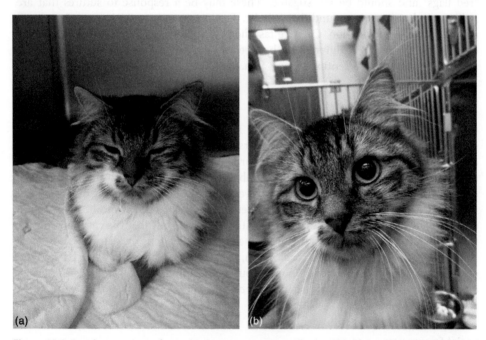

Figure 12.9 Facial expressions of pain: (a) demonstrates "partially closed/half closed eyes" and tension around the muzzle, the ears are also lower than normal. The presence of saliva falling from the mouth suggests the cat may be nauseous. (b) Shows the same cat after intervention; note the change in eye position and that relaxation of the muzzle alters the position of the whiskers. The dilated pupils are due to treatment with an opioid.

muzzle positions (*Figure* 12.3); flattened ears and a tense muzzle are indicators of pain. Adding the facial assessment to the scale made it more discriminatory and fewer cats were misclassified, which was a problem with the version published in 2014. *Figure* 12.9a shows the ear position and tense muzzle with whiskers pulled back in a cat prior to administration of a rescue analgesic. Compare this to the facial expression after intervention with an opioid (*Figure* 12.9b). A Feline Grimace Scale is undergoing development and validation and could be a novel and simple tool for pain assessment in cats.

The Overall Picture

With practice, it becomes easy to recognize several indicators of pain on the initial observation. The cat in *Figure* 12.10 has several facial features suggesting pain (ear position, eyes half closed, tense muzzle), it also looks hunched, tense and uninterested in its surroundings. The next step in assessing this cat is interacting with it to gather more information.

Appetite and Elimination Behaviors

Eating in a clinic environment is a positive sign of wellbeing. It is often assumed that if a cat is eating, it is unlikely to be in pain. However, taken in isolation, appetite or lack of appetite is not a sensitive indicator of pain. Cats in pain will eat, and there are many causes of inappetence or anorexia other than pain. Healthy cats have a decreased appetite and urinate and defecate less frequently than normal when first hospitalized; with time (2–3 days) these habits normalize. Demeanor also influences time to eating after surgery; twice as many cats with low demeanour scores ate by one hour after castration than those with high scores. Once again this shows the importance of factors other than pain that can influence behavior. A cat with a full stomach may not eat and this is not associated with pain. Failure to urinate or defecate may cause agitation and restlessness and confuse assessment. It may be that the litter box that has been provided is inappropriate (too small or difficult to access), they may have an aversion to the litter provided, or in the case of outdoor cats do not adjust quickly to using a litter box.

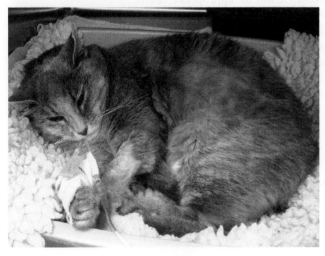

Figure 12.10 This cat shows several indicators of pain: its ears are down, the eyes are half closed, and the muzzle shows tension. The cat also appears tense and hunched and uninterested in its surroundings.

Other Factors to Consider in an Overall Assessment

Cats tend to spend a considerable amount of each day sleeping; however, when assessing sleep, the observer must differentiate normal restful sleep from so-called "feigned" sleep. Cats that are feigning sleep tend to be immobile and appear to be asleep for most of the time, with little or no time spent exploring their surroundings. In addition, they do not look relaxed and if disturbed, they may show an exaggerated startle response. Feigned sleep is thought to be a passive defense mechanism in stressful environments.

Cats are notorious for disliking bandages, restrictive dressings and Elizabethan collars, and these in themselves can alter behavior. Reluctance to move, abnormal postures, rolling around, and unwillingness to use a limb that has had an IV catheter placed in it, can all confuse the ability to assess pain.

Intervention Scores

The suggested score for intervention is > 7 out of a possible total of 30 for the UNESP-Botucatu MCPS and ≥5 out of 20 for the Glasgow rCMPS-F. Although using a validated scoring system is important, no cat should be denied analgesic therapy only on the results of a pain score; the final decision must be made based on an overall assessment and clinical judgment.

Using Response to Treatment as a Diagnostic Tool

Despite the advances in ability to recognize and assess pain in cats, there are many times when a clinician is not sure. In these cases, the benefit of the doubt should be given to the patient. In these situations, one approach is to use the response to analgesic intervention as a diagnostic tool.

- The patient's record is reevaluated, noting what caused the pain, when the cat was last given an analgesic, and whether it was an appropriate choice
- It may be that the cat requires another dose of an opioid sooner than expected or that it needs a higher dose or a different analgesic; this could be a different opioid, a different class of analgesic, or a combination of drugs or a nondrug therapy (e.g. icing) (Chapter 13)
- Following further intervention, the cat should be fully reassessed, and the pain score ought to be reduced. If it is not, then further investigation is warranted

Confounding Factors

Confounding factors that must be considered when assessing feline pain include:

- Demeanor or personality of the cat
- Fear and stress
- Disease
- Anesthetic drugs
- The observer
- Dysphoria, euphoria, and emergence delirium

Personality, Fear and Stress

Cats have different personalities, for example how a shy versus an outgoing confident cat interacts with its surroundings or people may influence assessment; this again emphasizes the importance of before and after evaluations. The influence of demeanor on pain scores has been discussed above. Fear, stress, and anxiety are negative emotions; therefore, in addition to pain each must be addressed and minimized in cats under our care. The psychological and physiological effects of these emotions can confuse clinical assessments. Distinguishing pain from fear, stress, anxiety, and dysphoria is challenging, but if the cause of changes in behavior can be determined, treatment plans can be optimized. Some of the postures adopted by cats that are fearful are similar to those adopted by cats in pain (*Figure* 12.11a, b). Determining if the cat is in pain will

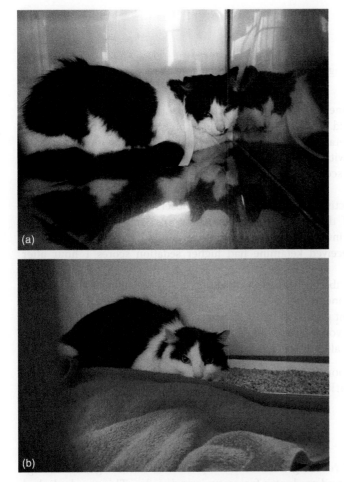

(a)

(b)

Figure 12.11 (a, b) Postures, ear position, and facial expressions (tension in the muzzle and whisker position) in fearful cats can be similar to painful cats. These images show two fearful cats, note the tense and crouched posture, flattened ears, eye position, and tension in the muzzle. For this reason, overall assessment must be made in context and using a composite scale.

require putting it in context (*has it had surgery or been injured?*), and further assessment such as palpation.

Disease

It is not clear how disease affects pain assessment especially given the variety of medical conditions. Pregnant cats, and those with upper respiratory tract disease (URTD) undergoing ovariohysterectomy required more rescue analgesia and had higher pain scores when compared with nonpregnant, healthy cats that underwent the same procedure. Pregnant cats require a larger abdominal incision to perform an ovariohysterectomy resulting in more trauma and inflammation and subsequent pain. Physical condition may affect pain assessment, for example, cats with URTD may exhibit postures and facial expressions similar to painful cats even after administration of opioids and NSAIDs.

Anesthetic Drugs

The effects of anesthetic drugs on behavior should be considered, especially in the early postoperative period.

- The influence of ketamine and alfaxalone on components of the UNESP-Botucatu MCPS have been reported. Cats were given dexmedetomidine, hydromorphone, and either alfaxalone or ketamine (randomized cross over study), intubated, and anesthesia maintained with isoflurane for 30 minutes. No surgery was performed and sedation and pain scores were recorded before and for up to 8 hours after anesthesia
- In the ketamine group, activity, attitude and comfort (observational items listed in the psychomotor section of this scale) were often above 0. Total scores reached or exceeded the suggested intervention level for up to 3 hours in some cats following anesthesia. Cats that received ketamine had higher sedation scores 1 hour after extubation
- Items listed in the pain subscale of the UNESP-Botucatu MCPS, including palpation, vocalization and miscellaneous behaviors, did not differ between treatment groups. One cat in each treatment group exceeded the subscale intervention value; this was a result of behaviour and vocalization. There was no response to palpation in either group emphasizing the value of this interaction whenever it is possible

This emphasizes the importance of interactive items and that pain tools are always evolving and may not work in a context other than the one in which they were developed.

The Observer

Female veterinarians and recent graduates are reported to use analgesics in dogs and cats more than males and graduates from previous decades. This may be linked to gender differences in discerning pain in animals as well as empathy for patients. A greater awareness of pain in animals through education and continuing education may explain the differences between older and newer graduates. Despite attempts to make pain scoring tools objective there may still be bias by observers using them.

Dysphoria and Euphoria

Cats can be described as dysphoric when they resent being handled, are restless or agitated, pace, and vocalize in a plaintive manner. This is distinct from euphoria, which is a positive emotional state defined as a cat that is calm and easy to handle and shows some or all of the following: purring, kneading with its forepaws, rolling, and rubbing its head and body against objects. Dysphoria and euphoria have both been described in cats following treatment with opioid drugs. If, after assessment, a cat is deemed comfortable but dysphoric, and an opioid has been used for analgesia, then administration of a sedative or tranquillizer is an appropriate intervention. If there is no improvement in behavior, partial reversal of the opioid or "waiting it out" are options. Reversal of μ opioid agonists can be achieved using butorphanol or diluted naloxone; both should be given very slowly (IV) until the desired effect is seen (e.g. cessation of agitation) (Chapter 13) .

Emergence Delirium

Emergence delirium is reported in preschool aged children in the early postanesthetic period. Due to variations in how this has been defined the reported incidence ranges from 10–80%. It has been described as a complex of perceptual disturbances and psychomotor agitation. Although short lived there is an increased risk of self-injury during this time. Emergence delirium may occur in conjunction with or independent from pain. "No eye contact", "no purposeful movement" and "no awareness of surroundings" are highly suggestive of emergence delirium in children. Rapid recovery from anesthesia, for example following the use of sevoflurane, and preoperative anxiety are predisposing factors.

Although there are no comprehensive reports describing emergence delirium in cats it undoubtedly occurs and can confound pain assessment. Anecdotally it seems to occur more often with fast recoveries, supporting the use of sedatives, tranquillizers and analgesics in balanced anesthetic protocols to allow for a slower and smoother recovery. In one study in children, each minute taken to recover from general anesthesia decreased the odds of emergence delirium by 7%. If it does occur, the cat should be wrapped in a towel and held if possible to protect it from self-harm; the episode may be short lived and self-limiting. If sedatives or analgesics have not been given they should be considered. Recovering cats in a quiet, warm, and dimly lit recovery area, and emptying the bladder before return of consciousness may decrease the incidence of suboptimal recoveries.

Using Pain-assessment Tools

- In general, evaluations should be made hourly for the first 4 to 6 hours after surgery or injury, provided the cat has recovered from anesthesia, has stable vital signs, and is resting comfortably. Many cats will show signs of pain as early as 30 minutes after extubation. Response to treatment and expected duration of action of the chosen intervention will help in determining the frequency of evaluations. Pain scores should be recorded in the cat's record
- If a cat is resting comfortably following the postoperative administration of buprenorphine, it may not need to be reassessed for 2 to 4 hours. Cats should be allowed to sleep following analgesic therapy; vital signs can often be checked without unduly disturbing them
- Animals are not awakened to check their pain status; however, this does not mean their scheduled analgesics should be withheld. Continuous, undisturbed observations, coupled with periodic interactive assessments are likely to provide more information than a cursory and occasional observation of the patient through the cage door
- In general, the more frequent the observations, the more likely subtle signs of pain or changes in the cat's behavior will be detected

Veterinary nurses and technicians play a vital role in pain assessment (*Box* 12.4)

Box 12.4: The importance of the entire animal care team in assessing pain

All veterinarians and animal care staff should be trained to assess pain in cats. The recognition, assessment, and treatment of pain are fundamental components of compassionate veterinary care. Several studies have highlighted the role of veterinary technicians and nurses as patient advocates. In a survey conducted in the United Kingdom, only 8.1% of veterinary practices used a pain scoring tool, yet 80.3% of nurses agreed these are clinically useful. Animal care staff are ideally suited to spearhead pain-assessment initiatives. They often admit the cat, interact with the cat and owner, carry out the initial preoperative assessment, and oversee the recovery phase of anesthesia so are most likely to observe changes in the cat's behavior.

Continued Assessment at Home

Despite advances in pain management, a better understanding of cats' needs, and identification of stressors in a hospital environment, most clinicians and cat owners agree that the home environment is, in many cases, the best place for cats to complete their recovery.

Although there is little information on changes in behavior in cats recovering at home, owners report decreases in activity and playfulness, an increase in time spent sleeping and changes in how the cat moves or its ability to jump. Owners also comment on changes in facial expression, interrupted stretching, crouched postures, interest in the wound, and aggression towards other cats in the household. These changes are more apparent after ovariohysterectomy than castration and can last for 1 to 3 days.

Owners have an important role to play and can help improve the postoperative care of cats. They know their cat best and are likely to pick up even subtle changes in behavior that are overlooked in a clinic setting. Educating owners on pain behaviors, and supplying them with pain assessment tools, is recommended.

Further Reading

Brondani, J. T., Luna, S. P., Minto, B. W., *et al.* (2013) Reliability and cut-off point related to the analgesic intervention of a multidimensional composite scale to assess postoperative pain in cats. *Arquivo Brasileiro de Medicina Veterinária e Zootecnia* **65**, 153–162.

Brondani, J. T., Luna, S. P., and Padovani, C. R. (2011) Refinement and initial validation of a multidimensional composite scale for use in assessing acute postoperative pain in cats. *American Journal of Veterinary Research* **72**, 174–183.

Brondani, J. T., Mama, K. R., Luna, S. P., *et al.* (2013) Validation of the English version of the UNESP-Botucatu multidimensional composite pain scale for assessing postoperative pain in cats. *BMC Veterinary Research* **9**, 143.

Buisman, M., Hasiuk, M. M., Gunn, M., *et al.* (2017) The influence of demeanor on scores from two validated feline pain assessment scales during the postoperative period. *Veterinary Anaesthesia and Analgesia* **44**, 646–655.

Buisman, M., Wagner, M. C., Hasiuk, M. M., *et al.* (2016) Effects of ketamine and alfaxalone on application of a feline pain assessment scale. *Journal of Small Animal Practice* **18**, 643–651.

Calvo, G., Holden, E., Reid, J., *et al.* (2014) Development of a behaviour-based measurement tool with defined intervention level for assessing acute pain in cats. *Journal of Small Animal Practice* **55**, 622–629.

Cambridge, A. J., Tobias, K. M., Newberry, R. C., *et al.* (2000) Subjective and objective measurements of postoperative pain in cats. *Journal of the American Veterinary Medical Association* **217**, 685–690.

Coleman, D. L., and Slingsby, L. S. (2007) Attitudes of veterinary nurses to the assessment of pain and the use of pain scales. *Veterinary Record* **160**, 541–544.

Darwin, C., Cummings, M. M., Duchenne, G., *et al.* (1872) *The Expression of the Emotions in Man and Animals.* John Murray, London.

Dobbins, S., Brown, N. O., and Shofer, F. S. (2002) Comparison of the effects of buprenorphine, oxymorphone hydrochloride, and ketoprofen for postoperative analgesia after onychectomy or onychectomy and sterilization in cats. *Journal of the American Animal Hospital Association* **38**, 507–514.

Dohoo, S. E., and Dohoo, I. R. (1996) Factors influencing the postoperative use of analgesics in dogs and cats by Canadian veterinarians. *Canadian Veterinary Journal* **37**, 552–556.

Hewson, C. J., Dohoo, I. R., Lemke, K. A. (2001) Factors affecting the use of postincisional analgesics in dogs and cats by Canadian veterinarians in 2001. *Canadian Veterinary Journal* 7, 453–459.

Holden, E., Calvo, G., Collins, M., *et al.* (2014) Evaluation of facial expression in acute pain in cats. *Journal of Small Animal Practice* 55, 615–621.

McCobb, E. C., Patronek, G. J., Marder, A., *et al.* (2005) Assessment of stress levels among cats in four animal shelters. *Journal of the American Animal Hospital Association* 226, 548–555.

Mellor, D., Patterson-Kane, E., and Stafford, K. (2009) Standardized behavioural testing in non-verbal humans and other animals. In *The Sciences of Animal Welfare* (eds. D. J. Mellor, E. Patterson-Kane, and K. J. Stafford). Wiley-Blackwell, Chichester, pp. 95–109.

Merola, I., and Mills, D. S. (2016a) Behavioural signs of pain in cats: an expert consensus. *PLoS One* 11 (2) e0150040.

Merola, I., and Mills, D. S. (2016b) Systematic review of the behavioural assessment of pain in cats. *Journal of Feline Medicine and Surgery* 18, 60–76.

Polson, S., Taylor, P. M., and Yates, D. (2012) Analgesia after feline ovariohysterectomy under midazolam-medetomidine-ketamine anaesthesia with buprenorphine or butorphanol, and carprofen or meloxicam: A prospective, randomised clinical trial. *Journal of Feline Medicine and Surgery* 14, 553–559.

Quimby, J. M., Smith, M. L., and Lunn, K. F. (2011) Evaluation of the effects of hospital visit stress on physiologic parameters in the cat. *Journal of Feline Medicine and Surgery* 13, 733–737.

Reid, J., Scott, E. M., Calvo, G., *et al.* (2017) Definitive Glasgow acute pain scale for cats: Validation and intervention level. *Veterinary Record* doi: 10.1136/vr.104208.

Robertson, S. A. (2016) Acute pain and behavior. In *Feline Behavioral Health and Welfare* (eds I. Rodan and S. Heath) Elsevier, St Louis, MO, pp. 162–183.

Slingsby, L. S., Jones, A., and Waterman-Pearson, A. E. (2001) Use of a new finger-mounted device to compare mechanical nociceptive thresholds in cats given pethidine or no medication after castration. *Research in Veterinary Science* 70, 243–246.

Smith, J. D., Allen, S. W., and Quandt, J. E. (1999) Changes in cortisol concentration in response to stress and postoperative pain in client-owned cats and correlation with objective clinical variables. *American Journal of Veterinary Research* 60, 432–436.

Steagall, P. V., Monteiro, B. P., Lavoie, A. M., *et al.* (2017a) Validation de la version francophone d'une échelle composite multidimensionnelle pour l'évaluation de la douleur postopératoire chez les chats. *Canadian Veterinary Journal* 58, 56–64.

Steagall, P. V., Monteiro, B. P., Ruel, H., *et al.* (2017b) Perceptions and opinions of Canadian pet owners about anesthesia, pain and surgery in small animals. *Journal of Small Animal Practice* 58, 380–388.

Väisänen, A. M., Tuomikoski, S. V., and Vainio, O. M. (2007) Behavioral alterations and severity of pain in cats recovering at home following elective ovariohysterectomy and castration. *Journal of the American Veterinary Medical Association* 231, 236–242.

Waran, N., Best, L., Williams, V., *et al.* (2007) A preliminary study of behaviour-based indicators of pain in cats. *Animal Welfare* **16(S)**, 105–108.

Williams, A. C., and Craig, K. D. (2016) Updating the definition of pain. *Pain* **157**, 2420–2423.

Zeiler, G. E., Fosgate, G. T., van Vollenhoven, E., *et al.* (2014) Assessment of behavioural changes in domestic cats during short-term hospitalization. *Journal of Feline Medicine and Surgery* **16**, 499–503.

13

Treatment of Acute (Adaptive) Pain

Paulo Steagall[1] and Polly Taylor[2]

[1]Université de Montréal, Saint-Hyacinthe, Canada
[2]Taylor Monroe, Little Downham, Ely, United Kingdom

Key Points

- Challenges and concerns in feline pain management. Epidemiological data on veterinary attitudes and perceptions about analgesic use in cats
- Pain is best treated using both analgesic drug administration and nonpharmacological (wound care, immobilization of fractures, environmental changes, physical support, fluid therapy) approaches together
- Principles of treatment in pain management range from prevention to multimodal analgesia
- Analgesics produce pain relief; however they may also cause adverse effects especially when specific contraindications are ignored
- Drug pharmacology, clinical effects, and potential adverse effects impact on the choice of appropriate drug and dosage

Introduction

Effective treatment is only achieved with proper assessment and recognition of acute pain in cats (Chapter 12). Lack of pain assessment lessens analgesic administration and contributes to inadequate treatment. This is a particular issue when pain is not included as the fourth vital sign, part of "Temperature, Pulse and Respiration" (TPR). The guidelines of the World Small Animal Veterinary Association (WSAVA) Global Pain Council (http://www.wsava.org/guidelines/global-pain-council-guidelines, accessed June 25, 2017), and the American Animal Hospital Association (AAHA) (https://www.aaha.org/public_documents/professional/guidelines/2015_aaha_aafp_pain_management_guidelines_for_dogs_and_cats.pdf, accessed June 25, 2017) provide open-access, comprehensive insights on pain management in small animals. Treatment of acute pain is one of the highlights of these two publications, which reveal the importance of the subject in feline medicine and surgery. Indeed, approximately 54% of cats presented as emergencies in a veterinary teaching hospital had signs of pain. Failure to address acute perioperative pain may lead to peripheral and central sensitization, and

Feline Anesthesia and Pain Management, First Edition. Edited by Paulo Steagall,
Sheilah Robertson and Polly Taylor.
© 2018 John Wiley & Sons, Inc. Published 2018 by John Wiley & Sons, Inc.

then maladaptive, persistent postsurgical pain (Chapters 11 and 14); this chapter includes therapies for treating acute pain but also highlights how these prevent long-term changes. Surgery produces nociceptive stimuli and inflammation that are perceived as pain by the conscious cat. It is therefore highly appropriate to administer analgesics to all cats undergoing a surgical procedure.

Challenges in Feline Pain Management

Historically, cats have received less pain relief when compared with dogs for the same surgical procedure. For example, castration was considered to be less painful in cats than in dogs. Prevalence of analgesic administration to "outpatients" was much higher in dogs than in cats. The cause of this difference was multifactorial and included fear of analgesic-induced adverse effects, lack of training in pain assessment and recognition, and the absence of validated instruments (tools) for feline pain assessment. There were several misconceptions (i.e. "morphine-mania", nonsteroidal anti-inflammatory drug (NSAID)-induced adverse effects) that prevented analgesic administration to cats. Nowadays, more cats receive analgesic treatment and there is a better understanding of feline pain management. Some reasons are listed below:

- Cat-specific clinical and experimental trials including a number of pharmacokinetic (PK)-pharmacodynamic (PD) studies have been published
- The subject is now of great importance in the veterinary curriculum and a crucial part of client services and communication
- Availability of approved analgesic drugs for the cat has increased
- Continuing education is now mandatory for most veterinarians. Pain management is a "hot topic" for inclusion in meetings across the world
- Studies on the attitudes and perceptions of veterinarians towards pain management show that postoperative analgesics are now more commonly administered to cats than in the past
- For example, most veterinarians in the United Kingdom now administer some sort of perioperative analgesia for routine canine and feline procedures. Most cats undergoing ovariohysterectomy in Canada receive analgesia before, after, or before and after surgery

These data are promising and reflect recent advances in feline pain management. However, there are still problems and challenges to be addressed. Many cats undergoing ovariohysterectomy still do not receive postincisional analgesia or pain medication once discharged from the hospital. Opioids and NSAIDs are administered less frequently for feline castration compared with the same type of surgery in dogs. In many countries analgesic administration is suboptimal. Veterinarians do not always have access to drugs such as opioids. Restricted financial resources are still a problem in many cases. Analgesics are often administered but are not necessarily the most appropriate choice for that particular condition. Prevalence of analgesic administration to "outpatients" is still higher in dogs than in cats. Finally, lack of staff compliance in administering analgesics in the hospital setting has been recognized as one of the causes of "oligoa-nalgesia": failure to recognize and provide analgesia to patients with acute pain.

These issues listed above prevent appropriate feline pain management. They should be identified and addressed on a case-by-case basis.

Principles of Pain Management

Pain management must be considered as a therapeutic strategy to re-establish organ function, mitigate debilitated body condition, accelerate hospital discharge, and minimize financial costs in addition to its benefits on patient welfare. *Box* 13.1 describes some of the most important principles in pain management for the treatment of acute pain in cats. *Table* 13.1 shows analgesic drugs and dosage regimens used for pain relief in cats.

Box 13.1: Principles of pain management

- Pain is considered to be the fourth vital sign. Assessment and treatment should be part of every patient's physical examination (Chapter 12)
- Nonpharmacological therapies are employed in all cases
- An analgesic plan (*Box* 13.3) should be developed for every medical condition and during the perioperative period. This includes administration of analgesics after hospital discharge
- Analgesic protocols should be prescribed on a case-by-case basis. Dosage regimens are adjusted based on assessment and any adverse effects. Duration of therapy should also be individualized
- Pain management is always best addressed using a preventive and multimodal analgesic approach (*Box* 13.2)
- The advantages and disadvantages of each class of analgesic including their adverse effects should be taken into consideration
- Hospitalization is recommended for invasive surgical procedures where the patient requires frequent assessment and treatment with, for example, opioid and ketamine infusions

---

In addition, there are some important concepts in the treatment of acute pain that constitute the basis for most therapies (*Box* 13.2).

Box 13.2: Concepts for the treatment of acute pain

- *Preemptive analgesia* is the administration of analgesics before the tissue insult (i.e. analgesic intervention before surgical incision), which should prevent the development of altered processing of afferent input, and amplification of postoperative pain
- This definition has now evolved to a broader concept since surgery alone is not the only trigger for central sensitization. Postoperative pain, inflammation, and additional nociceptive input can also induce long-term changes associated with peripheral and central sensitization. These changes cannot be controlled solely with preemptive administration of analgesics
- *Preventive analgesia* has now been used to describe all types of perioperative maneuvers and efforts to decrease postoperative pain. Analgesic treatment is administered at any time and for varying durations in the perioperative period to prevent central sensitization
- *Multimodal analgesia* is the administration of two or more analgesic drugs with different mechanisms of action. Such drug combinations may lead to synergism, allowing the use of lower doses of each and consequent prevention of adverse effects

---

Table 13.1 Suggested dosage regimens and routes of administration for drugs used in the treatment of acute pain in cats.

Drug	Doses (mg/kg), or otherwise indicated	Route	Comments
Opioids			
Morphine	0.2–0.5 q 4–6 hours	IM	Caution with IV administration due to histamine release (give slowly). May cause nausea and vomiting. Morphine (0.1 mg/kg) may be administered by the epidural route or intra-articularly as an adjuvant analgesic technique
Pethidine (meperidine)	3–5 q 1–2 hours	IM	Not suitable for IV administration due to histamine release
Methadone	0.3–0.5 q 4 hours	IM, IV, OTM	Has NMDA receptor antagonist properties
Oxymorphone	0.025–0.1 q 4–6 hours	IM, IV	May cause hyperthermia in cats.
Hydromorphone	0.025–0.1 q 4–6 hours	IM, IV	May cause nausea and vomiting
Tramadol	2–4 q 6–8 hours	IM, IV, PO	Noradrenaline (norepinephrine) and serotonin reuptake inhibitor in addition to its opioid-like effects
Fentanyl injectable	Bolus 1–3 µg/kg + CRI 5–15 µg/kg/hour	IV	High doses may produce dysphoria in awake patients Maximum decreases in MAC are observed at 10–15 µg/kg/hour
Remifentanil	4–6 µg/kg/hour (analgesia) 10–20 µg/kg/hour (anesthetic-sparing)	IV	Limited decreases in the minimum alveolar concentration (MAC) of inhalant anesthetics in cats (15–20%). Remifentanil does not require a bolus and is half as potent as fentanyl. Sympathetic stimulation may be observed at high doses
Butorphanol	0.2–0.4 q 1–2 hours	IM, IV	Limited analgesic efficacy only suitable for mild pain or for sedation. It can be used to reverse pure opioid agonist-induced respiratory depression (0.05 mg/kg IV) It can be used as a CRI for some types of visceral pain at 0.05 mg/kg/hour
Buprenorphine 0.3 mg/mL (Vetergesic®, Buprenex®, Temgesic®)	0.02–0.04 q 4–8 hours	IM, IV, OTM	Euphoria is commonly observed SC administration does not produce adequate analgesia

	Dose	Route	Notes
Buprenorphine 1.8 mg/mL (Simbadol®)	0.24 every 24 hours for up to 3 days	SC	Control of postoperative pain in cats – is designed for SC use. Good analgesia especially when administered with local anesthesia and NSAIDs
Naloxone (antagonist)	0.04 q 0.5–1 hours	IV	Commonly diluted and titrated to effect to reverse adverse effects. Naloxone is diluted with 5 mL of saline 0.9% and given at 0.5 mL/min until the side effects have subsided
NSAIDs [a]			
Meloxicam	0.2 or 0.3 followed by 0.05 mg/kg for 3–5 days	SC, PO	Can be administered at 0.05 mg/kg/day for control of postoperative pain
Robenacoxib	2 followed by 1–2 mg/kg during 3–5 days	SC, PO	Can be administered at 1 mg/kg/day for control of postoperative pain
Carprofen	4	SC	Single administration in cats
Tolfenamic acid	4	SC	Single administration in cats (not preoperative)
Ketoprofen	2	SC	Single administration in cats (not preoperative)
Local anesthetics (see Chapter 5)			
Bupivacaine	Doses should not exceed 2		Should never be administered IV due to cardiotoxicity
Lidocaine	Doses should not exceed 10		Can be administered at 1 mg/kg to treat ventricular dysrhythmias. CRI is not recommended due to cardiovascular depression (see text)

Notes: Dosage regimens for agonists of α_2-adrenergic receptors, ketamine and gabapentin are included in the text.
a) Suggested doses as these may vary according to country.

The use of multimodal analgesia has been endorsed by several professional organizations involved with anesthesiology and analgesia in humans, including the American Society of Anesthesiologists (ASA), and the International Association for the Study of Pain (IASP). Publications include the ASA acute pain management guidelines (http://anesthesiology.pubs.asahq.org/article.aspx?articleid=1933589, accessed June 25, 2017). Some of this information can be extrapolated to cats. For example, multimodal analgesic protocols involving local anesthetics can substantially decrease opioid requirements and their associated adverse effects. Gabapentin has now been administered to cats to minimize the development of persistent postsurgical pain (Chapter 14) especially when NSAIDs are contraindicated.

Pain management may be challenging in cats because assessment and recognition is difficult (Chapter 12). There is a plethora of painful conditions that may be encountered, and devising a good, individualized analgesic plan is not a simple undertaking. A good start is to ask three basic questions, taking into account that all surgery and many medical conditions and procedures induce pain and inflammation (*Box* 13.3).

Box 13.3: Three basic questions in the treatment of pain

- What is the most appropriate opioid for this case?
- Are there any contraindications to the administration of NSAIDs? (Since surgery will induce some degree of inflammation, NSAIDs are important in providing pain relief; the likely duration of treatment should be considered)
- Are there any local anesthetic techniques that could be applied to this case?

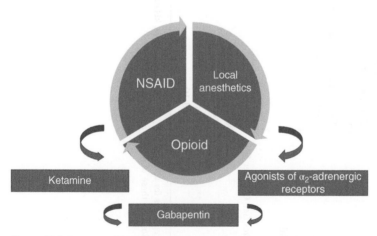

Figure 13.1 Drugs used for the treatment of acute pain. Opioids, local anesthetics, and nonsteroidal anti-inflammatory drugs are administered as the first line of treatment of acute pain. Adjuvant analgesic drugs (ketamine, gabapentin and dexmedetomidine) are administered for severe acute pain and prevention of persistent postsurgical pain.

A fourth question could be "Is there a need to administer adjuvant analgesics?" (e.g. ketamine, agonists of α_2-adrenoreceptors, tramadol). In summary, the first line of acute pain treatment involves nonpharmacological therapies, then administration of opioids, local anesthetics and NSAIDs, once contraindications have been excluded. The second line of treatment involves the addition of other analgesic therapies (*Figure* 13.1). Prescription of oral medication including NSAIDs, gabapentin, tramadol, and amantadine is crucial in severe acute pain control where it is particularly important to prevent persistent postsurgical pain after hospital discharge. Proposed dosing intervals and routes of administration must be thought out carefully to maximize the owner's compliance with the treatment they have to administer.

The main goals of acute pain therapy are to maximize analgesia and comfort, minimize adverse effects, and prevent a deleterious endocrine stress response. Treatment should also incorporate anxyolisis and muscle relaxation when needed to encourage a calm, quiet recovery.

Nonpharmacological Therapies in Acute Pain Management

Nonpharmacological therapies are used as adjuvants to complement the treatment of pain. In hospitalized human patients, nonpharmacological therapy in pain management can help to treat the affective and cognitive dimensions of pain. Some of these techniques used for treating chronic pain are presented in Chapter 15. In the acute setting, they include bandaging (wound care), cold therapy (*Figure* 13.2), nursing (i.e. positioning, fluid therapy, and nutrition), environment (i.e. dry, calm, quiet, and comfortable), and an area for cats that is separated from dogs (cat-friendly practice, Chapter 1). Such therapy is as important as drug administration and includes the concept of "tender, loving, care" (TLC) (*Figure* 13.3). Nonpharmacological techniques are cost effective and widely available. They can reduce stress, anxiety, inflammation, edema, tissue damage, muscle spasm and pain behaviors, and potentially accelerate

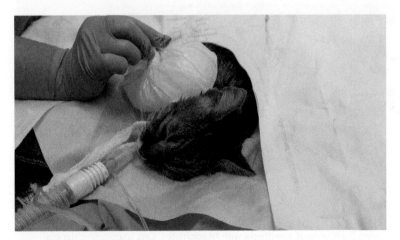

Figure 13.2 Nonpharmacological analgesia: cold therapy using an ice pack in a cat immediately after total ear canal ablation to reduce inflammation and edema.

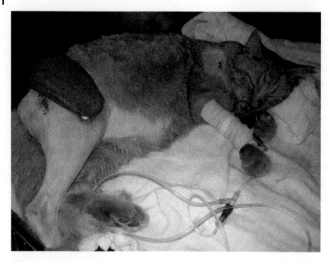

Figure 13.3 A cat sleeps comfortably after femoral fracture repair with an external fixator. "Tender, loving, care" (TLC) is provided by a quiet, clean environment with appropriate lighting, soft bedding, head support, bandaging, and human contact. Fluid therapy is administered in combination with analgesics for pain relief.

hospital discharge while improving comfort. Physical treatments have the potential to inhibit afferent nociceptive input and modulate the descending inhibitory system with the release of endogenous opioids.

In humans, nonpharmacological therapy improves activity and functional ability as well as reducing analgesic requirements and their consequent adverse effects. A similar benefit could be extrapolated to the cat even before controlled studies are published on the subject. A recent study showed that cats undergoing general anesthesia with classical music playing to them through headphones had lower respiratory rate and smaller

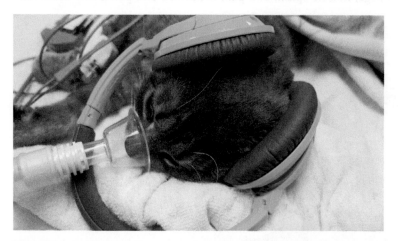

Figure 13.4 A cat recovers from general anesthesia with headphones. Cats undergoing general anesthesia with classical music provided via headphones had a low respiratory rate and small pupil diameter. Auditory sensory stimuli occur during anesthesia and influence autonomic nervous system responses.

pupillary diameter when compared with those hearing pop and heavy-metal music (*Figure* 13.4). This shows that auditory sensory stimuli processing is present even during general anesthesia, and the autonomic nervous system activity can be influenced by it. In humans, music reduces heart rate, blood pressure, respiration rate and distracts the patient by endorphin release, reducing pain perception.

Bandaging is an important part of wound care (*Figure* 13.3). It should be comfortable, clean, and changed according to need. Bandage material should be soft padded and appropriate to the wound. In cats, bandaging under anesthesia (without surgery) can induce an endocrine stress response as intense as that from anesthesia with surgery and greater than from anesthesia alone. Cats dislike bandages, and their appropriate management is important for the patient's welfare.

Cold treatment can easily be incorporated into postoperative care to reduce inflammation and edema (*Figure* 13.2). Cooling material (e.g. cold gel packages or ice packs) is applied for approximately 15–20 minutes around the wound. This can be carried out during recovery from anesthesia. Gauze should be placed between the skin and the cold source for hygiene and to prevent discomfort and skin damage. Nociceptive input around the wound will be diminished. Cold and ice applications have been shown to reduce pain in humans.

Positioning can be optimized by support from pillows, towels, and the use of pads to elevate a limb to lift it for instance to ameliorate blood flow, provide comfort, and prevent muscle spasm, which consequently reduces pain. This is particularly important in depressed cats. Unless they are sleeping, hospitalized cats should be gently stimulated to move and stretch when a caregiver is offering food or cleaning the litterbox, for example.

Pharmacological Therapy in Acute Pain Management

Opioids

Mechanism of Action

Opioid drugs bind to opioid receptors in the peripheral and central nervous system, which reduces the release of excitatory neurotransmitters and hyperpolarizes neuronal membranes. These effects decrease and inhibit nociceptive input without changes in proprioception. Opioids have a range of effects based on their receptor affinity, efficacy, potency and individual characteristics, and their use in feline practice has been reviewed in detail elsewhere (see list of further reading).

Clinical Use

Opioids are part of the first line of treatment in acute pain management. Full agonists of opioid receptors (e.g. morphine, hydromorphone, oxymorphone, meperidine (pethidine), methadone, fentanyl, remifentanil) provide dose-dependent analgesia (*Table* 13.1). They increase vagal tone, inducing bradycardia, without changes in systemic vascular resistance or myocardial contractility, offering hemodynamic stability. Sedation after opioid administration is particularly obvious in ill cats. These side effects are mild and easily treated, and the benefits of pain relief with opioids outweigh their side effects. Opioids can be administered using several different routes of administration (e.g. buccal, IV, IM, SC, epidural, intra-articular or transdermal), and by bolus injection or infusion.

Opioid administration decreases morbidity and mortality in dogs, and probably the same phenomenon occurs in cats. Opioids produce variable degrees of pain relief and decrease volatile anesthetic requirements; however this sparing effect is limited in cats compared with dogs. The use of opioids for balanced anesthesia is discussed in Chapter 6.

Agonists of κ-opioid receptors and antagonists of μ-opioid receptors (e.g. nalbuphine and butorphanol) provide limited analgesia, and are more commonly used for sedation when administered in combination with agonists of $α_2$-adrenergic receptors or acepromazine (i.e. neuroleptanalgesia, Chapter 3). Buprenorphine is a partial agonist of μ-opioid receptors and its use in feline practice has been reviewed in depth elsewhere (see further reading).

Changes in behavior (i.e. euphoria: purring, kneading with forepaws, rubbing on objects, "love bites") and mydriasis are commonly observed after opioid administration to cats. Dysphoria and excitement are rarely observed when recommended doses and intervals of administration are respected. The term "morphine mania" is a myth since adverse effects are not observed when clinical doses of opioids are given. Hyperthermia may be observed after administration of opioids especially hydromorphone in cats and is usually self-limiting. However, it can result in agitation, discomfort, and thrashing. Supportive care should be given and body temperature closely monitored in the postoperative period.

Doses and recommendations for opioid analgesics are presented in *Table* 13.1. Information on routes of administration and the various formulations of opioids suitable for feline practice is presented below:

- Except for morphine and meperidine (pethidine), the IV route of administration is usually preferred for opioids when an IV catheter is in place. Doses can be titrated to effect with rapid onset of action and immediate pain relief
- Opioid infusions are normally administered for dose-dependent analgesia and ease of titration. They are usually given to critically ill, hospitalized cats or patients undergoing invasive procedures with, for instance, multiple trauma, where pain is severe and difficult to control
- With the exception of a FDA-approved high-concentration formulation of buprenorphine hydrochloride (Simbadol™; 1.8 mg/mL) in the United States (*Table* 13.1), SC administration of opioids does not provide reliable analgesic effect in cats at clinical doses; the IV and IM routes are preferred
- SC administration of hydromorphone resulted in a higher prevalence of nausea and vomiting and inferior analgesia when compared with IV or IM administration
- Epidural administration of preservative-free morphine alone (0.1 mg/kg) or in combination with local anesthetics is an excellent technique for providing sustained perioperative analgesia for around 16–24 hours as part of multimodal analgesia
- Urinary retention is a common side effect when morphine is administered by the epidural route. Bladder expression is recommended at the end of surgery before patient extubation to avoid atony of the detrusor muscle
- Epidural analgesia is highly recommended for severe pain involving the thorax, abdomen and pelvic limbs
- Both buprenorphine and methadone can be administered by the buccal route (or oral transmucosal; OTM) to provide analgesia in cats. This method is an option for "hands-off" analgesia especially when administered as part of a multimodal protocol. Minimal restraint is required (*Figure* 3.3). However, clinical studies using buprenorphine showed that the IV and IM routes provide superior analgesia when compared with the OTM

- Cats have an alkaline buccal pH (8–9) which is similar to the pKa of opioids. This increases the nonionized portion of the drug and enhances absorption through the mucous membranes
- Sustained-release formulations of buprenorphine have been used in clinical practice, but there is only limited data on safety and efficacy
- Human fentanyl patches (12.5 or 25 µg/hour) have been used for postoperative pain control; however absorption variability, lower bioavailability when compared with dogs, and questionable analgesic efficacy have been reported in cats
- In theory, fentanyl patches should provide long-term analgesia (i.e. up to 72 hours); with a prolonged onset of action (7 hours), alternative analgesia should be provided in the interim. Accidental ingestion by children or animals, or human exposure to the patch is a source of liability, and patch use should be limited to hospitalized patients
- A transdermal patch of buprenorphine has been tested in cats; however, data are limited and insufficient for any recommendations for clinical use
- Intra-articular morphine is used for postoperative analgesia after joint surgery in humans, with the intention of preventing upregulation of µ-opioid receptors in the articular and periarticular tissues while the joint is inflamed. The technique is never used alone, only as part of a multimodal protocol
- Oral administration of opioids is not recommended in cats because of their low bioavailability, large individual variability, erratic gastrointestinal absorption, and limited analgesic effect
- Cats have marked variation in analgesic response to opioids as a result of different phenotype, age, PK, and physical conditions. In particular, some cats appear to be "opioid nonresponders": if an administered opioid does not produce any effect, a second, with activity at a different receptor should be given

Nonsteroidal Anti-inflammatory Drug (NSAID)

Mechanism of Action
Cyclooxygenase (COX) enzyme expression in cell membranes is inhibited by NSAIDs. The COX-1 isoform is a constitutive form of the enzyme found in many tissues. It regulates normal homeostasis by facilitating production of prostaglandins in the gastrointestinal mucosa, and by playing a role in platelet aggregation and renal blood flow. The COX-2 isoform is also constitutively expressed in a range of tissues and organs, including ovarian, CNS, and renal tissues; but it is primarily induced in larger quantities by damage or tissue injury as a proinflammatory enzyme. It is responsible for production of various eicosanoids, inflammatory mediators, which amplify nociceptive input and transmission to the spinal cord. NSAIDs also produce central analgesic effects as they penetrate the blood-brain barrier. Both forms of COX express physiological functions; *this explains why any NSAID can produce adverse effects whether they are nonpreferential COX inhibitors, preferential COX-2 inhibitors or COX-2 sparing drugs.*

Clinical Use
Nonsteroidal anti-inflammatory drugs are the most widely used analgesics in veterinary medicine due to their anti-inflammatory, analgesic, and antipyretic effects. They are noncontrolled substances that are key players in the treatment of acute pain in cats, used alone and in combination with opioids and local anesthetics. Nonsteroidal anti-inflammatory drugs exert a range of inhibition of both COX-isoforms and therefore can induce

adverse effects such as gastric irritation, protein-losing enteropathy, renal damage, and prolonged bleeding time by prevention of platelet aggregation. At least in dogs, liver-associated adverse effects are thought to be an idiosyncratic reaction to specific drugs rather than intrinsic hepatotoxicity. Adverse effects induced by NSAIDs occur when contraindications are not respected. Anorexia, diarrhea, vomiting and depression are usually the first signs of toxicity, and NSAID administration should be stopped immediately if any of these occur. Acute NSAID-induced renal injury in healthy cats after a single injection is a myth that should not be propagated. Notwithstanding their potential detrimental effects on bone healing, clinical use of NSAIDs in orthopedic surgery is unquestionably required for acute pain management. It is of note that in research studies, prevalence of NSAID-induced adverse effects is commonly no greater than in healthy cats receiving placebo. Key components of NSAIDs are described below.

- In many countries, NSAIDs are approved only for one or a few days of administration for treatment of acute pain. Labels vary among countries and veterinarians should be aware of the data sheet recommendations that apply locally
- For example, flunixin meglumine, carprofen, ketoprofen, meloxicam, robenacoxib and tolfenamic acid have been labeled for at least a single administration. The choice will vary according to the country. Some NSAIDs are labeled for treatment of upper respiratory tract disease but are more commonly used for postoperative pain control
- Oral administration and SC injection are the most common routes of administration, and both are effective. IV administration is recommended with some NSAIDs in some countries. Administration via different routes can result in a range of PK variation but the PD effect (i.e. control of inflammation and analgesia) is usually equivalent
- NSAID treatment of acute pain is convenient and practical because some have excellent palatability for oral administration; client compliance is also good because of easy administration intervals (every 24 hours). The corresponding injectable formulations allow intraoperative administration (IV and SC injection), and oral medication can be prescribed to continue treatment after hospital discharge
- The various NSAIDS are equally effective for postoperative analgesia after a single dosing. On the other hand, safety is an issue with continuous administration of some of these agents. Meloxicam and robenacoxib are safe for administration over several days in healthy patients undergoing soft tissue and orthopedic surgery
- Meloxicam is generally injected as a bolus (0.2 mg/kg SC) in the intraoperative period and continued for a further 3–5 days (0.05 mg/kg PO), depending on the procedure and country. Five-day therapy was superior to three-day therapy in cats undergoing onychectomy
- Robenacoxib is generally injected as a bolus (2 mg/kg SC) in the intraoperative period, and some studies have continued for up to 9 days (1 mg/kg PO) in the treatment of orthopedic pain. Oral administration should be after fasting or with a small amount of food to maximize bioavailability and peak plasma concentration. Duration of treatment will vary with the condition. The minimum effective dose is recommended
- For example, NSAIDs may be needed for only 48 hours (i.e. one dose in the intraoperative period and a second at 24 hours, given orally) after an ovariohysterectomy performed by an experienced surgeon, if administered in combination with opioids and intraperitoneal analgesia using bupivacaine. On the other hand, full-mouth dental extractions for treatment of feline chronic gingivostomatitis may require five to seven days of treatment
- Aspirin is used for feline arterial thromboembolism but no longer as an analgesic in cats because much better options are now available

- Client communication is important to avoid adverse effects
- Timing of NSAID administration is controversial (*Box* 13.4)

Box 13.4: Timing of NSAID administration

The timing of NSAID administration is controversial but it is reasonable to suggest that they can be administered when

- Blood pressure is monitored and under control
- Fluid administration has been initiated
- Contraindications have been excluded (gastrointestinal disease, NSAID intolerance, uncontrolled renal disease, hepatic disease, coagulopathies, hypovolemia and hypotension, concurrent NSAID or corticosteroid administration)

NSAIDs can generally be given preoperatively for routine neutering in young healthy cats without necessitating fluid therapy during anesthesia.

Healthy cats will benefit from therapy before surgery begins, and certainly before extubation and recovery from anesthesia. NSAIDs are often administered towards the end of the procedure so that patients will at least benefit from the analgesic and anti-inflammatory effects once they are conscious and can perceive pain.

Long-term administration of NSAIDs in cats may be required for severe acute pain and to prevent persistent postsurgical pain. Chapter 15 (*Box* 15.3) gives guidelines for the safe use of NSAIDs in cats. Chapter 15 also considers the advantages and disadvantages of NSAID therapy in cats with chronic kidney disease and degenerative joint disease.

Local Anesthetics

Mechanism of Action
The mechanism of action, psychochemical and PK-PD properties, toxicity, clinical use, and contraindications of local anesthetics are presented in Chapter 5.

Clinical Use
The value of local anesthetic techniques cannot be overemphasized.

- Local anesthetics are part of the first line of treatment in acute pain management, and there is rarely any contraindication for their administration (with the exception of epidural anesthesia) (Chapter 5)
- Maximum doses should always be calculated; negative aspiration of blood to avoid hematoma and accidental intravenous injections, and lack of resistance to prevent nerve damage must be confirmed before administration of a local anesthetic block
- A number of local anesthetic techniques for the head, thoracic and pelvic limbs, and trunk can be used to prevent and treat acute pain
- Local block provides muscle relaxation and analgesia, decreases opioid requirement, and produces a marked volatile anesthetic-sparing effect
- In feline practice, head blocks are commonly used in dentistry (Chapter 5)

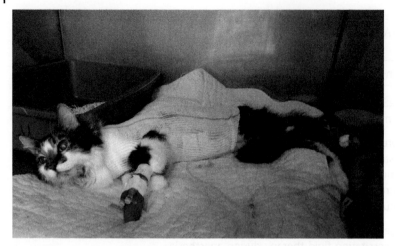

Figure 13.5 Lidocaine patches can be applied over wounds to provide local analgesia as part of a multimodal approach. A bandage is applied to secure the patch in place.

- Intraperitoneal analgesia and intratesticular anesthesia are particularly important in spay-neuter programs where opioids are not always available (Chapter 5)
- Contemporary loco-regional techniques (i.e. brachial plexus, sciatic, and femoral nerve blocks) can be performed using electrical nerve stimulators (*Figure* 5.4 and 5.7) or ultrasonography
- Anesthetic recovery is usually smooth when a local anesthetic block is effective, averting the need for large doses of opioids or sedatives in the perioperative period

Local anesthetics can be administered for treatment of acute pain using a range of routes of administration (e.g. transdermal and IV). Lidocaine patches (700 mg; 50 mg/g of adhesive) can be applied over a wound to provide local analgesia with minimum systemic absorption (*Figure* 13.5). The patch can be cut and adapted to the size of the patient and area of interest. A bandage can be applied to secure the patch in place. IV infusions of lidocaine produce perioperative analgesia in a number of species (Chapter 6). Although this decreases volatile anesthetic requirements in a plasma concentration-dependent manner, it causes significant cardiovascular depression and the technique is not recommended for pain management in cats.

Agonists of α_2-Adrenergic Receptors

Mechanism of Action
The mechanism of action, key pharmacological features, clinical use for sedation and chemical restraint, and contraindications of agonists of α_2-adrenergic receptors are presented in Chapter 3. The use of these drugs as part of anesthesia for spay-neuter programs is described in Chapter 4.

Clinical Use
Agonists of α_2-adrenergic receptors are used for sedation, muscle relaxation, and analgesia, and are commonly given in the premedication with an opioid analgesic.

They are potent adjuvant analgesics that can be administered to healthy cats in combination with local anesthetics, NSAIDs, and opioids. Agonists of α_2-adrenergic receptors play an important role in pain management for spay-neuter programs (Chapter 4). Administration of dexmedetomidine with buprenorphine enhanced antinociceptive activity when compared with either drug alone. These drugs can be given by a number of routes (e.g. epidural, buccal, IV), and will significantly reduce volatile anesthetic requirements. However, they may also delay anesthetic recovery, and reversal with an antagonist of α_2–adrenergic receptors (e.g. atipamezole, yohimbine) is recommended if recovery is prolonged, particularly in pediatric patients. Infusions of dexmedetomidine have not been thoroughly investigated in cats (Chapter 6), and their use is rarely required for pain management, particularly in the light of their cardiovascular depressant effects. Administration of agonists of α_2-adrenergic receptors is not recommended for balanced anesthesia if the goal is to improve hemodynamics.

Ketamine and Amantadine

Mechanism of Action
The mechanism of action, key pharmacological features, commercial preparations, clinical use for induction of anesthesia, and contraindications for ketamine are presented in Chapter 4.

Clinical Use
Low doses of ketamine given by infusion are used in acute feline pain management. Balanced anesthesia and analgesia with ketamine infusions (Chapter 6) are summarized in *Box* 13.5.

Box 13.5: Perianesthetic use of ketamine infusions for analgesia

- Constant rate infusions of remifentanil plus ketamine decreased isoflurane requirements by approximately 50% (expired concentrations of isoflurane approximately 0.7%) in healthy cats undergoing ovariohysterectomy when compared with saline. The combination should improve the quality of anesthesia
- Ketamine is administered as a bolus (0.5 mg/kg IV) followed by a constant rate infusion (10–30 µg/kg/minute IV). The reduction in isoflurane concentration may be critical in ill, painful cats, and is used as part of multimodal analgesia
- Remifentanil administered at 30 µg/kg/hour produced only a mild sparing effect on isoflurane concentration (15%, expired concentrations approximately 1%) when administered alone
- Based on human literature, lower doses of ketamine by infusion are administered to provide NMDA antagonism and an anti-inflammatory effect (2–10 µg/kg/minute) (Chapter 4, *Box* 4.3)
- Ketamine can be added to a crystalloid solution (60 mg of ketamine into a 500 mL bag, 10 µg/kg/minute) and administered at 5 mL/kg/hour, IV, throughout surgery using a fluid infusion device

---

Ketamine is commonly administered in combination with opioids and local anesthetics to prevent or treat central sensitization, hyperalgesia, and allodynia. It is used in critically ill patients, especially when NSAIDs are contraindicated and when cats are "opioid nonresponders" (see above). Ketamine is opioid sparing and does not produce behavioral changes at antihyperalgesic doses (2–10 µg/kg/minute); however, sedation and mood changes may be observed after bolus administration. The use of ketamine alone is not indicated since it does not produce clinically relevant analgesia.

Amantadine is another NMDA antagonist used for treatment of chronic pain (Chapter 15) and pain that is refractory to NSAID therapy; however, information is scarce, particularly in cats. The drug has been prescribed for pain control after hospital discharge, in combination with tramadol or NSAIDs, in acute feline pain management with a view to preventing the development of chronic pain.

Tramadol

Mechanism of Action
Tramadol hydrochloride is a phenylpiperidine analogue of codeine, with weak binding affinity to opioid receptors. It is a racemic mixture and is metabolized to both (+) and (−) enantiomer metabolites. The (+) enantiomer, O-desmethyltramadol (M1), has the greater affinity for the µ-opioid receptor and some serotonergic effects. Cats produce the (+) enantiomer faster than dogs (3.9-fold). Plasma concentrations of tramadol and the (+) enantiomer are dose dependent after oral administration. The (−) enantiomer inhibits noradrenalin reuptake. Cats produce the (−) enantiomer more slowly than dogs (4.8-fold). α_2-adrenergic receptor activation plays a significant role in spinal monoaminergic modulation of pain, and this probably contributes to tramadol's effects.

Clinical Use
In North America and some countries in Europe tramadol is primarily used for treatment of chronic pain (Chapter 15) but it has also a role in acute pain management. For example, it is commonly prescribed for continuous pain relief after hospital discharge, and is widely used in its injectable form in South America and parts of Europe. In this case, tramadol is commonly administered IV or IM with a sedative or tranquilizer (neuroleptanalgesia). In many countries, tramadol is the only opioid-like analgesic drug available in veterinary medicine.

Other than experience from use in clinical practice, there is limited information on the analgesic effects of tramadol in cats. Oral formulations of tramadol have poor palatability and this can limit its use even for short-term administration. Oral administration of 4 mg/kg induced thermal antinociception for 6 hours, and required frequent administration for a sustained effect. At doses of 1 mg/kg, subcutaneous tramadol had limited antinociceptive effects in cats. On the other hand, higher doses (2 mg/kg) every 8 hours resulted in postoperative analgesia in cats undergoing ovariohysterectomy. However, combinations of tramadol with an NSAID result in a superior analgesic effect over each drug alone. Clinical experience suggests that tramadol is an adjuvant analgesic and should be used in combination with other first line analgesics such as NSAIDs. Serotonin syndrome following tramadol overdose is described in Chapter 15.

Tapentadol

Mechanism of Action

Tapentadol is a novel atypical opioid drug with a dual mechanism of action. It is an agonist of μ opioid receptors and inhibits norepinephrine reuptake. Unlike tramadol, tapentadol is administered in the active form and does not require hepatic metabolism for an analgesic effect.

Clinical use

The efficacy of tapentadol is similar to morphine in the treatment of acute and chronic pain in humans. In cats, adverse effects after intravenous administration of tapentadol are similar to other species and include agitation, panting and salivation. These effects were not observed after oral administration of 25 and 50 mg of tapentadol in research cats. The higher dose of tapentadol (approximately 12 mg/kg) produced similar antinociception to IM buprenorphine (0.02 mg/kg). However, palatability was poor due to its bitter taste, and caused profuse salivation, which could limited its clinical use. Further studies using different formulations are needed before clinical use of tapentadol can be recommended.

Gabapentin

Mechanism of Action

Gabapentin is a lipophilic structural analogue of the inhibitory neurotransmitter γ-aminobutyric acid (GABA) which has been used for the treatment of chronic and neuropathic pain (Chapter 15). Its exact mechanism of action is unknown but it involves interaction with voltage-gated calcium channels binding to the $\alpha_2\delta$ subunit.

Clinical Use

A number of studies show that perioperative administration of gabapentin reduces acute postoperative pain in humans undergoing surgery. Current knowledge on the use of gabapentin for acute pain management in cats is scarce and based only on expert opinion and case reports. However, oral administration of gabapentin (two doses of 50 mg, 12 hours apart) in combination with IM buprenorphine (0.02 mg/kg) provided similar postoperative analgesia to SC meloxicam (0.2 mg/kg) and buprenorphine in a clinical trial involving 52 cats. Gabapentin is easy to administer, and a promising adjuvant analgesic for treatment of acute pain in cats because of its antihyperalgesic effects.

Further Reading

Aguiar, J., Chebroux, A., Martinez-Taboada, F., *et al.* (2015) Analgesic effects of maxillary and inferior alveolar nerve blocks in cats undergoing dental extractions. *Journal of Feline Medicine and Surgery* **17**, 110–116.

Benito, J., Monteiro, B. P., Beaudry, F., *et al.* (2016) Pharmacokinetics of bupivacaine after intraperitoneal administration to cats undergoing ovariohysterectomy. *American Journal of Veterinary Research* **77**, 641–645.

Benito, J., Monteiro, B., Lavoie, A. M., *et al.* (2016) Analgesic efficacy of intraperitoneal administration of bupivacaine in cats. *Journal of Feline Medicine and Surgery* **18**, 906–912.

Bortolami, E. and Love, E. J. (2015) Practical use of opioids in cats: A state-of-the-art, evidence-based review. *Journal of Feline Medicine and Surgery* **17**, 283–311.

Brondani, J. T., Loureiro Luna, S. P., Beier, S. L., *et al.* (2009) Analgesic efficacy of perioperative use of vedaprofen, tramadol or their combination in cats undergoing ovariohysterectomy. *Journal of Feline Medicine and Surgery* **11**, 420–429.

Cambridge, A. J., Tobias, K. M., Newberry, R. C., *et al.* (2000) Subjective and objective measurements of postoperative pain in cats. *Journal of American Veterinary Medical Association* **217**, 685–690.

Catbagan, D. L., Quimby, J. M., Mama, K. R., *et al.* (2011) Comparison of the efficacy and adverse effects of sustained-release buprenorphine hydrochloride following subcutaneous administration and buprenorphine hydrochloride following oral transmucosal administration in cats undergoing ovariohysterectomy. *American Journal of Veterinary Research* **72**, 461–466.

Doodnaught, G. M., Evangelista, M. C., and Steagall, P. V. (2017) Thermal antinociception following oral administration of tapentadol in conscious cats. *Veterinary Anaesthesia and Analgesia* **44**, 364–369.

Epstein, M. E., Rodanm, I., and Griffenhagen, G. (2015) 2015 AAHA/AAFP pain management guidelines for dogs and cats. *Journal of Feline Medicine and Surgery* **17**, 251–272.

Ferreira, T. H., Aguiar, A. J., Valverde, A., *et al.* (2009) Effect of remifentanil hydrochloride administered via constant rate infusion on the minimum alveolar concentration of isoflurane in cats. *American Journal of Veterinary Research* **70**, 581–588.

Ferreira, T. H., Rezende, M. L., Mama, K. R., *et al.* (2011) Plasma concentrations and behavioral, antinociceptive, and physiologic effects of methadone after intravenous and oral transmucosal administration in cats. *American Journal of Veterinary Research* **72**, 764–771.

Giordano, T., Steagall, P. V., Ferreira, T. H., *et al.* (2010) Postoperative analgesic effects of intravenous, intramuscular, subcutaneous or oral transmucosal buprenorphine administered to cats undergoing ovariohysterectomy. *Veterinary Anaesthesia and Analgesia* **37**, 357–366.

Hunt, J. R., Knowles, T. G., and Lascelles, B. D. (2015) Prescription of perioperative analgesics by UK small animal veterinary surgeons in 2013. *Veterinary Record* **176**, 493.

Lascelles, B. D., Court, M. H., and Hardie, E. M., *et al.* (2007) Nonsteroidal anti-inflammatory drugs in cats: A review. *Veterinary Anaesthesia and Analgesia* **34**, 228–250.

Lorenz, N. D., Comerford, E. J., and Iff, I. (2013) Long-term use of gabapentin for musculoskeletal disease and trauma in three cats. *Journal of Feline Medicine and Surgery* **15**, 507–512.

Mathews, K., Kronen, P. W., Lascelles, D., *et al.* (2014) Guidelines for recognition, assessment and treatment of pain: WSAVA Global Pain Council members and co-authors of this document. *Journal of Small Animal Practice* **55**, E10–E68.

Mira, F., Costa, A., Mendes, E., *et al.* (2016) Influence of music and its genres on respiratory rate and pupil diameter variations in cats under general anaesthesia:

Contribution to promoting patient safety. *Journal of Feline Medicine and Surgery* **18**, 150–159.

Pascoe, P. J., Ilkiw, J. E., Craig, C., *et al.* (2007) The effects of ketamine on the minimum alveolar concentration of isoflurane in cats. *Veterinary Anaesthesia and Analgesia* **34**, 31–39.

Perez Jimenez, T. E., Mealey, K. L., Grubb, T. L., *et al.* (2016) Tramadol metabolism to O-desmethyl tramadol (M1) and N-desmethyl tramadol (M2) by dog liver microsomes: Species comparison and identification of responsible canine cytochrome P-450s (CYPs). *Drug Metabolism and Disposition.* pii: dmd.116.071902.

Polson, S., Taylor, P. M., and Yates, D. (2012) Analgesia after feline ovariohysterectomy under midazolam-medetomidine-ketamine anaesthesia with buprenorphine or butorphanol, and carprofen or meloxicam: A prospective, randomised clinical trial. *Journal of Feline Medicine and Surgery* **14**, 553–559.

Pypendop, B. H., Siao, K. T., Ilkiw, J. E., *et al.* (2009) Effects of tramadol hydrochloride on the thermal threshold in cats. *American Journal of Veterinary Research* **70**, 1465–1470.

Simon, B. T., and Steagall, P. V. (2017) The present and future of opioid analgesics in small animal practice. *Journal of Veterinary Pharmacology and Therapeutics* **40**, 315–326.

Slingsby, L. S., Murrell, J. C., Taylor, P. M., *et al.* (2010) Combination of dexmedetomidine with buprenorphine enhances the antinociceptive effect to a thermal stimulus in the cat compared with either agent alone. *Veterinary Anaesthesia and Analgesia* **37**, 162–170.

Smith, J. D., Allen, S. W., and Quandt, J. E. (1999) Changes in cortisol concentration in response to stress and postoperative pain in client-owned cats and correlation with objective clinical variables. *American Journal of Veterinary Research* **60**, 432–436.

Smith, J. D., Allen, S. W., Quandt, J. E., *et al.* (1996) Indicators of postoperative pain in cats and correlation with clinical criteria. *American Journal of Veterinary Research* **57**, 1674–1678.

Steagall, P. V., Aucoin, M., Monteiro, B. P., *et al.* (2015) Clinical effects of a constant rate infusion of remifentanil, alone or in combination with ketamine, in cats anesthetized with isoflurane. *Journal of the American Veterinary Medical Association* **246**, 976–981.

Steagall, P. V., Benito, J., Monteiro, B. P., *et al.* (2017) The analgesic effects of gabapentin and buprenorphine in cats undergoing ovariohysterectomy: A randomised clinical trial. *Journal of Feline Medicine and Surgery (in press)*.

Steagall, P. V., and Monteiro-Steagall, B. P. (2013) Multimodal analgesia for perioperative pain in three cats. *Journal of Feline Medicine and Surgery* **15**, 737–743.

Steagall, P. V., Monteiro-Steagall, B. P., and Taylor, P. M. (2014) A review of the studies using buprenorphine in cats. *Journal of Veterinary Internal Medicine* **28**, 762–770.

Steagall, P. V., Pelligand, L., Giordano, T., *et al.* (2013) Pharmacokinetic and pharmacodynamic modelling of intravenous, intramuscular and subcutaneous buprenorphine in conscious cats. *Veterinary Anaesthesia and Analgesia* **40**, 83–95.

Steagall, P. V., Taylor, P. M., Brondani, J. T., *et al.* (2008) Antinociceptive effects of tramadol and acepromazine in cats. *Journal of Feline Medicine and Surgery* **10**, 24–31.

Steagall, P. V., Taylor, P. M., Rodrigues, L. C., *et al.* (2009) Analgesia for cats after ovariohysterectomy with either buprenorphine or carprofen alone or in combination. *Veterinary Record* **164**, 359–363.

Taylor, P. M., Kirby, J. J., Robinson, C., *et al.* (2010) A prospective multi-centre clinical trial to compare buprenorphine and butorphanol for postoperative analgesia in cats. *Journal of Feline Medicine and Surgery* **12**, 247–255.

Taylor, P. M., Luangdilok, C. H., and Sear, J. W. (2016) Pharmacokinetic and pharmacodynamic evaluation of high doses of buprenorphine delivered via high-concentration formulations in cats. *Journal of Feline Medicine and Surgery* **18**, 290–302.

Taylor, P. M., Slingsby, L. S., Pypendop, B. H., *et al.* (2007) Variable response to opioid analgesia in cats. *Veterinary Anaesthesia and Analgesia* **34**, A6–7.

Vettorato, E., and Corletto, F. (2016) Retrospective assessment of peripheral nerve block techniques used in cats undergoing hindlimb orthopaedic surgery. *Journal of Feline Medicine and Surgery* **18**, 826–833.

Wilson, D. V., and Pascoe, P. J. (2016) Pain and analgesia following onychectomy in cats: A systematic review. *Veterinary Anaesthesia and Analgesia* **43**, 5–17.

14

Assessment and Recognition of Chronic (Maladaptive) Pain

Beatriz Monteiro[1] and Duncan Lascelles[2]

[1]*Université de Montréal, Saint-Hyacinthe, Canada*
[2]*North Carolina State University, Raleigh, NC, United States*

Key Points

- Behavioral changes related to chronic pain
- Causes of chronic pain
- Owner's role in assessment of chronic pain
- Degenerative joint disease and osteoarthritis
- Persistent postsurgical pain

Introduction

Chronic pain reduces wellbeing, impacts on quality of life and induces behavioral changes that affect the owner–pet bond. The description of pain for an individual is personal and subjective in nature. Indeed, pain assessment in cats is a particular challenge that veterinarians face in patients with chronic disease. Cats do not always show clinical signs of pain in the same way as dogs. In addition, due to their small body size and ability to compensate for chronic painful musculoskeletal conditions, owners may not notice subtle changes in behavior, and thus will not seek help. Cats of any age can be affected by maladaptive pain, although middle aged to older cats are over-represented. Pain is now considered as the fourth vital sign in veterinary medicine, and its assessment should always be incorporated into clinical evaluation of all patients. Chapter 11 describes mechanisms of pain. Nevertheless, an overview of commonly used terms in this chapter is presented here.

- *Acute pain* is usually self-limiting, characterized by inflammation and nociception, and associated with potential or actual tissue damage. In contrast, chronic pain is not associated with normal healing and it persists beyond the expected course of an acute disease process with no clear endpoint. *Persistent postsurgical pain* is a condition where acute pain persists (abnormal healing) and has become maladaptive
- *Chronic pain* should not be considered a symptom, but rather a disease in its own right since it may be present in the absence of a primary cause. This occurs due to the plasticity of the central nervous system (CNS) in which nociceptive signal processing

Feline Anesthesia and Pain Management, First Edition. Edited by Paulo Steagall,
Sheilah Robertson and Polly Taylor.

within the spinal cord and higher centers is altered. This results in amplification of the signals, facilitated throughput, and even the generation of "pain signals" (nociceptive input) from the CNS itself
- The end result of these CNS changes is spontaneous pain, hyperalgesia (increased response to painful stimuli), and allodynia (pain from normally nonpainful stimuli) (Chapter 11). In chronic painful conditions, there is often an imbalance between the excitatory and inhibitory control of nociceptive input with consequent facilitation of excitatory transmission and reduced inhibitory transmission of pain. For example, there is decreased activation of the endogenous analgesic system and its ability to control painful stimuli

Clinical chronic pain is generally a mixture of different "types" of pain – inflammatory, neuropathic, and functional pain (*Box* 14.1). In many of these cases, the degree of pain does not necessarily correlate with the pathology due to neurobiological changes; these include altered:

- Transduction in the periphery
- Processing at the level of the spinal cord
- Descending inhibitory control

For these reasons, treatment of maladaptive pain can be difficult. For example, cancer patients may be affected by inflammatory and neuropathic pain, whereas cats with feline interstitial cystitis may present with a combination of inflammatory and functional pain. In both situations there may be varying contributions to the pain state from peripheral, spinal cord and higher center changes.

Box 14.1: Contributors to chronic (maladaptive) pain

- Inflammatory pain is associated with tissue injury, and direct stimulation and sensitization of nociceptors following activation of the inflammatory cascade. These changes result in the cardinal signs of inflammation (heat, pain, redness, swelling, and loss of function)
- Neuropathic pain is caused by a lesion or disease of the somatosensory system peripherally or centrally. The somatosensory system includes all structures allowing the perception of sensory information coming from the skin and the musculoskeletal system. Diagnosis of neuropathic pain includes assessment of nerve fibers involved in nociception and proprioception (Aβ, Aδ, C) using techniques such as quantitative sensory testing (QST), advanced imaging, and somatosensory evoked potentials
- Functional pain is not associated with any detectable inflammatory or neuropathic etiology. It is characterized by neurophysiological dysfunction with no detectable structural, metabolic or immunological cause

---

Inflammatory pain results from the release of nociceptive sensitizers (e.g. PGE2, nerve growth factor), and nociceptive activators. It is commonly associated with surgery-induced acute (adaptive) pain; however, several chronic painful conditions have a component of inflammatory pain. Degenerative joint disease (DJD), cancer, stomatitis,

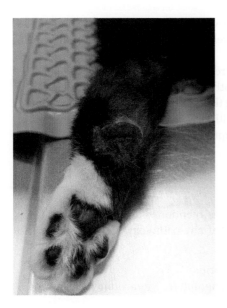

Figure 14.1 A tumor affecting the plantar aspect of the left pelvic limb of a cat. The tissue necrosis caused by the tumor results in inflammatory pain. This cat presented with the classical signs of inflammation including heat, redness and swelling of the area, pain on gentle palpation, and decreased function due to lameness of this limb. Neuropathic pain may also be present if a lesion of the somatosensory system occurs (e.g. compression of a nerve).

periodontal disease, pancreatitis, gastritis, inflammatory bowel disease and interstitial cystitis are some examples (*Figure* 14.1). A "new" category of inflammatory pain is referred to as "neuroimmune inflammation" in which glial and immune (toll-like receptors) cells can dramatically amplify pain leading to the development and maintenance of neuropathic pain (Chapter 11). Therefore, it is believed that some cases of neuropathic pain might be, at least in part, produced by an inflammatory component.

The development of *neuropathic pain* involves complex mechanisms including sensory aberrant ectopic activity, neuroplasticity, impaired endogenous inhibitory modulation and activation of the microglia (Chapter 11). Neuropathic pain may be caused by, for example, nerve compression or infiltration by cancers, or it may follow amputation involving nerve resection, or be associated with intervertebral disk impingement on the spinal cord or nerve roots. Growing evidence indicates that neuropathic pain is also present in many other conditions such as DJD. In humans, neuropathic pain is generally considered to cause severe and long-lasting pain which is less responsive to treatment with analgesics, and to cause greater impairment of mobility than other types of maladaptive pain. In cats, the hallmarks of a neuropathic component of chronic pain are:

- Malfunctioning and deterioration of the somatosensory system (i.e. abnormal processing of sensory information)
- Hyperalgesia
- Allodynia
- Spontaneous pain

However, these signs are not limited to neuropathic pain and may be observed in functional pain in which the etiology cannot be identified, and where neurobiological changes are not clearly related to disease or a lesion of the somatosensory system. In veterinary medicine, this terminology is new; however, functional pain can be seen in cats with interstitial cystitis, inflammatory bowel disease, and possibly orofacial pain syndrome.

The terms "chronic" and "maladaptive" pain are used interchangeably in this chapter, and the reader should understand that they both refer to a mixture of inflammatory, neuropathic and functional pain. Understanding the origin or cause of pain, which is not always known but underlies a particular condition, aims to help the veterinarian in directing what treatments should be used (Chapter 15).

Common Causes of Chronic Pain

Some chronic painful conditions have already been mentioned and the following list is not exhaustive. The clinician should consider that any pathology has the potential to cause maladaptive pain.

- Degenerative joint disease (DJD) and osteoarthritis (OA)
- Persistent postsurgical pain (e.g. limb or tail amputation, thoracotomy, chronic pain syndrome after onychectomy)
- Dental and oral disease (e.g. gingivitis, periodontitis, stomatitis)
- Feline orofacial pain syndrome
- Feline hyperesthesia syndrome
- Ocular conditions (e.g. corneal disease, uveitis, ulcers)
- Gastrointestinal conditions (e.g. megacolon, constipation, ileus, inflammatory bowel disease)
- Urogenital conditions (e.g. interstitial cystitis)
- Dermatological conditions (e.g. otitis, severe pruritus, burns, chronic wounds)
- Trauma
- Neoplasia (e.g. feline injection-associated sarcoma, oral squamous cell carcinoma)
- Chemotherapy-induced neuropathy, radiation-induced skin burns
- Diabetes-induced neuropathy
- Chronic kidney disease

Osteoarthritis refers to pathological changes in synovial joints that may be primary and idiopathic, secondary to trauma or abnormal developmental features. DJD is a general definition that encompasses OA and inflammatory arthropathies of synovial joints (including immune-mediated arthropathies), degenerative changes to fibrocartilaginous joints, and *spondylosis deformans* of the vertebral column. The term DJD is used in this chapter.

Clinical Signs

Table 14.1 shows common clinical signs and behavioral changes associated with chronic pain in cats.

Age-associated behavioral changes may overlap with chronic pain, and it is important to differentiate between the two with a rigorous and thorough clinical history and examination. Chronic pain must be ruled out before assuming that behavioral changes

Table 14.1 The most common clinical signs and changes in behavior associated with chronic pain in cats. These changes are generally subtle and may be inconsistent as signs can improve or deteriorate over time ("waxing-and-waning" effect). These clinical signs can be used together to assess quality of life.

Clinical signs	Behavior descriptors
Decreased mobility	Decreased ease and fluidity of movement compared with the past Difficulty when getting up or moving around after resting
Decreased ability to perform activities	Difficulty in performing routine activities such as playing with toys, hunting, or jumping up and down Instead of jumping directly onto a high vertical surface, the cat prefers to do this in stages using intermediate surfaces Instead of jumping directly down, the cat reaches down to shorten the jump or finds an intermediate surface to decrease the height of the jump
Isolation	Decreased interaction with owners and other pets Prefers to be alone
Depression	Lack of interest towards things that would normally interest the cat (toys, birds out side of the window, scratching posts, etc.)
Irritation	Complains/vocalizes/growls when picked up or handled Appears "grumpy" or short-tempered
Mood alteration	Change in temperament/demeanor (sadness, irritation, aggressiveness)
Decreased or increased grooming	Hair coat is not well groomed and can be greasy. Nails are dirty Increased grooming with possible alopecia at specific areas of the body indicating abnormal sensitivity (e.g. pain, numbness or tingling; hyperesthesia syndrome)[a] May resent being groomed
Inappropriate use of litter box	Difficulty in getting into or out of the litter box Inappropriate urination/defecation around the house
Appetite alteration	Decreased or increased appetite and/or water ingestion
Sensitivity to touch[a, b]	Resents simply being touched or petted
Acute and intermittent intense pain behaviors[a]	Suddenly screams, looks at a region of the body and starts licking it without a known cause Returns to normal behavior shortly after these episodes

Notes:
a) Observed in cats with neuropathic pain.
b) Observed in cats with allodynia.

are age-related only. Geriatric cats are likely to have DJD with or without chronic kidney disease. This population of cats should be closely examined for signs of pain.

The clinical signs depend on the primary cause of chronic pain, if there is one. In most cats, the signs are nonspecific and behavioral changes are subtler in nature when compared with dogs. For example, lameness is easily observed in canine patients with DJD. In cats, this is not commonly detected, and these individuals will normally show altered mobility and activity patterns that may only be noted in the home environment. Therefore, owners are crucial in the assessment and recognition of chronic pain and quality of life (QoL) in cats (*Box* 14.2).

Box 14.2: The role of the owner in assessment and recognition of chronic pain and quality of life in cats

There are currently no fully validated pain scoring systems for veterinarians to assess chronic pain in cats. Thus, most of the assessment is based on owner-reported signs. Client communication is important in diagnosis, and the first clinical consultation is usually time consuming when interviewing owners about the cat's behavior at home. Owners can normally detect deterioration of pain relief rather than efficacy *per se*, and the clinician must therefore plan carefully how to ask specific questions. The cat will be unlikely to display chronic pain-induced behavioral changes in the examination room. In many cases, the primary reason for the consultation is not actually related to pain. Nevertheless, the potential of a chronic pain component in the primary complaint must always be considered. Interestingly, owners will often notice changes in behavior in other cats following treatment of chronic pain in the first cat.

Implications for Quality of Life

In humans, the association between chronic pain and deleterious psychological effects is well recognized. These patients generally self-report suffering, anxiety, impaired mobility, depression, and isolation. It may be reasonable to assume that cats are similarly affected. Indeed, comparable behaviors are often perceived by their owners, which impact on the cat's health and welfare. A general QoL assessment can be made during a consultation and physical examination, and should include detailed history and investigation of specific clinical signs (*Table* 14.1).

Stepwise Approach for Assessment and Recognition of Chronic Pain in Cats in the Clinical Setting

- Discussion with the owner regarding behavioral indicators of chronic pain (*Table* 14.1)
- Low-stress physical examination (Chapter 1). A quiet room without "hiding places" in which the cat can become lodged is recommended. A surface that is soft and nonslip such as a yoga or baby's changing mat should be used. Restraint should be minimized, unless absolutely necessary
- A thorough evaluation focusing on body condition, the oral cavity, eyes, ears, skin, fur, paws and claws should be performed. Changes in grooming should be recorded (*Figure* 14.2). Thoracic auscultation and gentle abdominal palpation may reveal abnormalities and pain. Close monitoring of the cat's body language and facial expressions are important during assessment. The cat's temperament and resistance to manipulation should also be noted
- A cat's responses to painful stimuli will be affected by where they are (home versus clinic), and with whom (owner versus veterinarian). The presence of the owner in the examination room may or may not be helpful.

- If a body part is known to be painful, it should be the last to be examined. However, this must be balanced with the cat's tolerance to examination and manipulation. It may be necessary to divide the examination into several short periods
- Painful stimulation may elicit one or more of the following behaviors
  - Body tension, resisting manipulation
  - Vocalization (hiss, growl, howl)
  - Attempt to escape (avoidance)
  - Aggression (lash out, bite, scratch)
  - Hypersensitivity reactions (muscle and skin fasciculation, twitching)
- An orthopedic examination should follow, especially in geriatric cats that may be affected by DJD. Few cats will be willing to walk around the examination room and even if they do, lameness is unlikely to be seen. They may be encouraged to jump up and down, and over objects. Owners can be invited to submit "home videos" to the veterinarian to help with diagnosis
- Palpation of all joints and long bones is performed. Passive movement of joints (flexion and extension) may be performed under sedation if needed, however, this is likely to affect behavioral responses to pain. It is important to note that passive movement of joints does not accurately mimic their loading and movement during ambulation, just as in humans and dogs
- Neurological examination may help to identify cases of neoplasia and neuropathic pain, by revealing spinal conditions that can be a source of chronic pain
- Laboratory hematology is of limited value in diagnosing pain, but may point to underlying disease processes
- Radiographs may confirm the presence of DJD, neoplasia or megacolon, for example, but radiographic findings rarely correlate with pain in cats
- Other advanced imaging or laboratory evaluation may be useful on a case-by-case basis, but as with radiography, imaging findings do not correlate with pain

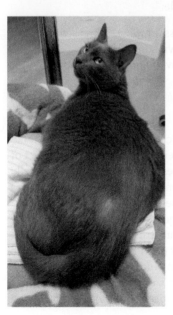

Figure 14.2 A 12-year-old male (neutered) cat with chronic lumbar pain. This cat resents being groomed and performs excessive grooming and self-plucking resulting in alopecia in the lumbar region. These behaviors are described to have had a "sudden onset", possibly indicating a neuropathic pain component. On physical examination, the cat reacts adversely to light touch and stroking the area, confirming the presence of allodynia.

The Concept of Analgesic Challenge

An "analgesic challenge" can be useful when chronic pain is suspected but not clear. In these cases, analgesics may be administered or prescribed; a decrease or resolution of clinical signs often confirms the diagnosis of chronic pain. In general, chronic pain is difficult to treat (compared with acute pain), and a lack of improvement with a single analgesic (e.g. a nonsteroidal anti-inflammatory drug (NSAID)) may not completely rule out the presence of chronic pain. An adjuvant analgesic may be added to the treatment (Chapter 15).

Assessing Chronic Pain in Specific Conditions

Degenerative Joint Disease and Osteoarthritis

Degenerative joint disease results from a combination of inflammatory, neuropathic, and functional components, albeit in unknown relative amounts. Plasticity of the nociceptive transmission system results in increased sensitivity, hyperalgesia, and allodynia. It is likely, as in humans, that the drivers of pain are a combination of peripheral sensitization, central sensitization, and decreased function of the endogenous analgesic system. In geriatric cats, the prevalence of DJD may be as high as 60–90%, and DJD is recognized as one of the main sources of chronic pain. In the axial skeleton, the lumbar and lumbosacral regions are most affected, whereas in the appendicular skeleton DJD is more prevalent in the hip, followed by stifle, tarsus, and elbow (*Figure* 14.3).

Clinical Signs

Impaired mobility is reported by owners and can include:

- Decreased mobility (decreased daily distance moved, less jumping, decreased height of obstacles, stiffness, and problems walking up and down stairs)
- Altered movement such as a decreased fluidity of movement
- Less grooming
- Hiding and decreased or altered socialization with other pets and household members
- Changes in litter box use

These changes are too subtle to be detected by the clinician or only relate to the home environment. Cats often "freeze" in the hospital environment due to stress. The impact of stress-induced analgesia is well described in prey species, and although not formally investigated in cats, it may be a component of their normal physiology. Hence, owners provide a more reliable perspective of the cat's everyday behavior. Although there are no pain scales for cats with DJD-related pain that have undergone complete validation, some owner-based and one veterinarian-based clinical instruments have been developed specifically for cats. The Feline Musculoskeletal Pain Index (FMPI) and the Client Specific Outcome Measures (CSOM) are the tools that have been studied most and investigate abnormalities related to mobility and self-maintenance, as well as social and exploratory behaviors. Questions are addressed towards the following specific behaviors: walking and

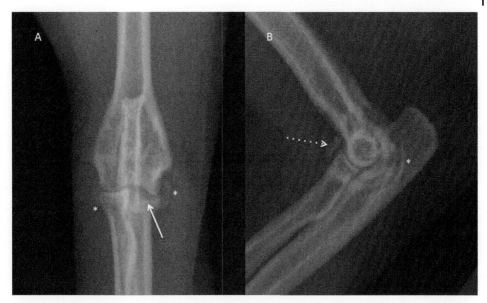

Figure 14.3 Radiographs of a cat with degenerative joint disease. Cranio-caudal (A) and lateral (B) radiographs of the elbow of a 10-year-old female (spayed) cat with osteoarthritis. Characteristic features are joint-associated mineralization (*), which on the medial aspect may be indicative of medial epicondylitis (where the ulnar nerve can be completely enclosed and flattened between the epitrochleo-anconeus muscle and new bone formation within the humeral head of the flexor carpi ulnaris muscle). The unevenly increased humero-ulna joint space (solid arrow) is probably associated with osteo-chondromatosis (osteochondral bodies within the joint, which have resulted in erosion of the joint surfaces). Although the presence of a sesamoid in the supinator muscle (dotted arrow) is a normal feature, its enlargement and uneven appearance is associated with osteoarthritis of the elbow joint.

running; playing and chasing objects; ability to jump up or down; height of jump; climbing and descending stairs; interaction with other pets; eating, grooming, and sleeping habits.

- The FMPI consists of a series of 17 questions. Its ability to detect cats with musculoskeletal pain and consequent effects of treatment has been demonstrated. It is available for use in clinical practice and is constantly being updated (https://cvm .ncsu.edu/research/labs/clinical-sciences/comparative-pain-research/clinical-metrology-instruments, accessed June 25, 2017)
- The CSOM consists of three to five activities that are unique to an individual cat and chosen by the owner following discussion with the veterinarian. These specific activities, including time and place (e.g. ability to jump onto the bed last thing at night), are graded according to the degree of impairment, and are followed over time
- The Montreal Instrument for Cat Arthritis Testing (MI-CAT(V)) has been developed for use by veterinarians. It focuses on mobility impairments that can be evaluated at a distance. It has undergone preliminary validation and reliability testing where gait and body posture allowed for distinction between cats with and without DJD

Table 14.2 Suggested numerical rating scale for changes in behavior during joint palpation in cats with suspected degenerative joint disease. Note: the change from baseline response (response without manipulation) is the most important aspect to assess.

Pain score	Behavior
0	No resentment (no change)
1	Mild withdrawal; mildly resists (slight change from baseline)
2	Moderate withdrawal; body tenses; may orient to site; may vocalize – increase in vocalization (moderate change from baseline)
3	Orients to site; forcible withdrawal from manipulation; may vocalize or hiss or bite (obvious change from baseline)
4	Tries to escape and prevent manipulation; bites, hisses; marked guarding of area (severe change from baseline)

Source: From Lascelles, B. D. X., Dong, Y., Marcellin-Little, D. J., *et al.* (2012) Relationship of orthopedic examination, goniometric measurements, and radiographic signs of degenerative joint disease in cats. *BMC Veterinary Research* **8**, 10–17.

Orthopedic Examination and Goniometric Measurements

Orthopedic examination in feline patients should consist of careful palpation of every appendicular joint as well as the axial skeleton while watching for pain responses (*Table* 14.2). Minimal restraint is applied. Additionally, each appendicular joint should be evaluated for crepitus, effusion, and thickening as these are other indicators of joint disease, although they do not necessarily relate to pain. Goniometry can be performed, but may prove to be difficult in awake cats. The temperament should also be assessed because a "grumpy" cat may be behaving that way due to chronic pain. Body condition score should be assessed and recorded for further monitoring.

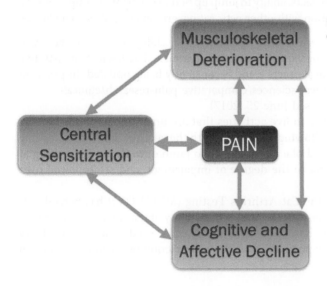

Figure 14.4 The progression of degenerative joint disease.

Clinical Signs versus Radiographic Signs

Radiographic signs of DJD do not necessarily correlate with clinical signs of pain. In cats, the best agreement between radiographic DJD and pain was found for the elbow and the lumbar and lumbo-sacral areas. In contrast, cats may have clinical evidence of DJD-induced pain without radiographic signs. This may be explained by lack of detail in radiographs that would enable detection of early changes in the joint. In humans, it has recently been suggested that pain may be more closely related to structures not assessed by radiographs, and magnetic resonance imaging is considered a more sensitive indicator of disease-induced pain. However, it is clear that as DJD progresses with ageing, radiographic severity becomes greater. *Box* 14.3 describes the progression of DJD and the importance of treating pain and increasing mobility while minimizing pathological changes associated with the disease (Chapter 15).

Box 14.3: The progression of degenerative joint disease

DJD-associated pain starts at the peripheral joint, and results in decreased ability to perform daily activities and decreased mobility. This initiates musculoskeletal deterioration due to decreased use and altered body carriage. Additionally, as explained in the text, this nociceptive input (pain input) into the system can result in sensitization and pain (somatosensory system deterioration). Heightened pain results in further negative effects on the musculoskeletal system (muscle deterioration, trigger point development, muscle pain) which in turn can result in a greater burden of pain as a result of decreased joint support. Thus, there is concurrent deterioration of the musculoskeletal system and the somatosensory system. Pain also has negative effects on cognitive function, and on affective systems, resulting in heightened fear, anxiety and poor sleep. These changes in turn feed back and heighten pain (e.g. anxiety amplifies pain, and pain in turn heightens anxiety). The inability to perform daily activities, resulting from pain and deterioration of the musculoskeletal system, also drives negative affective changes through decreased and altered interactions with the cat's environment. These two-way relationships between pain, central sensitization, musculoskeletal deterioration and cognitive/affective deterioration are illustrated in *Figure* 14.4.

With so many complex changes occurring, and multiple joints often involved, staging of the DJD patient may seem daunting. However, 'staging' is probably best performed by assessing the overall impact on the whole cat. A simple staging of the impact of DJD based on activity and mobility is proposed below.

- Stage 1: Early signs of activity impairment
- Stage 2: Intermittent signs of activity impairment
- Stage 3: Obvious activity impairment and some decrease in mobility
- Stage 4: Loss of mobility

In the future, treatment recommendations will take into account the 'stage' of DJD, and the stages will be sub-defined once central sensitization, cognitive decline and affective deterioration can be measured.

Other Conditions causing Chronic Pain

Some disease processes have the potential to cause chronic pain and are described below. For all these conditions, little is known about pain-induced behavioral changes and how to assess and recognize pain during physical examination. However, in most instances, the response to palpation of affected areas can be a useful indicator. Abnormally sensitive areas or areas with hyperesthesia may be identified with gentle to moderate stroking and palpation. The reaction evoked may be subtle, such as skin twitch, swallowing, turning to look at the area or trying to avoid or escape from the manipulation.

Neoplasia

Cancer is one of the main causes of mortality in veterinary patients, and pain is commonly a major component of the disease. Cancer-related pain may be caused by various mechanisms, with the location of the cancer as well as the type dramatically influencing the clinical signs. Inflammatory pain can be caused by tumor growth and destruction of adjacent tissues and structures (*Figure* 14.1). Visceral pain can be caused by visceral distension, and neuropathic pain can be caused by nerve compression or a primary tumor involving the nervous system with consequent lesions in the somatosensory system. Recent studies reveal that the tumor itself can contribute to the generation of pain via neuroimmune mechanisms. Even if the chronic pain is controlled, acute exacerbation of pain may occur if the tumor grows rapidly or becomes necrotic. Clinicians should also consider that patients with cancer are commonly affected by other painful comorbidities such as DJD or chronic kidney disease. Additionally, the cancer treatment itself may cause chronic pain such as persistent postsurgical pain, chemotherapy-induced neuropathy and radiotherapy-induced pain (*Figure* 14.5).

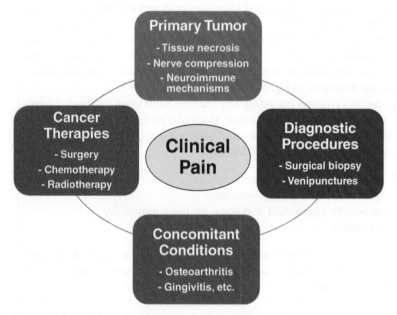

Figure 14.5 Multidimensional nature of pain in patients with cancer.

Persistent Postsurgical Pain

In humans, persistent postsurgical pain is the second largest cause of chronic pain after OA. Sensitization of the nervous system due to nerve injury induced by insufficient perioperative analgesia and extensive tissue injury are thought to be the main causes of persistent postsurgical maladaptive pain. Although this process can occur following any surgery, amputation and thoracotomy are classic examples of surgical procedures where extensive nerve damage is unavoidable. Spontaneous ectopic discharges from injured nerves result in significantly increased nociceptive input inducing neuroplasticity, central sensitization, and spontaneous pain. Inflammation resulting from the surgical trauma results in additional nociceptive input.

Amputation

The incidence of chronic pain following amputation in feline practice is unknown, whereas in humans, the condition often referred to as "phantom pain" may affect up to 80% of amputees. Clinical signs may develop within the immediate postoperative period or years after the procedure, and they are similar to those described for neuropathic pain (*Table* 14.1). Aggressive perioperative pain management is required for this procedure (Chapters 13 and 15).

Chronic Pain Syndrome after Feline Onychectomy

Feline onychectomy (i.e. the amputation of the third phalanx of each digit) is performed only in North America. Chronic pain syndrome can develop as a result of this procedure. A discussion of the ethical issues associated with this procedure is beyond the scope of this chapter. Diagnosis of the syndrome is based primarily on clinical signs and behavioral changes after ruling out DJD or other complications that could be corrected surgically. Behavioral changes associated with the syndrome include:

- Chronic lameness
- Licking and chewing at the feet
- "Walking as if on hot coals"
- Shaking and "flicking" of the paws
- Aversion to the feet being touched
- Reluctance to use the feet to play with toys or to cover urine and feces with litter
- Periods of suddenly sitting still
- Spontaneous vocalization "for no apparent reason"

Periodontal Disease

Periodontal disease characterized by inflammation of the gingiva or periodontal tissues is common in feline practice and is a source of chronic pain. Assessment of pain is difficult in these cases, but it may be assumed that if inflammation is present, pain is present. Dysphagia is the most common clinical sign, and some cats will frequently "paw against their mouth" during and after eating. Spontaneous vocalization with escape behavior and salivation may be observed. These behaviors normally disappear once the dental disease is treated (*Figure* 14.6).

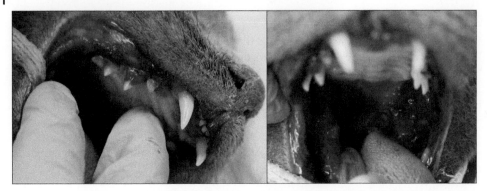

Figure 14.6 Cat with severe gingivostomatitis. This cat showed classical clinical signs of oral pain including pawing at the mouth while eating. These signs resolved completely following full-mouth tooth extractions. The cat is reported to have become more friendly after the procedure indicating an affective and emotional component of oral pain.

Feline Orofacial Pain Syndrome

Feline Orofacial Pain syndrome is a chronic condition with acute episodes (acute on chronic pain). The etiology is not fully understood but it is suspected to be a neuropathic pain disorder analogous to trigeminal neuralgia in humans. Nevertheless, discomfort appears to be limited to the oral cavity and lips and no other areas of trigeminal nerve innervation. The presentation is usually unilateral and the diagnosis is made by exclusion. Burmese cats appear predisposed. Affected cats should be assessed for concomitant oral lesions and possible environmental stressors, for example social incompatibility in a multicat household. Clinical signs may be triggered by mouth movement and include:

- Exaggerated licking and chewing movements
- Pawing at the mouth
- Anorexia or decreased appetite
- Mutilation of the tongue, lips, and buccal mucosa (severe cases)

Gastrointestinal Conditions

Any chronic disease affecting the gastrointestinal system and causing visceral distension, such as megacolon or constipation, should be considered painful. Inflammatory bowel disease is characterized by chronic intestinal inflammation and may occur concomitantly with pancreatitis or cholangiohepatitis. These inflammatory diseases have the potential to cause chronic abdominal pain. Assessment of these patients is based on the clinical history and response to abdominal palpation.

Interstitial Cystitis

Feline interstitial cystitis (FIC) is recognized as a chronic pain syndrome. Cats and humans are affected by this condition, which has many shared features between the species. The process by which chronic pain develops is not fully understood. Clinically, it has been noted that interstitial cystitis impacts on the QoL. In cats, several factors such as obesity, confinement, sedentary lifestyle, intercat aggression, and decreased water consumption have been proposed as potential contributors to development of the disease. Assessment of patients with FIC should comprise detailed history, consideration of possible environmental stressors, physical examination, urinalysis, and urine culture, as well as assessment of QoL. Although nonspecific for FIC, the most commonly observed clinical signs include:

- Dysuria
- Pollakiuria (excessive frequent urination)
- Hematuria (presence of blood in the urine)
- Periuria (urination in inappropriate locations)
- Overgrooming around the perineum
- Behavioral changes

Diabetes-induced Neuropathy

Prevalence of feline diabetes mellitus is increasing because of obesity and sedentary lifestyles; older neutered male cats are most frequently affected. Diabetes-induced neuropathy is a type of neuropathic pain characterized by demyelination of motor and sensory nerve fibers (Chapter 11). It affects approximately 10% of cats with this disease. Humans report numbness, tingling or allodynia, and emotional consequences include depression and decreases in QoL. It is now well recognized that diabetes mellitus in cats closely resembles human type-2 diabetes. It is reasonable to conclude that similar pain-induced behavioral changes occur in cats. Clinical signs are related to neuropathic pain (*Table* 14.1) and functional disability. These may include:

- Aversion to touching of the extremities
- Licking of the feet leading to discoloration of the fur (light-colored cats) (*Figure* 11.5)
- Pelvic limb weakness and difficulty in ambulating
- Impaired ability to jump

Further Reading

Bellows, J., Center, S., Daristotle, L., *et al.* (2016) Evaluating aging in cats: How to determine what is healthy and what is disease. *Journal of Feline Medicine and Surgery* **18**, 551–570.

Benito, J., Hansen, B., DePuy, V., *et al.* (2013) Feline Musculoskeletal Pain Index: Responsiveness and testing of criterion validity. *Journal of Veterinary Internal Medicine* **27**, 474–482.

Bennett, D., Ariffin, S. M. Z., and Johnston, P. (2012) Osteoarthritis in the cat. 1. How common is it and how easy to recognise? *Journal of Feline Medicine and Surgery* **14**, 65–75.

Bennett, D., and Morton, C. (2009) A study of owner observed behavioural and lifestyle changes in cats with musculoskeletal disease before and after analgesic therapy. *Journal of Feline Medicine and Surgery* **11**, 997–1004.

Buffington, C. A. (2011) Idiopathic cystitis in domestic cats: Beyond the lower urinary tract. *Journal of Veterinary Internal Medicine* **25**, 784–796.

Clarke, S., and Bennett, D. (2006) Feline osteoarthritis: A prospective study of 28 cases. *Journal of Small Animal Practice* **47**, 439–445.

Grubb, T. (2010) Chronic neuropathic pain in veterinary patients. *Topics in Companion Animal Medicine* **25**, 45–52.

Gruen, M. E., Griffith, E., Thomson, A., *et al.* (2014) Detection of clinically relevant pain relief in cats with degenerative joint disease associated pain. *Journal of Veterinary Internal Medicine* **28**, 346–350.

Gruen, M. E., Griffith, E., Thomson, A. E., *et al.* (2015) Criterion validation testing of clinical metrology instruments for measuring degenerative joint disease associated mobility impairment in cats. *PLoS One* **10**, e0131839.

Guillot, M., Moreau, M., Heit, M., *et al.* (2013) Characterization of osteoarthritis in cats and meloxicam efficacy using objective chronic pain evaluation tools. *Veterinary Journal* **196**, 360–367.

Hardie, E. M., Roe, S. C., and Martin, F. R. (2002) Radiographic evidence of degenerative joint disease in geriatric cats: 100 cases (1994–1997). *Journal of the American Veterinary Medical Association* **220**, 628–632.

Kerwin, S. (2012) Orthopedic examination in the cat: Clinical tips for ruling in/out common musculoskeletal disease. *Journal of Feline Medicine and Surgery* **14**, 6–12.

Klinck, M. P., Monteiro, B. P., Lussier, B., *et al.* (2017) Refinement of the Montreal Instrument for Cat Arthritis Testing, for use by Veterinarians: detection of naturally occurring osteoarthritis in laboratory cats. *Journal of Feline Medicine and Surgery* DOI: 10.1177/1098612X17730172

Lascelles, B. D. (2010) Feline Degenerative Joint Disease. *Veterinary Surgery* **39**, 2–13.

Lascelles, B. D., Dong, Y., Marcellin-Little, D. J., *et al.* (2012) Relationship of orthopedic examination, goniometric measurements, and radiographic signs of degenerative joint disease in cats. *BMC Veterinary Research* **8**, 10–17.

Lascelles, B. D., Hansen, B. D., Roe, S., *et al.* (2007) Evaluation of client-specific outcome measures and activity monitoring to measure pain relief in cats with osteoarthritis. *Journal of Veterinary Internal Medicine* **21**, 410–416.

Lascelles, B. D., Henry, J. B. 3rd, Brown, J., *et al.* (2010) Cross-sectional study evaluating the prevalence of radiographic degenerative joint disease in domesticated cats. *Veterinary Surgery* **39**, 535–544.

Mathews, K., Kronen, P. W., Lascelles, D., *et al.* (2014) Guidelines for recognition, assessment and treatment of pain: WSAVA Global Pain Council members and co-authors of this document. *Journal of Small Animal Practice* **55**, E10–68.

Perry, R., and Tutt, C. (2015) Periodontal disease in cats: Back to basics – with an eye on the future. *Journal of Feline Medicine and Surgery* **17**, 45–65.

Rios, L., and Ward, C. (2008) Feline diabetes mellitus: Diagnosis, treatment, and monitoring. *Compendium: Continuing Education for Veterinarians* **30**, 626–639.

Robertson, S. A. and Lascelles, B. D. (2010) Long-term pain in cats: How much do we know about this important welfare issue? *Journal of Feline Medicine and Surgery* **12**, 188–199.

Rusbridge, C., Heath, S., Gunn-Moore, D. A., *et al.* (2010) Feline orofacial pain syndrome (FOPS): A retrospective study of 113 cases. *Journal of Feline Medicine and Surgery* **12**, 498–508.

Slingerland, L. I., Hazewinkel, H. A., Meij, B. P., *et al.* (2011) Cross sectional study of the prevalence and clinical features of osteoarthritis in 100 cats. *Veterinary Journal* **187**, 304–309.

Taylor, P. M., and Robertson, S. A. (2004) Pain management in cats-past, present and future. Part 1. The cat is unique. *Journal of Feline Medicine and Surgery* **6**, 313–320.

Zamprogno, H., Hansen, B. D., Bondell, H. D., *et al.* (2010) Item generation and design testing of a questionnaire to assess degenerative joint disease-associated pain in cats. *American Journal of Veterinary Research* **71**, 1417–1424.

15

Treatment of Chronic (Maladaptive) Pain

Beatriz Monteiro and Eric Troncy

Université de Montréal, Saint-Hyacinthe, Canada

Key Points

- Analgesic drugs used in the treatment of chronic pain
- Nonpharmacological techniques in the treatment of chronic pain
- General recommendations in degenerative joint disease-related pain
- The role of the owner in chronic pain
- The importance of environmental enrichment

Introduction

Chronic (maladaptive) pain causes suffering and reduces quality of life (QoL) in cats. Treatment often involves a *multimodal approach* including both administration of analgesic drugs and application of nonpharmacological therapies. The environment in which the cat lives is also important. It should be predictable, provide comfort and mental and physical stimulation, and interactions with family members. Continuous *tender loving care* will play a role in the cat's welfare and reinforce the human-animal bond.

Appropriate assessment of chronic pain is paramount for adequate treatment (Chapter 14). Normally, identification of a primary cause (e.g. gingivitis, otitis) will facilitate diagnosis and treatment. In some cases, a primary, single cause or condition cannot be identified (e.g. interstitial cystitis) and in others there is no cure (e.g. degenerative joint disease (DJD), some cancers). Pain and discomfort may eventually become severe and refractory to standard analgesic treatment.

The following principles should be considered when treating chronic pain in cats, and may explain why response to treatment varies greatly among individuals:

- Clinical reasoning is the thought process involved in identifying the etiology and structural anatomical sources of pain. It requires an understanding of the pathophysiology of the painful condition (Chapter 11) to allow for a mechanism-based therapeutic approach. The mechanism and type of pain (e.g. nociceptive, neuropathic, inflammatory, mixed) is potentially identified and an analgesic drug chosen based on

Feline Anesthesia and Pain Management, First Edition. Edited by Paulo Steagall, Sheilah Robertson and Polly Taylor.
© 2018 John Wiley & Sons, Inc. Published 2018 by John Wiley & Sons, Inc.

its mechanism of action. However, this is not always easy and it is often necessary to choose a therapy and assess the response before deciding on a longer term treatment (an "analgesic challenge," Chapter 14)

• Psychosocial reasoning is related to the owners' emotions, behaviors, attitudes, and coping skills regarding their pets' pain. The owner's perceptions can sometimes be extrapolated as the cat's perceptions, by proxy

Client Communication: A Crucial Component of Treatment for Chronic Painful Conditions

Owners play an important role in the diagnosis and treatment of chronic pain (Chapter 14) because "trial and error" is often required in terms of finding a strategy that works best for managing the cat's pain (*Box* 15.1). The emotional burden of chronic pain for both the cat and the owner must not be underestimated. The owner-cat bond can be challenged, especially when grooming and elimination habits have changed. Euthanasia is a treatment option and should be considered in cases of poor prognosis, scheduling and financial constraints, and lack of response to therapy.

Box 15.1: Planning the treatment protocol with the owner

The owner must understand that complete resolution of clinical signs is rarely achieved and that the main goal of treatment is to improve comfort and QoL. A long-term treatment protocol should be based on reasonable expectations in consultation with the owners during the first visit. Treatment should take into account ease of drug administration, palatability, scheduling, and the cat's tolerance. Owners are integral to the treatment process and are responsible for:

• Enriching the environment
• Frequent administration of analgesic drugs
• Monitoring efficacy and adverse effects

Challenges in the Treatment of Chronic Pain in Cats

The following list includes some of the major challenges faced when treating chronic pain in cats:

• Difficulties in recognizing and assessing chronic pain in cats, resulting in inappropriate and ineffective treatment
• Fear of adverse effects with long-term administration of analgesic drugs
• Lack of pharmacokinetic (PK) and pharmacodynamic (PD) cat-specific data
• Individual variability in response to treatment
• Ineffective response to solely drug therapy
• Treatment cost
• Owners' compliance, time commitment, and expectations

Table 15.1 The most common pharmacological options used in the multimodal treatment of chronic pain in cats. Drug regulations, labeling, and scheduling vary among different countries.

Drug name	Treatment protocol	Observations
Amantadine	3–5 mg/kg PO every 12 to 24 hours	Information on safety and efficacy is not available
Amitriptyline	1–4 mg/kg PO every 12 to 24 hours	AE: Sedation GR: Doses may be started at the low end and slowly increased. Variable efficacy
Buprenorphine (1.8 mg/mL)	0.24 mg/kg SC every 24 hours up to 3 days	SE: Few studies indicate efficacy (antinociception) and safety AE: Euphoria has been observed (rolling, kneading with thoracic paws and purring) GR: This high-concentration formulation can be used "off-label" in cats with severe chronic pain or when pain flares up
Fluoxetine	0.5–1.5 mg/kg PO every 24 hours	Information on safety and efficacy is not available
Gabapentin	5–10 mg/kg PO every 8 to 12 hours	SE: Efficacy in feline DJD following 3 weeks of treatment (10 mg/kg PO every 8 hours) AE: Sedation and ataxia GR: Doses should be gradually increased to avoid profound sedation, especially in cats with renal disease. Higher doses have been reported and are generally limited by the severity of adverse effects. Important: treatment should not be stopped abruptly. It must be tapered down gradually to avoid breakthrough pain
Grapiprant	2 mg/kg PO every 24 hours	SE: Efficacy data are not available. A few reports indicate a good tolerance following 28 days of administration AE: Unknown
Meloxicam	0.1 mg/kg PO once, followed by 0.05 mg/kg PO every 24 hours	SE: Dose-dependent efficacy and good tolerance in cats with feline DJD AE: See *Box* 15.2 GR: Administration of the minimum effective dose should be attempted in long-term treatment
Pamidronate	1–2 mg/kg IV every 21 to 28 days	SE: Efficacy studies are not available. A few reports in cats with bone-invasive squamous cell carcinoma or metastatic bone tumor indicate good tolerability AE: Gastrointestinal upset and neutropenia have been observed only in cats undergoing concomitant chemotherapy
Piroxicam	1 mg/cat (~0.3 mg/kg) PO every 24 hours	SE: Some reports describe its administration in cats with various carcinomas and sarcomas with unclear efficacy and acceptable tolerance AE: See *Box* 15.2. Vomiting, melena, and anemia have been reported in long term treatment GR: Administration every 2–3 days should be attempted in long term treatment. Piroxicam can be chosen over other NSAIDs for its anticancer activity; however, it should not be used in other chronic painful conditions
Robenacoxib	1–2.4 mg/kg PO every 24 hours	SE: Good tolerance in cats with feline DJD AE: See *Box* 15.2 GR: Administration of the minimum effective dose should be attempted in long-term treatment
Selegiline	0.5–1 mg/kg PO every 24 hours	Information on safety and efficacy is not available
Tramadol	2–5 mg/kg PO every 8 to 12 hours	SE: Efficacy in feline DJD following 2 weeks of treatment (3 mg/kg PO every 12 hours) AE: Sedation, vomiting, euphoria, and constipation may occur

Notes: PO – oral administration; AE – adverse-effects; SE – scientific evidence in chronic pain; GR – general recommendations.

Table 15.2 Suggested treatment for some chronic painful conditions in cats including "off-label" regimens. Nonpharmacological options should be considered for all cases.

Condition	Suggested pharmacological treatment	Suggested nonpharmacological treatment	Comments
DJD-related pain	NSAID Tramadol Gabapentin Antidepressants	Physical activity and weight control Implement environmental enrichment Chondroprotective agents Physical therapy and rehabilitation, Acupuncture, TENS	In mild cases, analgesics are avoided As severity increases, more adjuvants are added
Cancer-related pain	NSAID as needed Gabapentin if neuropathic pain Antidepressants Amantadine Buprenorphine in the case of breakthrough pain	Any nonpharmacological treatment may be applicable depending on the case	Treat primary cause if possible
Periodontal disease	NSAID as needed Gabapentin if there is nerve involvement	Provide soft food; add water to the kibble	Treat the primary cause if possible
Interstitial cystitis	NSAIDs None in acute cases Amitriptyline in chronic cases	Reduce environmental stressors and implement environmental enrichment	Concomitant urinary-tract infection should be investigated and addressed
Chronic pancreatitis	Low-dose NSAIDs (contra-indicated if concomitant inflammatory intestinal disease) Gabapentin Tramadol	Nutritional management: highly digestible diet with high fiber and limited fat Administration of pancreatic enzyme supplement	Treat primary cause if possible Consider the use of proton pump inhibitors
Chronic wounds	NSAIDs Adjuvants if needed: tramadol, amitriptyline	Bandages and wound care	Treat primary cause if possible (i.e. surgery, antibiotics, etc.)
Chronic otitis	NSAIDs Gabapentin if there is nerve involvement	Ear cleaning	Treat primary cause
Feline orofacial pain syndrome	Gabapentin until resolution of clinical signs; consider adding amitriptyline if not successful NSAID Antidepressants Amantadine	Reduce environmental stressors and implement environmental enrichment	Oral lesions (e.g. fractured tooth or tongue mutilation) may be present and should be addressed
Diabetes-induced neuropathy	Gabapentin until resolution of clinical signs; consider adding amitriptyline if not successful	Weight control	Diabetes must be carefully monitored
Chronic pain syndrome after feline onychectomy	Amantadine for 3–4 weeks NSAID: doses should be gradually decreased every 4 days for a total of 15–20 days Gabapentin until resolution of clinical signs; consider to add amitriptyline if not successful Buprenorphine for 2–4 days	Provide soft surfaces in areas where the cat likes to walk around Check for the preferred type of litter box Reduce environmental stressors and implement environmental enrichment	Radiographs should be performed to check if there are bone fragments and surgery is required Similar recommendations in cases of persistent post-surgical pain after procedures such as amputation and thoracotomy

Notes: NSAID: nonsteroidal anti-inflammatory drug; TENS: transcutaneous electrical nerve stimulation.

Pharmacological Therapy

Recommended doses for the most commonly used analgesics for treatment of chronic pain in cats are given in *Table* 15.1 and *Table* 15.2. Some of these recommendations are based on personal experience and anecdotal reports due to the lack of large, robust, prospective clinical studies.

Drug Administration

- The oral route (PO) is most convenient for long-term treatment
- Most medications are well tolerated if given with canned food. However, the unpalatability of some analgesic medications (e.g. tramadol and amitriptyline) may limit their clinical use (*Figure* 15.1 and *Box* 15.2)
- NSAIDs such as meloxicam and robenacoxib are highly palatable and well tolerated
- Medication administered by the oral route may be available as pills, tablets, and liquid or spray formulations
- The SC route is a potential route of administration although few injectable options exist for long-term treatment
- Sustained release formulations of some drugs are now available and may be convenient for long-term treatment; however, data on safety and efficacy are lacking in cats

Opioids

- Opioids are the cornerstone of acute pain management (Chapter 13); however, their efficacy has not been demonstrated in chronic pain. Orally administered opioids have low bioavailability, and most are controlled drugs with potential for abuse
- A high concentration of buprenorphine (1.8 mg/mL, Simbadol®) is available in the United States. It may provide up to 24 hours of postoperative analgesia in cats (0.24 mg/kg) and is labeled for three consecutive days of use. This formulation is not licensed for long-term administration but could be an "off-label" option for cats with severe chronic pain as part of a multimodal approach, or when pain flares up ("acute on chronic" pain)

Local Anesthetics

- The pharmacology of local anesthetics is discussed in Chapter 5. Transdermal lidocaine patches may be an option for some types of pain (e.g. subcutaneous mass, chronic wound). The PK of a 700 mg lidocaine patch have been described in healthy cats with intact skin, and systemic uptake is minimal
- Local anesthetic techniques may be applied in cases of severe, postsurgical or breakthrough pain in the hospital setting

Box 15.2: The issue of medicating cats

Common methods of oral delivery of medication

Medicating cats for chronic conditions can be quite challenging. The most common methods used by owners include force-pilling or hiding the medication within highly palatable food (*Figure* 15.1). Force-pilling is made by placing the medication deep in the oral cavity with either the fingers or with a pet-piller device. However, cats generally resent being restrained for force-pilling and have a natural discriminatory ability when it comes to eating, resulting in difficulties in administering the medication.

Possible consequences of force-pilling

Although some owners and cats can be trained to allow stress-free administration of medication using force-pilling, this method can be an additional environmental stressor for others. It can disturb the human-animal bond and therefore it should be avoided. This is important in conditions in which stress plays a role in the pathophysiology of pain (e.g. idiopathic cystitis). In addition, force-pilling may result in the medication becoming trapped in the esophagus causing esophagitis or esophageal stricture.

What do owners think?

A recent e-survey involving owners of cats showed that medication labeled for use in the species and formulations such as solutions and suspensions are more likely to be accepted by the cat when compared with non-labeled medication (odds ratio: 4.9) and formulations such as tablets or capsules (odds ratio: 4.8), respectively. Adverse effects and the "individual behavior of the cat" (e.g. resisting medication, salivation) were the most common reasons for lack of compliance to treatment.

Cat-friendly medications

As medications that are developed for cats are made available, acceptability and compliance is expected to increase. An award called "Easy to Give" is offered annually by the International Cat Care to pharmaceutical companies who produce medications in a format that is easy for owners to administer.

General recommendations

- Pilling should always be followed by positive reinforcement (e.g. treats, petting)
- If force-pilling is absolutely necessary, it should be followed by oral administration of a small amount of soft food
- Unpalatable medications (e.g. tramadol, amitriptyline) may be inserted into small capsules or compounded in palatable flavors
- The website of the International Cat Care (www.icatcare.org, accessed June 26, 2017) has detailed recommendations and step-by-step videos teaching how to administer oral medication to cats
- Veterinary technicians are valuable for discussing these issues with owners and emphasizing the importance of stress-free administration of medication

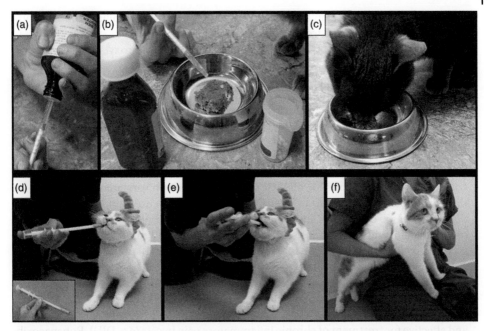

Figure 15.1 Different methods for administering medication to cats (*Box* 15.2). The top pictures show the preferred method, without any physical contact. The bottom pictures show the "force pilling" method with the use of a pet-piller device. In some cats this latter approach can be quite stressful. Note how the white cat depicted in these pictures tries to escape the administration by walking backwards. Top pictures: Gabapentin compounded in a palatable liquid formulation is withdrawn (a). A pill of amitriptyline is hidden within tasty soft food and liquid gabapentin is added to the mixture (b). A cat eats his meal with hidden medication (c). Bottom pictures: Pet-pillar device prepared with a capsule of tramadol (d) (corner). The medication is administered by placing one hand in the cat's neck while the other hand gently inserts the device through the side of the cheek pouch (d). The device is advanced as the cat opens the mouth and the medication is administered by pushing onto the plunger (e). The cat is petted immediately afterwards for positive reinforcement (f).

Nonsteroidal Anti-inflammatory Drugs (NSAIDs)

- These act by inhibiting expression of cyclooxygenase (COX) enzymes in cell membranes (Chapter 13), and have both peripheral and central actions
- Meloxicam has high bioavailability following PO and SC administration
- Robenacoxib has moderate and high bioavailability following PO and SC administration, respectively
- Piroxicam has high bioavailability and a long terminal half life following PO administration
- NSAIDs accumulate in inflammatory exudate, so analgesic effects may last for up to 24 hours after a single dose despite relatively short half lives
- Many NSAIDs are metabolized in the liver via glucuronidation making them potentially toxic to cats. Meloxicam utilizes oxidative pathways and has been successfully used long term in cats

- Meloxicam and robenacoxib are excreted predominantly via the biliary route (fecal), with a minor contribution from the kidneys (urine)
- Excretion of piroxicam in humans is primarily through hydroxylation with some glucuronidation. There is little equivalent information for cats

Clinical Use

- Indications: treatment of inflammatory pain (e.g. DJD-related pain, cancer pain, gingivostomatitis, otitis, interstitial cystitis, chronic wound)
- NSAIDs are the first line of treatment for cats with DJD. These drugs decrease pain and improve activity, mobility, and QoL in this population
- Labeled recommendations for meloxicam and robenacoxib vary among countries. In the United States meloxicam is labeled for treatment of acute pain (single injectable dose), whereas in other areas, including Europe and Australia, it is labeled for treatment of acute pain and chronic musculoskeletal disorders (0.1 mg/kg on the first day, followed by 0.05 mg/kg PO every 24 hours; continued dosing). Robenacoxib is labeled for treatment of acute pain only, with a maximum duration of treatment in the United States of 3 days and 6 days in other countries (including Europe and Australia)
- Despite labeling variations, both meloxicam and robenacoxib have undergone several investigations in the research and clinical settings. Meloxicam has been shown to be safe and effective for treatment of chronic inflammatory pain in cats (e.g. DJD). Robenacoxib has been shown to be safe in cats with DJD, although efficacy studies are lacking
- NSAID-induced adverse effects should not be underestimated. Guidelines for safe administration are provided in *Box* 15.3. The Association of American Feline Practitioners (AAFP) and the International Society of Feline Medicine (ISFM) have published an extensive review on the subject as well as client brochures for owner education (http://www.catvets.com/guidelines/practice-guidelines/nsaids-in-cats, accessed June 25, 2017)
- In general, the lowest effective dose should be administered while monitoring for adverse effects. For example, meloxicam was safe, palatable, and effective when administered to cats with DJD at 0.01–0.03 mg/kg for up to 9 months. Adverse effects included vomiting and diarrhea in a small number of individuals. No significant changes in serum creatinine were detected
- Long-term safety of meloxicam and robenacoxib have been reported in cats with concomitant DJD and chronic kidney disease (*Box* 15.4)

Clinical Use in Cancer Pain

- Nonsteroidal anti-inflammatory drugs also have anticancer properties, especially in tumors overexpressing COX-2. Their administration in cats with cancer should always be considered, unless otherwise indicated. These drugs are commonly used in oncology, including for squamous cell carcinoma, adenocarcinomas (e.g. nasal, mammary, anal gland, vulvar), transitional cell carcinoma, pulmonary carcinoma, soft-tissue sarcoma, fibrosarcoma, and osteochondrosarcoma
- Piroxicam is a nonselective NSAID with chemopreventative and antitumor effects. This drug is commonly administered with other cancer therapies. Piroxicam can be used for both its analgesic and anticancer effects in oncology patients; however, their

use might result in increased incidence of adverse effects when compared with meloxicam and robenacoxib. Piroxicam is not labeled for use in cats
- Chronic administration of piroxicam (0.3 mg/kg PO every 24 hours) for at least 1 month was generally well tolerated in cats with cancer. Gastrointestinal clinical signs were more prevalent in cats receiving concomitant chemotherapy

---

Box 15.3: Guidelines for the safe use of NSAIDs in cats

Adverse effects induced by NSAIDs are thought to be related to their COX-1 inhibition. In general, COX-1 activity has cytoprotective effects in the gastrointestinal tract (secretion of gastric mucus and production of bicarbonate), kidneys (maintenance of renal blood flow under hypotensive conditions), and platelet aggregation (production of thromboxane). The most common clinically detectable adverse effects include anorexia, vomiting, diarrhea, and lethargy. Hepatic adverse effects are thought to be an idiosyncratic reaction to specific drugs rather than intrinsic hepatotoxicity. The following should be considered when NSAIDs are administered on a long-term basis:

- Patient selection
  - Complete history
  - Check for pre-existing diseases
  - Check for current medication and possible interactions
- Client communication
  - Handouts for owner education and monitoring of clinical signs
  - What to expect: possible clinical signs such as anorexia, depression, vomiting, and diarrhea
  - How to proceed: stop medication if clinical signs develop and contact the veterinarian
- Monitoring
  - Via telephone interview or physical examination during re-evaluation
  - Hematology: although not specific, liver and renal enzymes may be monitored for trends
- Dosage may be tailored to the individual, and the minimum effective dosage should be given for long-term therapy
- A minimum washout of 5–7 days is recommended when switching between NSAIDs to prevent inadvertent NSAID cross-toxicity. Analgesia can be provided using a different class of drug during this period.

Contraindications

- History of gastrointestinal disease
- History of NSAID intolerance
- Uncontrolled renal or hepatic disease (*Box 15.4*)
- Anemia
- Coagulopathies
- Hypovolemia or hypotension
- Concurrent corticosteroid administration including topical treatments
- Administration in close temporal relationship with other NSAIDs

NSAID-induced adverse effects are observed when dosage regimens are not respected.

Box 15.4: Cats with chronic pain and concomitant chronic kidney disease (CKD): administration of NSAIDs

Rationale

NSAIDs are generally contraindicated in cats with renal disease due to inhibition of both COX enzymes and consequent negative effects on the maintenance of renal perfusion (vasodilation of renal artery) during hypovolemia or hypotension. However, it is common that cats with chronic painful conditions are also affected by CKD (approximately 70% of cats with DJD have CKD).

Controversy

Growing evidence indicates that meloxicam and robenacoxib can safely be administered to cats with chronic painful conditions and stable CKD. It has been hypothesized that improved mobility and overall QoL subsequent to pain relief result in better appetite and increased water consumption. Another possibility is that NSAIDs may have a direct anti-inflammatory effect on the kidneys, leading to less deterioration of renal function.

Evidence in cats with chronic pain

Retrospective case-control study: cats with CKD receiving meloxicam (0.02 mg/kg/day) for a median duration of 467 days, and cats with CKD not receiving a NSAID. The cats in the first group (NSAID) showed smaller increases in blood creatinine concentration over time when compared with the cats in the second group (no NSAID). There was no difference between groups in urine specific gravity. Retrospective study: cats without CKD and with stable CKD (IRIS stage II and III) that had been under continuous treatment with meloxicam (0.02 mg/kg/day) for at least 6 months. There was no difference between groups in longevity. Prospective clinical study: cats with CKD and cats without CKD receiving robenacoxib (1–2.4 mg/kg/day) or placebo treatment for 28 days. There was no difference between groups in the frequency of reported adverse events, body weight changes, serum and urine chemistry, or hematological variables.

Evidence in healthy normovolemic cats

Prospective study: cats with surgically-induced decreased renal mass and consequent CKD (IRIS stage II and III) receiving meloxicam, acetylsalicylic acid, or placebo treatment for 7 days. There was no decrease in glomerular filtration rate following any of the treatments.

Evidence in humans

Systematic review: population of 12 418 study subjects and 23 877 controls. The study aimed to evaluate the role of NSAIDs in the development of nephropathy. Eight out of nine reports failed to identify an increased risk of chronic renal impairment with heavy NSAID consumption.

Conclusions

Nonsteroidal anti-inflammatories can be administered to cats with concomitant chronic painful conditions and CKD provided their overall clinical status is stable. Moreover, if these cats undergo anesthesia, maintenance of normal hydration, circulating blood volume and blood pressure are important.

Tramadol

- Tramadol has a dual mechanism of action. It has weak affinity for μ-opioid receptors and acts as a serotonin and noradrenergic reuptake inhibitor. The latter effects are related to activation of the endogenous descending inhibitory pain pathways, which modulate central sensitization
- In humans, the analgesic effects are primarily due to the active metabolite O-desmethyl-tramadol, which has an opioid effect
- In cats, tramadol has high bioavailability (93 ± 7%) after oral administration; O-desmethyl-tramadol follows tramadol's disposition profile and both are dose dependent
- The analgesic profile of tramadol in cats is thought to be superior to that in dogs, due to a longer elimination half life and higher concentrations of the active metabolite. The rate of formation of O-desmethyl-tramadol from tramadol in the cat liver is faster than that in dogs (3.9 fold)
- The terminal half life of O-desmethyl-tramadol after IV (2 mg/kg) and oral (5 mg/kg) administration in cats is 261 ± 28 and 289 ± 19 minutes, respectively
- An injectable formulation of tramadol is available in some countries; however, the oral route is preferred for long-term administration
- Tramadol is bitter, often results in profound salivation, and is resented by most cats

Clinical Use

- Indications: conditions characterized by central sensitization (e.g. DJD-related pain, cancer-related pain). Tramadol has a synergistic effect when administered with NSAIDs and is normally administered as part of a multimodal protocol
- Antinociceptive studies suggest that a dosage regimen of 4 mg/kg, PO, every 6 hours would be ideal. However, such regimens may decrease owner compliance. The magnitude and duration of antinociception appear to be dose dependent in cats; higher doses produce prolonged and sustained antinociception
- Sedation may be observed and dose adjustments can be made accordingly. However, clinical experience suggests that sedation normally subsides following the first days of administration
- In cats with DJD-related pain, tramadol (3 mg/kg, PO, every 12 hours) increased activity and mobility, and decreased central sensitization when compared with placebo
- Further studies may clarify the ideal dose and dosing interval for treatment of chronic pain. Based on currently available PK and PD data, 2–5 mg/kg, PO, every 8 to 12 hours is recommended
- Tramadol may be partially antagonized by naloxone in cases of intoxication (administered IV to effect)
- In many countries, tramadol is now a controlled substance (usually schedule IV)

Contraindications

- Tramadol must not be administered in combination with serotonin reuptake inhibitors including monoamine oxidase inhibitors and tricyclic antidepressants due to the risk of serotonin toxicity

- Serotonin toxicity is a clinical syndrome characterized by autonomic dysfunction, neuromuscular abnormalities and changes in mentation that may occur when multiple serotonergic agents are administered, or in cases of overdose
- The diagnosis of serotonin toxicity is based on the exposure to serotonergic agents associated with clinical signs. Possible clinical signs in cats include: change in mental status, ataxia, agitation, tremor, myoclonus, seizures, hyperreflexia, tachycardia, hypertension, hyperthermia, nausea, vomiting, diarrhea, and abdominal pain
- Treatment of serotonin syndrome involves ceasing administration of serotonergic medications and giving supportive treatment including fluid therapy, analgesics and antagonists of 5-hydroxytryptamine (HT)2 receptors (e.g. cyproheptadine, chlorpromazine). The long-term prognosis after serotonin toxicity is good to excellent
- Toxicity has been reported in a cat following tramadol overdose (80 mg/kg) due to a prescription error resulting in serotonin syndrome. This cat developed neurological signs (agitation followed by severe depression), hypersalivation, hypertension, tachycardia, tachypnea, constipation, and abdominal pain. Treatment comprised fluid therapy, buprenorphine, cyproheptadine and microenema, and the cat recovered fully within 7 days

Gabapentin

- Gabapentin was developed as an anticonvulsant and produces analgesia by reducing neuronal excitability and blocking calcium channels. It decreases excitatory neurotransmitter release and increases concentrations of GABA, an inhibitory neurotransmitter
- Gabapentin has high oral bioavailability in cats with a mean half life of 2.8 hours. In humans, gabapentin is eliminated unchanged by renal clearance

Clinical Use

- Indications: neuropathic pain, for instance persistent postsurgical pain (e.g. after amputation, chronic pain syndrome after feline onychectomy), feline orofacial pain syndrome, diabetes-induced neuropathy, DJD-related pain, cancer-related pain
- Administration of gabapentin (10 mg/kg PO every 12 hours) for 2 weeks in a clinical trial in cats with clinical and radiographic signs of DJD improved owner-assessed mobility scores. However, decreased activity, measured with accelerometers, was observed when compared with placebo, probably resulting from sedation, a known potential side effect of gabapentin
- In research cats with DJD-related pain, gabapentin (10 mg/kg PO every 8 hours) decreased central sensitization and improved levels of activity when compared with placebo treatment
- Recommended dosage regimens have not been determined. Doses up to 50 mg/kg PO every 12 hours have been reported anecdotally. This emphasizes the need for individualized therapy based on the degree of pain, response to therapy and development of adverse effects
- Although adverse effects such as sedation generally subside within a few days of starting gabapentin administration, it may be reasonable to initiate treatment at low doses and increase it slowly (e.g. weekly) until an analgesic response is observed. This

approach may avoid profound sedation and ataxia, which could be discouraging for the owner. Moreover, this approach should be used in cats with renal disease who may have impaired clearance and increased incidence of adverse effects
- Treatment for chronic conditions should be discontinued gradually to avoid break-through pain. This may be achieved by slowly decreasing the dose or dosing intervals over the course of a few weeks
- An analgesic trial of 3–6 weeks is recommended and may be required before any effect is apparent

Contraindications

No serious contraindications have as yet been reported for cats. See paragraph above on the use of gabapentin in cats with chronic kidney disease.

Amitriptyline

- Amitriptyline is a tricyclic antidepressant. It produces analgesia via serotonin and norepinephrine reuptake inhibition, N-methyl D-aspartate (NMDA) antagonism, and blockade of calcium channels
- A PK study in cats (5 mg/cat PO or transdermal) revealed poor transdermal absorption when compared with oral administration

Clinical Use

- Indications: neuropathic pain; it may "boost" the endogenous descending inhibitory pathways and reverse central sensitization
- In cats with chronic interstitial cystitis that had failed other treatments, amitriptyline (10 mg/day PO every 24 hours) for 12 months completely resolved the clinical signs in 9/15 patients during treatment. Response to treatment was usually observed after 7 days. Reported adverse effects included sedation, weight gain, and decreased grooming. However, another study reported conflicting results. Cats with acute interstitial cystitis treated with amitriptyline (5 mg/day PO every 24 hours) for 7 days did not show any benefit when compared with placebo
- Since interstitial cystitis is a syndrome resulting from several different mechanisms rather than a disease with a single cause, some cats may still benefit from treatment with amitriptyline (in association with environmental enrichment)
- The emotional component of depression in chronic pain may be targeted by amitriptyline, although efficacy data are not available for cats
- Other examples of tricyclic antidepressant drugs include imipramine and clomipramine
- There are anecdotal reports describing the use, in cats, of other antidepressants such as serotonin-specific reuptake inhibitors (fluoxetine), serotonin and norepinephrine reuptake inhibitors (venlafaxine and duloxetine), and monoamine oxidase inhibitors (selegiline), but information about these medications is very limited
- An analgesic trial of 3–6 weeks is recommended and may be required before any effect is apparent

Contraindications

Amitriptyline should be administered with caution in combination with drugs that affect serotonin uptake or metabolism due to the risk of serotonin toxicity; this includes monoamine oxidase inhibitors and tramadol.

Amantadine

- Amantadine was originally used as an antiviral agent. The drug is a NMDA receptor antagonist and increases dopamine concentration in the CNS
- Amantadine (5 mg/kg PO and IV) has high oral bioavailability in cats. Its efficacy has not been documented in this species but it shows potential for pain therapy

Clinical Use

- Indications: conditions characterized by central sensitization (e.g. DJD-related pain, cancer-related pain)
- Amantadine should be administered in combination with other analgesics (i.e. multimodal analgesia) including opioids, NSAIDs, tramadol, and amitriptyline. It is not used as a "stand-alone" treatment for chronic pain
- Amantadine significantly improved physical activity when compared with placebo in dogs with OA that were treated concurrently with meloxicam. This might be an option when pain is refractory to NSAID therapy
- An analgesic trial of 3–6 weeks is recommended and may be required before any effect is apparent

Contraindications

Currently unknown.

Emerging Analgesic Modalities

- *Anti-nerve-growth factor monoclonal antibodies*: nerve-growth factor is pronociceptive and may contribute to peripheral and central sensitization. Species-specific antibodies that target nerve growth factor are currently under investigation for treatment of DJD in cats. Early reports indicated adequate safety and efficacy for up to 6 weeks after a single SC injection in cats with naturally occurring disease
- *Stem-cell therapy*: stem cell therapy has well-documented anti-inflammatory and immunomodulatory effects. Mesenchymal stem cells can differentiate into a variety of cell types. They are collected from the bone marrow or adipose tissue, for example, isolated and transplanted to tissues in need of regeneration. This therapy has been under investigation in humans with DJD, and there are several other potential applications such as gingivostomatitis, a severe oral inflammatory disease. A recent study involving a small number of cats with severe refractory gingivostomatitis reported the IV administration (two injections, one month apart) of autologous

mesenchymal stem cell therapy. Oral biopsies and clinical evaluation before and after treatment showed complete remission or substantial clinical improvement in five out of seven cats. The impact of pain in these cats was not systematically evaluated, although it may be presumed that pain and discomfort were reduced with reduced inflammation. Further research may confirm the applicability of this treatment in the management of pain in cats with chronic inflammatory conditions such as DJD or gingivostomatitis

- *Piprants*: piprants are prostaglandin receptor antagonists, a new class of selective compounds. They are differentiated from NSAIDs in that they act further down the inflammatory cascade by selectively antagonizing the prostaglandin E2 EP4 receptor; thus maintaining normal activity of COX enzymes. The EP4 receptor has been identified as the primary receptor involved with pain and inflammation in DJD. Grapiprant is a new analgesic and anti-inflammatory drug in the piprant class that is labeled for the control of pain and inflammation associated with DJD in dogs. This drug was safe and effective when administered long term in the target population (2 mg/kg PO every 24 hours, for 28 days). Moreover, the daily administration of grapiprant of doses up to 15 mg/kg for 28 days was well tolerated in research cats. Efficacy and safety data in cats with DJD may be available in the near future

Other Analgesics

- *Pregabalin*: an anticonvulsant with a mechanism of action similar to gabapentin. Data from cats are not available but it has potential benefit for treatment of maladaptive pain. Cost could be a limitation
- *Tapentadol*: a centrally acting analgesic with a dual mechanism of action (μ opioid receptor agonist and noradrenaline reuptake inhibitor). In humans, it is often used for treatment of chronic pain as it has fewer adverse effects than opioids. In cats, tapentadol produced short term (approximately 2 hours) thermal antinociception (50 mg/cat); however, it was reported to be highly unpalatable, which could be a limitation in the clinical setting
- *Codeine*: its analgesic effects appear to depend on metabolites such as codeine-6-glucuronide, norcodeine, and morphine. Codeine did not produce thermal antinociception in cats. Its role in treatment of chronic pain remains unknown. Some codeine formulations are combined with acetaminophen (paracetamol) which is contraindicated in cats due to the risk of toxicity
- *Maropitant*: a central inhibitor of emesis and a neurokinin (NK)-1 receptor antagonist that blocks the effects of substance P, a major pain neurotransmitter. In sevoflurane-anesthetized cats, administration of maropitant decreased the minimum alveolar concentrations of sevoflurane during ovarian ligament stimulation. Similar findings are reported in dogs. Although maropitant is effective in treating or preventing vomiting, and has anesthetic-sparing effects to visceral stimulation, its analgesic effects per se remain controversial
- *Bisphosphonates* (e.g. pamidronate, zoledronate, tiludronate): these inhibit bone resorption due to osteoclast activity and produce analgesia for bone-cancer pain. Some studies reveal a good therapeutic profile in dogs with osteosarcoma, especially when combined with NSAIDs. Tiludronate has shown some efficacy in experimental OA

in dogs. Although there are no studies investigating the analgesic effects of bisphosph-onates in cats, its administration is justifiable in terms of similar cancer biology across mammalian species. In a retrospective pilot study involving cats with invasive bone cancer, administration of pamidronate (1–2 mg/kg IV every 21 to 28 days) was feasible and safe; no discomfort was observed during or after IV administration and no adverse effects were observed, except in cats undergoing concomitant chemotherapy

Nonpharmacological Treatment

The benefits of nonpharmacological treatment should not be underestimated. Although there is less scientific evidence on the efficacy of these techniques in veterinary patients, their importance in treatment of chronic pain in humans has been increasingly recognized. These techniques should be used in combination with pharmacological treatment (integrative medicine) with the ultimate goal of improving QoL.

Physical Activity and Weight Control

Physical deconditioning results from a sedentary lifestyle leading, among other changes, to a decrease in lean body mass. Physical deconditioning makes a major contribution to chronic pain and is therefore an important therapeutic target. It may also be a consequence of chronic pain and the whole process becomes a vicious cycle (Chapter 14). Sedentary lifestyle and obesity are now common in animals, and treatment should include changing the attitude towards physical activity. Regular exercise is beneficial for both physical and mental health of the patient and for treatment of chronic pain.

Environmental Enrichment

- A critical component in treatment of chronic pain as it increases activity and decreases pain
- Environmental enrichment is low cost and easy to implement. Owners should be encouraged to be creative and allow cats to choose their preferred environmental enrichment
- Detailed description of all environmental needs of cats is published elsewhere (http://www.catvets.com/guidelines/practice-guidelines/environmental-needs-guidelines, accessed June 25, 2017). Owners should provide multiple environmental resources that stimulate interest and physical activity such as scratching, playing, hunting, and chasing (*Figure* 15.2)
- Scratch posts (vertical, horizontal, diagonal) should be available in different parts of the house. These must provide good stability, have a wide base, and allow the cat to stretch fully. Owners must be educated that scratching behavior is part of the nature of the cat, and scratch posts may increase the level of activity and at the same time decrease destruction of household items
- Toys (e.g. wrapping tapes, artificial prey, feathers) should be offered. These should stimulate hunting behaviors such as stalking, chasing, pouncing, and biting. They should be rotated around the house to maintain interest
- Food can be hidden within different toys to encourage foraging and hunting behavior
- Elevated surfaces, ramps, and stairs offer opportunities for playing and jumping

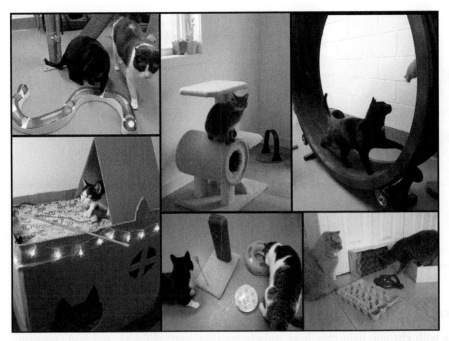

Figure 15.2 Commercially available and homemade options for environmental enrichment. It can be seen how they provide excellent opportunities for playing and exercising, resulting in increased physical activity, weight control, and mental stimulation. Food is hidden within some toys to stimulate hunting behavior. Scratch posts are important for scratching and stretching. Other toys or condos (jumping/ scratching playground) stimulate running or jumping.

Weight Control

- Obesity negatively affects musculoskeletal health due to increased loading forces on joints, but also due to increased circulating proinflammatory cytokines (i.e. chronic low-grade inflammation). The latter is a metabolic consequence of obesity since adipose tissue is capable of secreting cytokines and proinflammatory proteins, and plays a role in the development of DJD
- Weight control can be achieved with restricted-calorie diets and increased physical activity
- Research in dogs shows that decreased food intake is associated with decreased progression of OA. A weight control program in dogs with OA decreased lameness, and improved objective variables measured using kinetic gait analysis. Similarly, decreased kinetic measures have been observed with weight gain
- Cats may be at increased risk of hepatic lipidosis if weight loss occurs too quickly. Therefore, a nutritional dietary program should be set up and carefully monitored

Physical Therapy, Massage, Acupuncture, and Transcutaneous Electrical Nerve Stimulation (TENS)

These modalities are said to increase blood flow to the areas of attention as well as increasing the activity of descending inhibitory pain pathways.

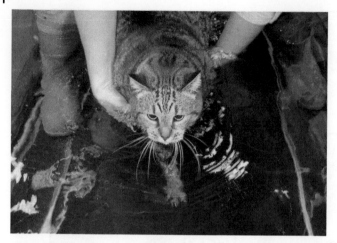

Figure 15.3 An obese and geriatric female cat undergoing physical therapy (water treadmill) for management of DJD. Exercise helps with weight loss and muscle strength, contributing to the multimodal management of chronic pain.

Physical Therapy and Massage

- Cats with chronic pain may have muscle wasting, joint stiffness, and body tension. Physical therapy aims to prevent and treat these conditions in a controlled fashion.
- Stretching and exercises to enhance joint range of motion (ROM) and muscle strength are performed
- Several techniques are available, including passive ROM, treadmill activities, water exercise (*Figure* 15.3) and stair exercise. These should be performed or supervised by individuals with appropriate training in physical therapy and rehabilitation
- Research in pediatric patients indicates that massage significantly reduces the degree of stress, pain, and discomfort
- Massage techniques as well as passive ROM exercises can be taught to owners and may be used to alleviate muscle pain. A rubber brush (also known as "zoom groom") can be used both for massage and as an aid with grooming in cats that are unable to do this

Acupuncture

- Acupuncture needles are inserted into anatomically predefined points (acupoints), which may be also stimulated by digital pressure (acupressure) or electric current (electro-acupuncture)
- The mechanism of action is not fully understood, but may be related to the effects of neuromodulation due to neuronal gating and release of endogenous opioids. Acupuncture can indeed be antagonized by naloxone
- Acupuncture has been recognized by the US National Institutes of Health as a modality for treatment of chronic pain. It inhibits nociceptive transmission and inflammation, produces muscle relaxation, and decreases joint compression. It also restores blood flow, improving oxygen and nutrient distribution to the affected site. The efficacy of acupuncture has been demonstrated in human and canine patients with chronic pain

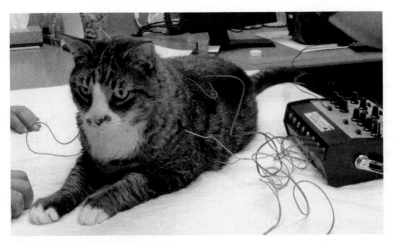

Figure 15.4 A cat undergoing electro-acupuncture therapy session for management of chronic pain. Needles are inserted in acupoints and connected to an electric current. The cat is relaxed (body position and facial expression) and accepts the treatment willingly.

- Acupuncture treatment is minimally invasive and generally well tolerated by most patients (*Figure* 15.4); some cats become relaxed and may sleep during treatment
- In chronic pain states, 3–5 sessions are required before clinical improvement can be detected, and as seen with pharmacological treatment, not all cats will respond. Acupuncture should be performed cautiously in cats with neuropathic pain since needle insertion can induce pain if allodynia and central sensitization are present
- Acupuncture can be recommended in a range of maladaptive conditions such as DJD-related pain, intervertebral disc disease and secondary muscle stiffness, radiation-induced neuropathic pain, bone-cancer pain and visceral pain secondary to intestinal bowel disease
- Treatment should be performed by certified, trained acupuncturists

Transcutaneous Electrical Nerve Stimulation

- Electrodes (patches) are placed over the shaved skin of a painful area and electrical impulses are used to stimulate the area, resulting in analgesia, increased blood flow, and decreased muscle stiffness
- Protocols include sensory-level TENS (high frequency, low intensity) and motor-level TENS (low frequency, high intensity). A combination of both protocols (i.e. mixed frequency) is usually applied to prevent adaptation and accommodation to a set protocol
- The mechanism of action of TENS is not fully understood, but conditioned pain modulation (i.e. the CNS modulates or "filters" its response to incoming electrical activity) may be involved. In this case, stimulation of cutaneous structures may reduce transmission of nociceptive input from the spinal cord to the brain based on the "gate control theory"

- May be used in cats with maladaptive pain such as chronic musculoskeletal pain and neuropathic pain
- Contraindicated in patients with a pacemaker and over open wounds or healing skin

Monitoring for Treatment Efficacy

Monitoring is based on routine assessment of owner-observed behavior and lifestyle changes. Treatment of chronic pain should restore, at least in part, the natural behavior of the cat; for example improving activity, sociability, and wellbeing. Analgesic drug-induced adverse effects should also be monitored and evaluated; they form the basis of decisions whether the treatment protocol should be maintained or altered.

Degenerative Joint Disease (DJD)

Treatment of DJD-related pain should employ a multimodal approach and is dependent on the severity of the disease and feasibility of the treatment (*Figure* 15.5).

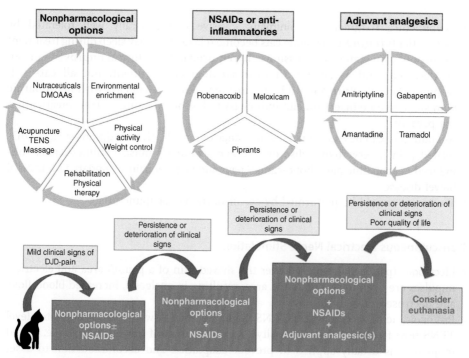

Figure 15.5 Multimodal approach for the management of DJD in cats based on the severity of clinical signs. Treatment options are added according to the progression of the disease. Ideally, cats with mild DJD should be managed without the administration of analgesics. As the disease progresses, NSAIDs are added to the treatment. Finally, in cats with severe DJD, adjuvant analgesics are added to the protocol. Several options (pharmacologic and nonpharmacologic) can be used in a "trial-and-error" manner. *Notes:* DMOAAs = disease-modifying osteoarthritic agents; TENS = transcutaneous electrical nerve stimulation.

Analgesics

Degenerative joint disease produces pain secondary to joint inflammation, amplified nociceptive input and central sensitization. Clinically, cats with DJD are less active and have poor QoL.

- Long-term therapy with NSAIDs increases activity and mobility without adverse effects (see above; *Table* 15.1)
- Some cats with DJD may have central sensitization and allodynia. Pain becomes refractory to treatment with NSAIDs and nonpharmaceutical therapies. Drugs such as gabapentin, amantadine, tramadol or amitriptyline may be considered. With the exception of tramadol and gabapentin, most adjuvant analgesics have not been systemically investigated in cats with DJD-related pain. Nevertheless, they have been widely used with apparent good therapeutic and safety profiles

Physical Activity and Weight Control

The role of increased activity and weight control in the treatment of DJD-related pain cannot be overemphasized. Increased mobility is beneficial for bone and joint health, muscle tone, and consequent joint stability. In humans, an intensive lifestyle intervention characterized by weight loss and exercise may prevent development of joint pain in patients at risk.

Nutraceuticals

Nutraceuticals are products derived from food sources that are purported to provide extra health benefits other than nutrition. They are administered orally and are increasingly being used in animals.

- Cats with DJD that were fed a supplemented joint diet were more active than cats fed a standard diet. The supplemented diet was high in fish oil-derived eicosapentaenoic acid (EPA) and docosahexaenoic acid (DHA), and was supplemented with green-lipped mussel extract and glucosamine with chondroitin sulfate
- Recent reviews on the use of nutraceuticals in dogs and humans recommend their use in management of DJD-related pain despite the lack of high-quality studies
- Cats with mild DJD may benefit from these diets in combination with weight control and environmental enrichment. Cats with moderate to severe DJD may also require treatment with analgesics

Chondroprotective Agents

Chondroprotective agents, or disease-modifying osteoarthritic agents, are precursors of cartilage matrix. They favor matrix synthesis and repair articular cartilage. They are generally considered most effective in the earlier stages of OA.

- *Glucosamine and chondroitin sulfate*: these are popular chondroprotective agents. However, there is limited information on their efficacy in both humans and animals. Administration of oral chondroprotective agents for 30 days was safe in cats based on

clinical pathology. In cats with DJD-related pain, treatment with glucosamine and chondroitin sulfate was not superior to meloxicam. Although, there are no known contraindications to their administration, chondroprotective agents can become expensive for long-term administration, and this must be taken into consideration in the treatment protocol since their efficacy is questionable
- *Polysulfated glycosaminoglycan* (PSGAG): inhibits certain catabolic enzymes that are overexpressed in DJD-joints due to chronic inflammation. Known by the commercial name of Adequan®, this drug is FDA approved for use in dogs and horses with strong evidence of efficacy. Little is known about its use in cats, but general recommendations include SC administration (1–5 mg/kg every 4 days for 6 doses)
- *Pentosan polysulfate*: a semisynthetic glycosaminoglycan that inhibits and modulates proinflammatory mediators. Known by the commercial name of Cartrophen Vet®, and available in many countries, this drug is labeled for management of DJD in dogs with unclear evidence of efficacy. A few reports describe its use in cats with interstitial cystitis, with no clinical success. In cats with DJD, its use is anecdotal (3 mg/kg SC every 5–7 for 4 doses), and its analgesic effects remain to be investigated

In summary, there is no "one-size-fits-all" treatment for every maladaptive condition. Treatment should be tailored to each individual and may be changed and adapted according to acceptance by the patient, response to therapy, development of adverse effects, and patient-owner compliance. There is little scientific evidence for most of the treatment options presented in this chapter. A treatment plan will be decided in conjunction with the owner, considering all available pharmacological and nonpharmacological options, as well as financial and time constraints. The treatment of any maladaptive painful condition will be constantly changed and adapted to the patient (i.e. personalized medicine).

Further Reading

Arzi, B., Mills-Ko, E., Verstraete, F. J., *et al.* (2016) Therapeutic Efficacy of Fresh, Autologous Mesenchymal Stem Cells for Severe Refractory Gingivostomatitis in Cats. *Stem Cells Translational Medicine* **5**, 75–86.

Bennett, D., Zainal Ariffin, S. M., and Johnston, P. (2012) Osteoarthritis in the cat: 2. How should it be managed and treated? *Journal of Feline Medicine and Surgery* **14**, 76–84.

Chew, D. J., Buffington, C. A., Kendall, M. S., *et al.* (1998) Amitriptyline treatment for severe recurrent idiopathic cystitis in cats. *Journal of the American Veterinary Medical Association* **213**, 1282–1286.

Corti, L. (2014) Nonpharmaceutical approaches to pain management. *Topics in Companion Animal Medicine* **29**, 24–28.

Ellis, S. L., Rodan, I., Carney, H. C., *et al.* (2013) AAFP and ISFM feline environmental needs guidelines. *Journal of Feline Medicine and Surgery* **15**, 219–230.

Gowan, R. A., Baral, R. M., Lingard, A. E., *et al.* (2012) A retrospective analysis of the effects of meloxicam on the longevity of aged cats with and without overt chronic kidney disease. *Journal of Feline Medicine and Surgery* **14**, 876–881.

Greene, S. A. (2010) Chronic pain: Pathophysiology and treatment implications. *Topics in Companion Animal Medicine* **25**, 5–9.

Grubb, T. (2010) Chronic neuropathic pain in veterinary patients. *Topics in Companion Animal Medicine* **25**, 45–52.

Gruen, M. E., Thomson, A. E., Griffith, E. H., *et al.* (2016) A feline-specific anti-nerve growth factor antibody improves mobility in cats with degenerative joint disease-associated pain: A pilot proof of concept study. *Journal of Veterinary Internal Medicine* **30**, 1138–1148.

Guillot, M., Moreau, M., Heit, M., *et al.* (2013) Characterization of osteoarthritis in cats and meloxicam efficacy using objective chronic pain evaluation tools. *Veterinary Journal* **196**, 360–367.

Herron, M. E., and Buffington, A. T. (2010) Environmental Enrichment for Indoor Cats. *Compendium on Continuing Education for the Practicing Veterinarian* **32**, E4.

King, J. N., King, S., Budsberg, S. C., *et al.* (2015) Clinical safety of robenacoxib in feline osteoarthritis: Results of a randomized, blinded, placebo-controlled clinical trial. *Journal of Feline Medicine and Surgery* **18**, 632–642.

KuKanich, B. (2013) Outpatient oral analgesics in dogs and cats beyond nonsteroidal antiinflammatory drugs: An evidence-based approach. *Veterinary Clinics of North America Small Animal Practice* **43**, 1109–1125.

Lamont, L. A. (2008) Adjunctive analgesic therapy in veterinary medicine. *Veterinary Clinics of North America Small Animal Practice* **38**, 1187–1203.

Lascelles, B. D. (2005) Feline Degenerative Joint Disease. *Veterinary Surgery* **39**, 2–13.

Lascelles, B. D., DePuy, V., Thomson, A., *et al.* (2010) Evaluation of a therapeutic diet for feline degenerative joint disease. *Journal of Veterinary Internal Medicine* **24**, 487–495.

Marshall, W. G., Hasewinked, H. A. W., Mullen, D., *et al.* (2010) Effect of weight loss on lameness in obese dogs with osteoarthritis. *Veterinary Research Communications* **34**, 241–253.

Mathews, K., Kronen, P. W., Lascelles, D., *et al.* (2014) Guidelines for recognition, assessment and treatment of pain: WSAVA Global Pain Council members and co-authors of this document. *Journal of Small Animal Practice* **55**, E10–68.

McNamara, P. S., Barr, S. C., Erb, H. N., *et al.* (2000) Hematologic, hemostatic, and biochemical effects in cats receiving an oral chondroprotective agent for 30 days. *Veterinary Therapeutics* **1**, 108–117.

Monteiro, B. P., Klinck, M. P., Moreau, M., *et al.* (2016) Analgesic efficacy of an oral transmucosal spray formulation of meloxicam alone, or in combination with tramadol, in cats with naturally occurring osteoarthritis. *Veterinary Anaesthesia and Analgesia* **43**, 643–651.

Monteiro, B. P., Klinck, M. P., Moreau, M., *et al.* (2017) Analgesic efficacy of tramadol administered orally for 2 weeks in cats with naturally occurring osteoarthritis. *PlosOne* **12** (4), e0175565.

Rausch-Derra, L. C., and Rhodes, L. (2016) Safety and toxicokinetic profiles associated with daily oral administration of grapiprant, a selective antagonist of the prostaglandin E2 EP4 receptor, to cats. *American Journal of Veterinary Research* **77**, 688–692.

Robertson, S., and Lascelles, D. (2010) Long-term pain in cats – how much do we know about this important welfare issue? *Journal of Feline Medicine and Surgery* **12**, 188–199.

Sivén, M., Savolainen, S., Räntilä, S., *et al.* (2017) Difficulties in administration of oral medication formulations to pet cats: An e-survey of cat owners. *Veterinary Record* **180**, 250.

Sul, R. M., Chase, D., Parkin, T., *et al.* (2014) Comparison of meloxicam and a glucosamine-chondroitin supplement in management of feline osteoarthritis. A double-blind randomised, placebo-controlled, prospective trial. *Veterinary and Comparative Orthopaedics and Traumatology* **27**, 20–26.

Index

Feline Anesthesia and Pain Management, First Edition. Edited by Paulo Steagall,
Sheilah Robertson and Polly Taylor.
© 2018 John Wiley & Sons, Inc. Published 2018 by John Wiley & Sons, Inc.

Printed and bound by CPI Group (UK) Ltd, Croydon, CR0 4YY

03/04/2025

14653336-0001